Pediatric Audiology

Edited by

FREDERICK N. MARTIN

THE UNIVERSITY OF TEXAS

PRENTICE-HALL, INC. *Englewood Cliffs, New Jersey 07632*

Library of Congress Cataloging in Publication Data

Main entry under title:

Pediatric audiology.

    Includes bibliographies and index.
    1. Hearing disorders in children. 2. Hearing
disorders in children—Diagnosis. 3. Children, Deaf.
I. Martin, Frederick N.
RF291.5.C45P43   617.8'9   77–18086
ISBN 0-13-655472-5

To Cathy, my wife, who read and criticized;
To David, my son, who typed and filed;
To Leslie Anne, my daughter, for her loving nature;
and to my parents, for all they have done,
this book is dedicated.

© *1978 by Prentice-Hall, Inc., Englewood Cliffs, N.J. 07632*

Printed in the United States of America

10 9 8 7 6 5 4 3 2 1

Prentice-Hall International, Inc., *London*
Prentice-Hall of Australia Pty. Limited, *Sydney*
Prentice-Hall of Canada, Ltd., *Toronto*
Prentice-Hall of India Private Limited, *New Delhi*
Prentice-Hall of Japan, Inc., *Tokyo*
Prentice-Hall of Southeast Asia Pte. Ltd., *Singapore*
Whitehall Books Limited, *Wellington, New Zealand*

Contents

iii

3 Management   309

4 The Public Schools   387

Contributing Authors

Charles I. Berlin, Ph.D.
Professor, Physiology and Otorhinolaryngology
Director, Kresge Hearing Research Laboratory
Louisiana State University Medical Center
New Orleans, Louisiana

Francis Irving Catlin, M.D., Sc.D.
Professor, Otorhinolaryngology and
* Communicative Sciences*
Baylor College of Medicine
Houston, Texas

Patricia R. Cole, Ph.D.
Co-Director, Austin Speech, Language and Hearing Center
Austin, Texas

Robert T. Fulton, Ph.D.
Professor, Audiology
University of Kansas Medical Center
Kansas City, Kansas

Victor P. Garwood, Ph.D.
Professor, Speech Communication and Otolaryngology
University of Southern California
Los Angeles, California

Cornelius P. Goetzinger, Ph.D.
Professor, Audiology
Director, Audio-ENG Clinic
University of Kansas Medical Center College of
* Health Sciences and Hospital*
Kansas City, Kansas
Consultant-Psychologist, Kansas School for the Deaf
Olathe, Kansas

William R. Hodgson, Ph.D.
Professor, Speech and Hearing Science
University of Arizona
Tucson, Arizona

Frederick N. Martin, Ph.D.
Professor, Speech Communication
The University of Texas
Austin, Texas

Stephen P. Quigley, Ph.D.
Professor, Education and Speech and Hearing Science
University of Illinois
Urbana-Champaign, Illinois

Audrey Simmons-Martin, Ed.D.
Professor, Speech and Hearing
Washington University
Director, Early Education
Central Institute for the Deaf
St. Louis, Missouri

Kathryn S. Stream, M.A.
Clinical Audiologist, Otolaryngology
University of Texas Medical Branch
Galveston, Texas

Richard W. Stream, Ph.D.
Associate Professor, Otolaryngology
University of Texas Medical Branch
Galveston, Texas

Wendel K. Walton, Ph.D.
Educational Consultant, State of Connecticut
Hartford, Connecticut

Wesley R. Wilson, Ph.D.
Associate Professor, Speech and
*   Hearing Sciences*
Seattle, Washington

Mary Lovey Wood, Ph.D.
Co-Director, Austin Speech, Language and Hearing Science
Austin, Texas

Preface

While the primary role that audiologists should play in the overall management of hearing-impaired patients is not entirely agreed upon, surely it must be agreed that the needs of children must be uppermost. Unless the problems of children who are born with or acquire hearing losses are recognized early, their attainment of future success is in jeopardy. If these children are to receive every possible benefit, the talents of experts must be utilized in diagnosis and management.

The authors bring to this book a great deal of sophistication in dealing with problems of hearing loss among children. Each has a significant amount of clinical experience with children and is a recognized scholar. For this reason I have asked the authors to depart from the traditional third person in their writing and to clearly identify in the first person their philosophies, theories, and even their biases. The book chapters, however, are so constructed as to make the reader aware of differences between the author's personal opinion and statements of the literature. Although following the general chapter format, each author has written in his own style and from his own experiences. The general guidelines they have followed were proposed so that the book would conform to a clear, readable, and uniform pattern.

The reader may note that the personal pronoun "he" is used throughout this book. This was done at my request; if epithets of "male chauvinist" are to be hurled they must be directed toward Austin, Texas. This decision was not made lightly, but only after conference with my colleagues in linguistics and with the editors of national journals. It was my final conclusion that the pronoun "he" would be used in its generic rather than its sexual sense and would include all human beings.

The purpose of this book is to provide information for persons who work or plan to work at the professional level with hearing-impaired children. Each author was advised to assume no knowledge on the reader's part beyond the basic audiology course and to take the reader as far as possible in each particular subject within the alloted space.

I wish to extend my sincerest appreciation to the authors for the spirit and enthusiasm they brought to their respective chapters, to my colleagues who advised me throughout the formative stages of the book, to Brian Walker, Speech Editor at Prentice-Hall, who took a strong and personal interest in this project and lent a great deal of support and guidance, and to my family for their love and understanding.

Frederick N. Martin

The child who is normal, and easy to teach,
Will need and deserve our care.
But the child with a problem has further to reach,
And should get a more bountiful share.

A.J.S.

Causes and Effects

Before remedial work can begin with the hearing-impaired child, the professional worker must understand the causes of hearing impairment, the effects of such impairment on the development of speech and language, and the psychological implications of hearing loss. The three chapters in Part I deal with causes and effects of hearing loss in children.

In Chapter 1, Dr. Catlin outlines hearing impairments in children from a hierarchical viewpoint according to age at the onset of medical conditions affecting hearing and frequency with which they occur. This allows the reader to view the etiologies and incidences of hearing loss from a useful and sensible angle. Dr. Quigley, in Chapter 2, discusses the language and speech difficulties of the hearing-impaired child, first tracing the development of language in a normal child, then contrasting it with the language development difficulties encountered by the severely hearing-impaired, moderately hearing-impaired, and mildly hearing-impaired child. In Chapter 3, on psychological implications of hearing impairment, Dr. Goetzinger considers the ways that hearing loss in children can affect their educational and psychological development.

CHAPTER ONE

Etiology and Pathology of Hearing Loss in Children

FRANCIS I. CATLIN

INTRODUCTION

Audiology, like medicine, is an applied science, but there is an art to applying scientific knowledge and principles to ameliorate hearing disorders. That it parallels the management of disease in medicine, in which facts and principles precede applications, is not surprising. One conclusion is obvious: The audiologist should understand the nature and causes of different hearing disorders before attempting to work with the hearing-impaired child at the professional level.

In the United States, significant bilateral hearing impairment is found in about 8 children per 1,000 between the ages of 6 and 16; profound hearing loss—or deafness—in about 2 per 1,000. The onset of hearing impairment may be prenatal (prior to labor and delivery), perinatal (during labor and birth), or postnatal (after birth). In general, the period of onset is a useful way to approach the etiology of childhood hearing loss and is the method used in this chapter.

During the past two and a half decades we have gained a better understanding of the etiological and pathological factors of hearing loss in children. Significant changes in the relative incidences of the various etiologies producing deafness and hearing impairment have resulted from the introduction and use of antibiotics, antiallergic drugs, and anti-inflammatory agents and from changing methods for determining the character and nature of hearing impairment. The impact of such developments is discussed in succeeding sections of this volume.

CHAPTER OBJECTIVES

The purpose of this chapter is to acquaint the reader with the various etiologies associated with hearing loss in children. Included are brief descriptions of the underlying pathologies. The etiological factors have been classified according to a chronological sequence and in order of relative incidence. Further information about the pathological processes can be found in the suggested readings at the end of the chapter. This chapter is designed to furnish the specialist who treats disorders of children with information about the relative incidence, clinical features, and prognosis for each etiological factor.

INCIDENCE OF HEARING LOSS

How hearing loss and deafness are defined determine their apparent prevalence and incidence. Therefore, these definitions are important; unfortunately, they are not easy to agree on.

Because of objections to computational methods, a functional description for deafness was adopted by the National Association of the Deaf (NAD). It defines the deaf as "all non-institutionalized residents of the United States who have lost or never had the ability to hear and understand speech, even when amplified, this loss having been suffered prior to 19 years of age" (Schein and Delk, 1974).

This population, labelled *pre-vocationally deaf,* forms the basis for the National Census of the Deaf Population (NCDP) of 1971. It includes the prelingual, perilingual, and postlingual deaf (i.e., those whose deafness occurred before, during and after the acquisition of language comprehension and use). Table 1-1 is taken from this census and shows the prevalence and prevalence rates for hearing impairment as reported by Schein and Delk (1974).

These data suggest a considerable increase in the prevalence of deafness since the 1930 census, with the current rate for all ages at 873 per 100,000. The prevalence rate for deafness beginning in the prelingual period (prior to age 3) is 100 per 100,000, about half the prevalance rate for prevocational deafness (prior to age 19).

Other data from the NCDP study indicate that almost 75% of those individuals who were deaf by age 19 had lost their hearing before age 3, and that more

TABLE 1-1. Prevalence and Prevalence Rates for Hearing Impairments in the Civilian Non-institutionalized Population by Degree and Age at Onset: United States, 1971.

Degree	Age at Onset	Number	Rate/ 100,000
All hearing impairment	All ages	13,362,842	6,603
Significant bilateral impairment	All ages	6,548,842	3,236
Deafness	All ages	1,767,046	873
	Prevocational*	410,522	203
	Prelingual†	201,626	100

Source: Schein and Delk, 1974.

*Prior to 19 years of age

†Prior to 3 years of age

TABLE 1-2. Prevalence and Prevalence Rates for Significant Bilateral Hearing Impairment and Deafness in the Civilian Noninstitutionalized Population: United States, 1971

Age in Years	Significant Bilateral Hearing Impairment		Prevocational Deafness	
	Number	*Rate/100,000*	*Number*	*Rate/100,000*
All ages	6,549,643	3,237	410,522	203
Under 6	56,038	262	8,071	38
6 to 16	384,557	852	86,278	191
17 to 24	235,121	862	46,154	169

Source: Adapted from Schein and Delk, 1974, p. 29.

than half became deaf during the first year of life. About 12% became deaf after age 6.

To describe the hearing disorders less severe than deafness, as defined above, the NCDP study also reviewed a group that included both those defined as deaf and those having lesser degrees of loss. This groups was labelled as having "significant bilateral hearing impairment," a term encompassing losses in both ears, the better ear having some difficulty hearing and understanding speech. Table 1-2 shows a comparison by age of the prevalence of significant bilateral hearing impairment and deafness for persons under 24 years old.

The large increases in rates for both classifications of hearing loss found in children from age 6 to 16 as compared to children under 6 may be attributed to several factors, including the rubella epidemic of 1963/64 as well as the problems encountered in defining hearing loss in younger children.

In general, prevalence data support the impression that significant hearing loss and deafness tend to occur early in life. The prevalence of hearing impairment shows a gradual increase with age until the sixth decade is reached. Deafness, on the other hand, tends to occur early in childhood; about 50% of the cases occur within the first year of life. A review of some of the more important of the etiologies for hearing impairment will be presented in the following sections of this chapter.

Some mention has been made earlier of the overall incidence of significant hearing inpairment and of deafness as defined by NCDP, Catlin (1975) compared the percentage distribution of reported causes of deafness as listed in various health surveys of the United States and of Great Britain from 1920 through 1971. These data are illustrated in Fig. 1-1, which presents information from the United States census of 1920 (Best, 1943), collated distributions of congenital and prelingual deafness from 1940 through 1960 (Marcus, 1970), the etiological experience for deafness in Great Britain in 1964 (Fraser, 1964), and the NCDP data in 1971 (Schein and Delk, 1974). The reader must be cautioned about the danger in comparisons of this kind, because of the differ-

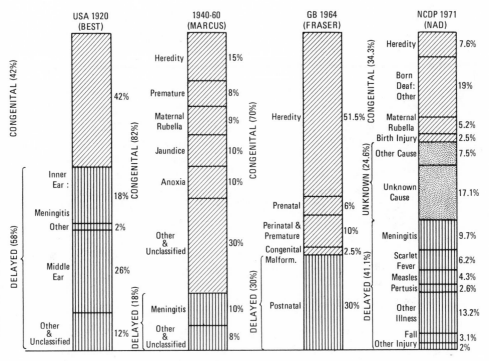

Fig. 1-1. Percent Distribution of Reported Causes of Deafness

ences in methodology and diagnostic criteria—including definitions of "hearing loss," "deafness," and etiological categories—among these studies. Nevertheless, most authors tend to classify etiologies of hearing impairment by time of onset, the most popular being (1) congenital or prenatal, (2) perinatal, (3) delayed or postnatal, and, if the author is completely honest uncertain or unknown. Congenital, perinatal, and postnatal factors may all combine to produce hearing impairment; nevertheless, a brief look at published incidence data by time of onset is appropriate.

Incidence of Congenital Onset

The incidence of a congenital onset for deafness ranges from 34.3% in the NCDP study to 82% in the Marcus (1970) survey. However, in the latter study, 30% of the "congenital" category is listed as due to "other or unclassified" causes. It is likely, therefore, that the true incidence of congenital causes is nearer 35 to 55%.

The NCDP data indicate that 7.6% have an "obvious" hereditary basis for their deafness, whereas 19% were "born deaf" of other causes. Prematurity is probably included in the "born deaf: other" category in this study. The proportion of prematurity amounts to 10% in the Fraser study and 8% in the Marcus review. The NCDP survey attributes 5.2% to maternal rubella and 2.5% to birth injury.

Incidence of Delayed Onset

Incidence figures for delayed onset range from 18% to 58%. The low figure is found in the Marcus survey, which lists two categories: meningitis, 10%; "other and unclassified," 8%. The highest incidence is taken from the 1920 Census (Best, 1943) in which a high proportion of meningitis (18%) and middle-ear disease (26%) are mentioned.

The NCDP data list meningitis as the most common single etiological factor for delayed onset; scarlet fever, measles, and pertussis together form an infectious disease category of 13.1%. Injuries make up 5.1%; other illnesses, 13.2%. Deafness from meningitis was reported to be 18% in 1920, dropped to 10% in the 1940–60 studies, and remained near that level in 1971.

Incidence of Unknown Onset and/or Cause

In the 1920 census, 12% were listed in an "other and unclassified" category. Marcus's analysis of the 1940–60 studies assigns two "other and unclassified" categories: congenital onset, 30%; and delayed onset, 8%. Fraser's data of 1964 include only known causes. The NCDP study of 1971 lists deafness of unknown time of onset at 24.6%. Within this grouping are 7.5% from "other cause" and 17.1% of "unknown cause." Thus, it would appear that no specific cause can be assigned in at least 12 to 30% of deaf children. If lesser degrees of hearing impairment are included, the higher figure appears to be more accurate (Shimizu, 1976).

PRENATAL ETIOLOGIES

Hearing Loss of Congenital Onset

In the NCDP survey, about one-third of deaf respondents indicated that they were born deaf. Nearly one in three stated that they inherited their hearing loss. As Dublin (1976) has so aptly put it: "Congenital, genetic, and hereditary factors may be combined in the production of hearing loss, and their respective participation may not always be separable. Complexity is the rule rather than the exception" (page 105). Approximately 75% have inherited recessive deafness. Only about 20% of inherited deafness occurs through dominant transmission of the trait. About 6% of the recessive cases show a sex-linked inheritance, and 91% of deaf children have parents with normal hearing (Schein and Delk, 1974).

Patterns of Inheritance. Most people have the ability to hear. This ability is a genetic trait. Some people do not have this ability; they have a trait for deafness or hearing impairment. When a person is unable to hear, the cause may be inherited, or it may be environmental. Therefore, some knowledge about hereditary factors is advisable.

Like other inherited traits, hearing impairment (including deafness) is transmitted either by the ordinary, paired chromosomes (autosomal) or by the sex chromosomes (X-linked). At the risk of unnecessary repetition, a review of single gene inheritance seems appropriate at this time. (A gene it will be remembered is a factor in the chromosome which carries an hereditarily transmissible characteristic.)

Autosomal Dominant Inheritance. In this condition, there is at least one dominant gene for hearing loss in one of the ordinary paired chromosomes. Possession of a single dominant gene is enough to cause the trait. A hearing-impaired parent in this instance will have one normal gene and one gene for hearing loss. Such a parent is hearing-impaired himself and will transmit either a gene for hearing loss or a gene for normal hearing to a child. Typically, for each pregnancy the chances for the child to have the trait are about 50%. Males and females are equally affected. The trait is carried vertically from one generation to the next. Failure of hearing loss to occur at all in a person with the gene for the loss is spoken of as "lack of penetrance." Autosomal dominant disorders often vary in severity among those affected: this phenomenon is described as "variable expressivity."

Autosomal Recessive Inheritance. In recessive hearing impairment, the gene for hearing loss is recessive to the gene for normal hearing. Parents of children with autosomal recessive inheritance usually have normal hearing, but they are carriers (heterozygotes) who possess one gene for hearing loss and one for hearing (one normal gene being sufficient). If both parents are carriers, the probability is only 1 in 4 that the child will receive the defective gene from each parent and exhibit hearing loss. Parental consanguinity (blood relationship) may increase the probability and should be considered. Although two deaf parents who have the same recessive gene should technically produce only hearing-impaired children, normal-hearing children are often produced because many different recessive genes can affect hearing impairment.

X-linked Inheritance. X-linked inheritance is a special type of recessive inheritance. In its most common form, the mother, on one of her two X chromosomes, carries the gene for X-linked hearing loss. Because X-linked traits are often recessive, the matching gene on the other X chromosome usually allows for normal hearing. The mother would have normal hearing, but each son has a 50% possibility of inheriting hearing loss. Each daughter of a carrier mother stands a 50% chance of inheriting the affected chromosome and of being a carrier of the X-linked trait; that is, she is capable of transmitting it to *her* sons. An affected male will transmit the X-linked trait for hearing loss to all of his daughters, making them carriers, but to none of his sons, since he can contribute only Y chromosomes to them.

Females may manifest X-linked disorders in modified form since they are heterozygous and one X chromosome may be randomly "dominant." This is called the Lyon hypothesis. An affected female can result from the union of an affected male and female heterozygote, but this is rare.

Trisomy Hearing Impairment. Some types of genetically determined sensori-neural hearing loss result from chromosomal abnormalities in which an extra chromosome is found within a pair, called trisomy. Such conditions are not necessarily hereditary. Recognized autosomal trisomy syndromes include the Trisomy 13, Trisomy 18, and Trisomy 21 (Down's syndrome). Anomalies of the inner ear, internal auditory canal, and central pathway may occur. Two children with Trisomy 13 showed no auditory reponses, and multiple anomalies have also been reported with this disorder. Malformed ears have been found at autopsy in Trisomy 18. Most of these patients usually die before age 2. In Trisomy 21, or Down's syndrome, there is evidence of an increased incidence of sensorineural hearing impairment ranging from 10% to over 50%; however, these children are very susceptible to upper respiratory infections. As a result, conductive hearing impairment is reported in 3 to 20%, and mixed in an additional 10 to 20% (Glousky, 1966; Fulton and Lloyd, 1968).

The incidence of hereditary deafness varies in reported studies from 11 to 60%. Such variance is due, in part, to the relative distribution of transmission factors, including dominant genes, recessive genes, sex-linked genes, multifactor genetic properties, mutations, or gross chromosomal abnormalities such as those previously mentioned.

More than 90 types of hereditary deafness syndromes have been described by Konigsmark and Gorlin (1976). Eight categories of genetic and metabolic deafness are recognized. The hearing loss may be congenital, of early onset, or of late onset. Examples of each category are:

I. Genetic hearing loss with no associated abnormalities. This group comprises the majority of congenital hereditary deafness syndromes. Konigsmark and Gorlin report at least 16 types, including:

1. Dominant congenital severe sensorineural deafness.
2. Dominant progressive early-onset sensorineural hearing loss.
3. Otosclerosis (Conductive or mixed loss, uncommon below age 15).
4. Recessive congenital severe sensorineural deafness.

5. Recessive congenital moderate sensorineural hearing loss.
6. X-linked congenital sensorineural deafness.
7. X-linked early-onset sensorineural deafness.
8. X-linked moderate sensorineural hearing loss.

II. Genetic hearing loss with external ear abnormalities. External ear changes make these syndromes easier to diagnose. The hearing loss may be congenital or slowly progressive. About 11 syndromes are known, including:

1. Atresia (closure) of the external auditory canal and conductive hearing loss.
2. Ear malformations, persistent periauricular pits (depressions around the external ear), sinuses or nodules, and mixed hearing loss.
3. Preauricular pits, persistent branchial (Gill) clefts or fistulas, and sensorineural hearing loss.
4. Malformed low-set ears and conductive hearing loss.
5. Small external ear, meatal atresia and conductive hearing loss.
6. Lop ears, small lower jaw, and hearing impairment of mixed type.

III. Genetic hearing loss associated with eye disease. Usher syndrome is the most common disorder among the 25 syndromes reported in this category. In addition to hearing loss in association with eye disease, some of these syndromes involve the nervous system; others include diabetes mellitus.

1. Usher syndrome: Autosomal recessive. Congenital moderate to severe sensorineural hearing loss, vestibular hypofunction, and slowly progressive retinitis pigmentosa, (an infection of the retina with degeneration of the nerve elements). Some patients show mental deficiency and later psychosis. May be a syndrome of genetic heterogenicity. Expressivity can be quite variable. Comprises 5–10% of congenital deafness.
2. Alström syndrome: Probably autosomal recessive. Transient early obesity, atypical retinal degeneration with loss of central vision, adult diabetes mellitus, and progressive sensorineural hearing loss, the latter starting about age 7 and progressing during the second and third decades. Vision and hearing deteriorate progressively.
3. Cockayne syndrome: Autosomal recessive. Cachectic (emaciated) dwarfism with senile appearance, mental deterioration, and moderate sensorineural hearing loss. Hearing is usually normal at birth but deteriorates during childhood.
4. Refsum's syndrome: Autosomal recessive. Progressive atypical

retinal scarring (retinitis pigmentosa) with constricted visual fields and night blindness, hypertrophic peripheral neuropathy, mild cerebellar ataxia and nystagmus, and progressive sensorineural hearing loss in about half of those affected. The hearing loss most often begins in the second or third decade of life and progresses slowly, the higher frequencies being most affected.

5. Cryptophthalmia syndrome and mixed deafness: Autosomal recessive. Unilateral or more often bilateral extension of the forehead skin to completely cover the eye or eyes, variable fusion of fingers and/or toes (syndactyly), coloboma (notching) of the nostrils, various urogenital anomalies, and mixed deafness with atresia of the external auditory canals.

6. Optic atrophy, juvenile diabetes, and sensorineural hearing loss: Autosomal recessive. Childhood onset of progressive visual loss due to optic atrophy, diabetes mellitus with onset in the first or second decade, and progressive sensorineural hearing loss. The hearing difficulty may be noted in the first several years of life; it becomes gradually worse, resulting finally in bilateral symmetrical moderate-to-severe sensorineural hearing impairment in the second decade. The hearing impairment is more marked in the higher frequencies.

IV. *Genetic hearing loss associated with musculoskeletal disease.* About 33 syndromes exhibit hearing loss and musculoskeletal abnormalities. The hearing deficit may be conductive, mixed, or sensorineural. Several more prominent examples include:

1. Otopalatodigital (OPD) syndrome: X-linked recessive inheritance. Pugilistic facies (broad nasal root; hypertelorism or great width between the eyes; frontal and occipital bossing or protuberance; and soft mandible), cleft palate, growth retardation, abnormalities of hands and feet that include widely spaced first and second digits and shortened great toes, a wide variety of skeletal abnormalities, mild mental retardation, and a moderate conductive hearing loss.

2. Klippel-Feil anomalad and abducens paralysis with retracted spinal bulb and sensorineural or conduction deafness: Multi-factorial inheritance. Fusion of cervical vertebrae, abducens (VIth cranial nerve) palsy with retracted spinal bulb (Duane syndrome), occasional cleft palate and/or wryneck (torticollis—abnormal position of the neck), and severe congenital sensorineural or conductive hearing loss.

3. Crouzon syndrome—craniofacial dysostosis: Autosomal dominant inheritance. Premature fusion of cranial bones (craniosynostosis), ocular hypertelorism, shallow orbits and exophthalmos, beaked

nose, maxillary hypoplasia with relative mandibular prognathism (projecting jaws) and occasional bilateral atresia of the external auditory canals, ossicular anomalies, and mixed hearing loss. About one-third of patients exhibit hearing loss, mostly conductive.

4. Osteogenesis imperfecta: Autosomal dominant inheritance. Osteogenesis imperfecta (brittle bones) with frequent fractures, blue sclerae, and mild to moderate conductive hearing loss in 30–60% of patients.

V. Genetic hearing loss and integumentary (skin) system disease. At least twenty syndromes have been described with skin, nail, or hair changes associated with a severe, usually congenital, hearing loss. Except for the Waardenburg syndrome, which accounts for about 2% of the congenitally deaf (1:42,000 births) most of these syndromes have been described in only one or a few families.

1. Waardenburg syndrome: Autosomal dominant transmission with variable expressivity. Lateral displacement of eyes (medial canthi and lacrimal points). Broad nasal root in about 75%. Hyperplasia of medial eyebrows in about 50%. Heterochromia of the iris and loss of pigment epithelium of optic fundus (base of the eye) in about 25%. White forelock in about 20%. Skin pigmentary changes, including smooth, light-colored patches (vitiligo) and spotty hyperpigmentation in less than 15%. Cleft lip and/or palate in less than 5%. Vestibular hypofunction in about 75%. Congenital mild to severe unilateral or bilateral sensorineural hearing loss in about 50%.

VI. Genetic hearing loss with renal disease. About ten syndromes have been described, the most common being Alport Syndrome, which accounts for about 1% of genetic deafness.

1. Alport Syndrome: Autosomal dominant inheritance with males being more severely affected. Nephritis (inflammation of the kidney) and sensorineural hearing loss. Progressive nephritis with uremia (retention of blood in the urine). Hematuria (excretion of blood in the urine) is often a presenting sign during the first years of life, but more often it appears in the first or second decades with associated asymptomatic urinary albumin and pus. Hypertension and renal failure occur during the teen years, especially in males. Ocular-lens abnormalities including lenticonus (abnormalities of the lens) or cataracts are found in about 10% of cases. Progressive sensorineural hearing loss, especially in the middle to high frequencies, usually appears in the second decade of life. The hearing loss remains relatively mild with marked variation in the degree of deafness. About 55% of males and 45% of females are affected.

2. Lemieux-Neemeh syndrome (Charcot-Marie-Tooth syndrome, nephritis, and sensorineural deafness): Probably autosomal dominant inheritance. Nephropathy similar to that of Alport syndrome, Charcot-Marie-Tooth syndrome, and progressive sensorineural hearing loss beginning in childhood.

3. Macrothrombocytopathia, nephritis, and sensorineural deafness: Dominant inheritance, probably autosomal. Poor prognosis with death from renal failure in the third decade in some patients. Renal disease resembling that seen in Alport syndrome, giant platelets with low circulating blood platelets (thrombocytopenia) and moderate to severe sensorineural hearing impairment, more marked in the higher frequencies. The onset of hearing impairment is usually between the ages of 3 and 10.

4. Infantile renal tubular acidosis and congenital sensorineural deafness: Autosomal recessive. A specific deficiency of carbonic anhydrase B (an enzyme that catalyzes the reaction of oxygen and carbon dioxide) has been demonstrated in affected individuals. Infantile renal tubular acidosis with hyperchloremia (increase of sodium chloride in the blood). An inability to acidify the urine normally, growth retardation, and congenital profound sensorineural hearing impairment that is more pronounced in the higher frequencies.

5. Adolescent or young adult renal tubular acidosis and slowly progressive sensorineural hearing loss: Autosomal recessive. Characterized by mild renal tubular acidosis with onset in adolescence or early adulthood and slowly progressive sensorineural hearing impairment. The hearing loss is moderate in degree and more marked in the higher frequencies.

6. Nephritis, urticaria (rash), amyloidosis (deposits of brown-staining protein), and sensorineural deafness (Muckle-Wells syndrome): Autosomal dominant transmission with variable expressivity. Adolescent onset of recurrent episodes resulting in nephropathy and uremia, and childhood onset of progressive sensorineural deafness that advances to severe loss in the third and fourth decades of life.

VII. *Genetic hearing loss with nervous system disease.* About 14 syndromes have been reported, most of these within a family or two. Most common is acoustic neuroma and neural deafness; several other syndromes of this category are outlined.

1. Acoustic neuroma and neural deafness: This syndrome, with its dominantly transmitted bilateral acoustic neuromas, should be distinguished from neurofibromatosis (multiple neuro-fibroma with

skin pigmentation). About 4% of persons having acoustic neuromas have this syndrome. Autosomal dominant transmission. Slow to rapid progression of neural hearing loss, neurologic deficit due to acoustic neuromas beginning early in adult life, and vestibular dysfunction. The average of onset is 20 years; rarely, it begins in infancy. Hearing loss is noted in the second or third decade and usually progresses to total deafness within 5 to 10 years.

2. Ataxia, hypogonadism (decreased gonadal internal secretion), mental retardation, and sensorineural deafness—Richards-Rundle syndrome: Autosomal recessive transmission. Progressive severe mental deterioration, early onset of progressive mild ataxia and horizontal nystagmus, muscle wasting—particularly involving the distal extremities—absent development of secondary sex characteristics, reduced urinary hormonal secretion of estrogen, pregnanediol, and total neural 17-ketosteroids (products of adrenal cortical or gonadal steroids) and early onset of severe progressive hearing loss noted at about age 2, although partial hearing is maintained for several years before severe deafness supervenes.

3. Sensory radicular (root) neuropathy and progressive sensorineural deafness: Many affected families exhibit the characteristic neurological alterations but do not manifest deafness. Autosomal dominant transmission. Progressive sensory loss with lightning pains that involve the distal extremities and begin in the second or third decade, loss of spinal cord dorsal root ganglia, particularly in the lower thoracic and lumbar areas, and sensorineural hearing loss beginning at about the time of the sensory loss (age 15 to 36) and with slow progression to severe deafness within 10–20 years.

4. Bulbopontine paralysis with progressive sensorineural hearing loss: Autosomal recessive. Childhood onset (second decade of life) of slowly progressive bulbar paralysis with weakness of facial muscles, lips, tongue, larynx, and muscles of mastication, depressed vestibular function, and progressive sensorineural hearing loss—frequently the first symptom of the disease—beginning between 10 and 35 years of age. Several patients exhibited auditory hallucinations.

VIII. *Genetic hearing loss with metabolic and other abnormalities.* Over 16 syndromes have been placed in this category. A few are fairly common; most are rare single-gene disorders or are the result of chromosomal aneuploidy.

1. Goiter and profound congenital sensorineural deafness—Pendred syndrome: Accounts for about 10% of congenital deafness and results from an inborn error of the thyroid hormone (thyroxine).

Autosomal recessive. Goiter developing prior to adolescence, and symmetric, generally severe, congenital sensorineural hearing loss which progresses slightly during childhood.

2. Mucopolysaccharidoses: Disorders of metabolism of the mucus-forming elements due to at least seven recessive enzyme deficiencies, autosomal except for the X-linked Hunter syndrome. The clinical findings in Hurler and severe Hunter syndromes include severe mental deterioration, defection ossification (dysostosis multiplex), and enlargement of liver and spleen. The Maroteaux-Lamy syndrome includes severe dysostosis and enlarged liver and spleen without mental deterioration. The Morquio syndrome is characterized by severely deforming skeletal maldevelopment (dysplasia). The Sanfillipo A and B syndromes are fatal disorders exhibiting severe mental deterioration with only mild involvement of other body structures. A wide spectrum of hereditary expression is seen with most of these enzyme deficiencies; i.e., both the severe Hurler and the mild Scheibe exhibit enzyme deficiency. Most Hurler syndrome patients probably have some degree of progressive conductive hearing loss. In the Scheibe syndrome, some 10–20% may exhibit hearing loss in middle age. Hunter syndrome has been accompanied by hearing impairment in about 50% of cases. The loss is usually not severe and may be of mixed type. In the Sanfillipo syndrome, hearing loss has been rarely reported; most patients with Morquio syndrome exhibit a moderate hearing impairment of mixed type beginning in the second decade of life. About one-quarter of patients with Maroteaux-Lamy syndrome show a hearing loss that is probably conductive and that appears at about 6–8 years of age following frequent bouts of otitis media.

3. Mannosidosis: Autosomal recessive. Coarse facies, short neck, recurrent upper respiratory infections, kyphoscoliosis (spinal curvature), mild hypotonia (decreased muscle tension), protuberant abdomen, inguinal and/or umbilical hernia, progressive mental retardation, mild dysostosis multiplex, reduced mannosidase (enzymatic) activity in liver, plasma, and leukocytes, vacuolated (abnormal) lymphocytes, and severe high-frequency sensorineural hearing impairment.

4. Congenital sensorineural deafness with electrocardiographic abnormalities, fainting spells, and sudden death—Jervell and Lange-Nielsen syndrome: Estimated to occur at a rate of three to four cases per million births. Autosomal recessive. Congenital severe sensorineural hearing loss, abnormal electrocardiogram findings, and

recurrent Stokes-Adams attacks beginning in early childhood and occasionally resulting in sudden death.

5. Turner syndrome: Characterized by short stature, sexual infantilism, streak gonads, elevated urinary gonadotropin (gonad-stimulating hormone) levels, various physical stigmata—such as pterygium colli (a congenital band of connective tissue from the mastoid region to the clavicle), cubitus valgus (inward deviation of the forearm when extended), short fourth finger, osteoporosis (bone rarefaction), and increased cutaneous nevi (moles). Sex chromosomal studies may show negative nuclear sex chromatin or other abnormalities of sex chromatin pattern. Sensorineural or conductive hearing loss, or both, are found. Otitis media has been reported in 50-68% of cases; conductive or mixed hearing loss, however, is less common and is reported in 20-35% of the individuals. Sensorineural loss with recruitment was reported in about 65% of cases, generally as a bilaterally symmetrical dip in the audiogram near 2000 Hz. No striking progression of hearing loss has been reported. Severe deafness in Turner syndrome is noted in only about 10% of cases.

Pathological Maldevelopment. Structural lesions producing hearing impairment may be produced by (1) failure of development, (2) interruption of development and/or (3) damage to tissues already developed. The majority of hereditary hearing losses of congenital onset show no abnormality except in the organ of hearing. Most congenital abnormalities occur in the membranous labyrinth. The auditory ossicles are seldom abnormal in an otherwise normal ear. When a middle-ear deformity is present, the stapes, which develops from different embryological origins than the malleus and incus, is usually involved. Malformations of the malleus and incus are occasionally present. Fraser (1964) attributes 2.5% of severe childhood deafness to congenital malformations; Shimizu (1976) reports an incidence of 3% of children with hearing loss.

Six types of inner ear congenital anomaly have been described (Lindsay, 1973; Dublin, 1976) which are related to the stage of development at the time of occurrence of the disorder. These may overlap to some extent.

Type I. The Michel type is probably caused by failure of the otic vesicle (the embryonic cells forming the inner ear) to separate from the neural ridge or to develop. The inner ear completely fails to develop and the petrous part of the temporal bone may be absent or contracted.

Type II. The Mondini-Alexander type has been described as a flattened cochlea with development of the basal coil only, and with similar malformation of the vestibule. Labyrinthine development appears to have been interrupted at the sixth or seventh week of gestation. The utricle, saccule, and semicircular canals may be normal or abnormal, and the malformation may be bilateral or unilateral.

Type III. The Bing-Siebenmann type shows further development of the inner ear than Type II. The condition may be due to failure of development, or to degeneration. The petrous bone and bony labyrinth are fully developed, but the membranous inner ear is malformed.

Type IV. The Scheibe, or cochleo-saccular, type is the most common congenital abnormality (70% of cases) and may be familial or sporadic. Here, development of the ear has progressed further and, as in the Bing-Siebenmann type, the cochlear canal may be dilated rather than collapsed, suggesting that the changes could be developmental rather than degenerative. The bony labyrinth is fully formed, and the membranous utricle and semicircular canals are functioning normally. In the cochlea and saccule, the organ of Corti, and the macula are represented by a mound of undifferentiated cells. The tectorial membrane is malformed, and there is degeneration of the stria vascularis. The degree of development may vary in different parts of the cochlea.

In many cases of the Bing-Siebenmann and Scheibe types, reference is made to lack of pigment in various organs of the body. In addition, some categories that have accompanying malformations other than the inner ear are recognized (Dublin, 1976).

Type V. The Siebenmann type shows malformations of middle ear and external ear canal.

Type VI. This type exhibits microtia and atresia of the external meatus.

Maternal Viral Infections

The first 28 days of fetal life form a crucial time of very rapid fetal growth and development during which more than 70% of long-term neurological handicaps originate (Hardy, 1973, quoting Masland). A significant portion of these handicaps appear to begin with fetal infection acquired during pregnancy in the period immediately before or after birth.

The maternal infection may be clinically evident or subclinical, with atypical characteristics, or it may not be apparent at all. The cause of the infection may be viremia, commonly of two or three weeks duration, or the infection may persist for longer periods of time.

Fetal infection occurs by one or more of the following routes: (1) transplacental passage of virus, (2) extension up the birth canal with infection of the membranes, or (3) direct contact or contamination during the birth process. There are documented instances of fetal infection and disease following maternal infection with rubella, cytomegalovirus (CMV), herpes virus (hominis), chicken

TABLE 1-3. Adverse Effect of Prenatal Rubella Upon Hearing in 94 Liveborn Babies by Gestational Age at the Time of Maternal Illness

Weeks Gestation	No. Infants	No. Impaired	% Impaired
0 - 8	50	43	86%
9 - 12	14	12	85%
13 - 20	15	8	53%
21 - 35	15	3	20%
Total:	94	66	70%

Source: Adapted from Hardy, 1973, p. 234.

pox vaccinia (varicella), and poliomyelitis. Measles and influenza have also been incriminated but insufficient evidence is available to permit assessment of the precise risk for these agents (Hardy, 1973).

Rubella. The pathogenesis of congenital rubella and, to a lesser extent, CMV infection appears to result from two aspects of the infectious process. The first is the specific fetal anomaly or teratogenic effect, presumably resulting from loss of critical cells during the period of organogenesis. For rubella, the effect upon hearing is most evident when infection occurs during the first eight weeks of gestation, however, it is still found when infection occurs during the second and even the third trimester of pregnancy, as shown in Table 1-3 (Hardy, 1973). The second aspect of the infectious process reflects the continued presence of a chronic viral infection which may persist throughout fetal life and often for months after birth. This second set of effects is predominant in children whose mothers contract rubella after the tenth week of gestation (especially during the second trimester), but it also occurs concomitantly with the teratogenic effects which result from early infection. In some of the less severely affected infants, the result of chronic infection may not be apparent until early childhood.

For these reasons, rubella, as a cyclical viral disease, is a leading cause of prenatal hearing impairment. The virus enters by the maternal nose or mouth and is transmitted to the embryo. Maternal immunity does not prevent the fetus from attack by the virus (McCracken, 1963; Skinner, 1961). The prevalence of post-rubella pathology in post-rubella children averages 35%. Hearing impairment is a major residue, occurring in 12 to 50% (average: 33%). There is a 71.7% prevalence rate for multiple disabilities, especially cerebral palsy. Thus, rubella-deafened children may possess traits often attributed to brain damage and may exhibit restlessness, hypersensitivity, distractibility, impulsiveness, and/or instability.

The use of maternal viral culture and antibody testing in the Collaborative Perinatal Research Project, in a series of 165 laboratory-documented cases of prenatal rubella, has shown that 49% presented typical clinical findings, and 51%

TABLE 1-4. Maternal History—Offspring Hearing Test Results

Maternal Rubella	Hearing Test Viral Positive		Hearing Test Serology Positive	
	Passed	Failed	Passed	Failed
1st Trimester	3	14	14	22
2nd Trimester	2	1	10	7
3rd Trimester	0	0	4	4
No history of clinical rubella	8	2	51	23

Source: Brookhouser and Bordley, 1973.

were of subclinical type. The hearing-test results in relation to maternal history are depicted in Table 1-4 (Brookhouser and Bordley, 1973).

The failure rate for hearing tests in the viral-positive infants was 56.6%; the rate for the group with positive serology only was 41.5%. When maternal rubella occurred during the third trimester, no viral-positive infants were reported but half of those with positive serology failed the hearing tests. When there was no associated history of clinical rubella, 10 viral-positive and 74 serology-positive infants were found. Of the latter group, 30% failed the hearing tests. In this series, hearing loss was the only defect in 36 infants (22%) with positive laboratory studies, but most exhibited other abnormalities.

In general, the hearing loss is found to be sensorineural in character, but the severity of the loss varies greatly among patients and, to a lesser degree, between the ears of each patient. The audiograms tend toward a "belly-type" curve with greatest loss in the mid-frequency range of 500-2000 Hz. Serial audiograms in Houston (Alford, 1968) and Baltimore (Bordley and Alford, 1970) show a progressive decrease in hearing sensitivity in about 25% of patients, although a current follow-up of the Houston children at 11 years of age suggests that the incidence of hearing impairment is much higher and that the number of children showing progressive loss of hearing has also increased.[1]

In a review of 3,033 children with hearing loss who were tested at a major medical center from 1965-1974, Shimizu (1976) found an average incidence of prenatal rubella etiology in 7.6%. The incidence fluctuated greatly, however, from year to year, ranging from as high as 45.6% in 1964 to 33.3% in 1965 to nearly none in 1970.

The pathological findings of the rubella-infected ear are usually a cochleosaccular change of the Scheibe type with partial collapse of Reissner's membrane and adherence of this membrane to the stria vascularis and organ of Corti. Abnormalities of the tectorial membrane as well as collapse of the saccule have

---

[1]Personal communication from Dr. M.M. Desmond, Baylor College of Medicine, Houston, Texas, 1976.

been noted in some instances. The relation of such findings to hearing status have been discussed by Brookhouser and Bordley (1973).

Cytomegalovirus. Cytomegalovirus (CMV) is the commonest known microbiological cause of brain damage in infancy (Stern et al., 1969). CMV infection is especially common during pregnancy, and becomes progressively more common from trimester to trimester (Reynolds et al., 1973). The incidence of viral excretion by pregnant women is reported among various ethnic groups to be 3 to 6% for urinary excretion and 4 to 28% for cervical discharge (Montgomery, 1972). In Australian studies, 27% of apparently healthy but seropositive postpartum women show virolactia (Hayes et al., 1972).

Intra-uterine CMV infection is most likely to damage the fetus, but infection acquired during birth or in the immediate postnatal period may also be harmful (Sells et al., 1974). Hearing impairment has been reported in 50% of 19 children, ages 21 to 77 months, with subclinical congenital infection (Dahle et al., 1974). The hearing losses ranged from a slight high-frequency impairment to a profound unilateral loss. Viruria (active viruses excreted in the urine) was found in 90% of the children below age 3; in older children the incidence dropped to 12.5%. Hanshaw (1973) comments that mild degrees of mental retardation and minimal cerebral dysfunction, loss of hearing, and more subtle changes such as learning disability may not become apparent until late postnatal life. It appears that because the hearing loss is progressive, it is not immediately detected in some cases. Indirect evidence for progression of hearing impairment is cited by Dahle et al. (1974) in the analysis of the level of the hearing impairment to the age at time of testing. Dahle noted that both the incidence and the severity of hearing impairment increased with age.

Strauss and Davis (1973) report that 1 to 2% of consecutive autopsies of infants show diffuse CMV disease. Severe forms of CMV infection can produce microcephaly (small head size), hydrocephaly (increased intracranial fluid), spasticity, mental retardation, and chorioretinitis (inflammation of the choroid and retina) as well as jaundice, petechiae (small skin hemorrhages), and visceral involvement. The temporal bone findings are those of an endolymphatic labyrinthitis secondary to the viremia via the stria vascularis. Inclusion-bearing cells (cells containing virus) are seen in the superficial lining cells of the stria, Reissner's membrane, the limbus spiralis, saccule, utricle, and semicircular canals. Increased labyrinthine fluid, or hydrops, has been reported in the cochlear apex, utricle, and saccule; however, such histopathologic findings have been reported only for severe forms of the disease.

Kernicterus. This condition was originally described by gross anatomical findings—namely, the icteric (jaundice) staining of certain nuclei of the brain with microscopic evidence of necrosis (death) of ganglion cells in the stained area. At various times the term has been applied to the clinical condition known as erythroblastosis fetalis, which may occur because of Rh-factor differences between mother and child, but which may also occur in ABO incompatibility. The Rh factor is a genetically-determined clumping, or agglutination, factor which is found in the erythrocytes of 85% of the population. Theoretically, erythro-blastosis-possible combinations could occur in 1 out of 12 pregnancies in which an Rh-negative female mates with an Rh-positive male; actually, kernicterus from this cause is observed in only 1 out of 20 such pregnancies. The risk increases with each pregnancy and with inappropriately matched blood trans-fusion. The overall incidence of kernicterus is about 1 per 200 births. Current methods of detection and medical management have greatly reduced the propor-tion of kernicterus due to Rh incompatibility. The condition results in staining of all nuclei, metabolic disturbances from liver damage, agglutination of erythro-cytes in brain capillaries, and hypoxemia from anemia, plus the other factors previously listed. Most infants sustain brain damage, which may be evidenced by language disorders, cerebral palsy, distractibility, hyperactivity, inconsistent behavior, emotional lability, temporal rigidity, lack of inhibition and/or compul-siveness. A high incidence of hearing impairment, usually of sensorineural type, has also been reported.

PERINATAL ETIOLOGIES

Kernicterus

Of equal importance is the recognition that kernicterus need not result from maternal iso-immunization at all but can occur in a variety of seemingly unre-lated conditions in the newborn. Kernicterus has been observed in congenital hemolytic anemias such as hereditary spherocytosis and others; in association with the administration of certain preparations of vitamin K, tranquilizers, hypo-tensive drugs, and/or sulfonamides; in mature and, particularly, in premature infants with sepsis (poisoning from products of infection, including CMV); in association with pulmonary and/or cerebral hemorrhage, and with hypoxia. In some instances, the extent of increased blood destruction appears to be negligible.

Kernicterus is now known to occur in familial nonhemolytic jaundice, neo-natal hepatitis, and sometimes, in the absence of any associated pathologic condition, 'functional immaturity of the liver' (so-called physiological jaundice) occurs. Zuelzer and Brown (1961) have commented about several factors which seem important for the development of kernicterus; namely, the affinity of skin and fat to act as reservoirs for bilirubin (the principal pigment of liver bile), the permeability of the blood-brain barrier and, perhaps, the functional and develop-mental status of the brain.

Marcus (1970), in his survey of studies that had been made between 1940 and 1960, concluded that about 10% of severe hearing loss is related to neonatal jaundice, but Shimizu (1976) noted only a 1.5% incidence of prelingual hearing loss for hyperbilirubinemia (excessive amounts of bilirubin in the blood). These value differences may reflect the multifaceted etiology of kernicterus, for, as Crosse (1961) has shown, the incidence of kernicterus is increased by many factors, including low birth weight, marked prematurity, birth asphyxia, low body temperature, and excessive intake of vitamin K; to these can be added the administration of certain drugs and exchange transfusion.

Hymen et al. (1969) reported the following abnormalities in 405 infants followed for four years with a history of neonatal hemolytic disease or hyper-bilirubinemia (indirect bilirubin of 15 mgm or greater). Fifteen percent had one or more of the following: sensorineural hearing loss, athetosis, strabismus, minimal cerebral dysfunction syndrome, or miscellaneous problems (impaired mentality, psychotic behavior, or spontaneous nystagmus). Hearing impairment was found in 4.2%, or 17, of the 405 infants. This included: 4 with mild loss, 8 with moderate to severe loss, and 2 profoundly deaf children; 3 with profound loss in one ear and normal hearing in the other ear. The only impairment was hearing loss in 10 of the 17 (59%). Sensorineural hearing loss was observed in 13% of prematures in comparison to 3.5% of term babies. Athetosis was found in 7% of the 405 infants studied, seizures in 5%, minimal cerebral dysfunction in 4.9%, strabismus in 2.7% and miscellaneous central nervous system (CNS) problems (mostly impaired mentality) in 1.7%.

Hyman adds that all infants who had marked neurological abnormalities as neonates showed CNS abnormalities at follow-up. Such abnormalities were found at follow-up in 29% of infants initially suspected of having CNS damage and in 12% of prematures in whom CNS damage was not initially suspected. The author further notes that these CNS abnormalities could not have been diagnosed during the neonatal period.

Kernicterus is an excellent illustration of the interrelatedness of congenital, perinatal, and postnatal causes of hearing impairment. For instance, kernicterus frequently occurs in the premature infant whose hyperbilirubinemia and/or anoxia may be prenatal and/or neonatal in origin.

Prematurity

Prematurity is probably the most commonly mentioned perinatal cause of hearing loss. Shimizu (1976) notes that the risk of hearing loss in premature infants is 35 times greater than in the average newborn population. There appears to be little agreement concerning the relative incidence of hearing loss from prematurity: Fraser (1964) indicates about 10%; Marcus (1970), 8%; and Shimizu (1976), 3.3%. These apparent discrepancies may be caused, in part, by differences in the definitions and criteria each employed. Shimizu notes that

20% of 101 premature infants with confirmed hearing impairment weighed between 2000 and 2500 grams at birth; he recommends that birth weights up to 2500 grams be considered "at risk" until proven otherwise.

Prematurity, with or without other factors, carries a high risk for central nervous system problems. Grewar (1961) comments that 0.2% of nonerythroblastotic premature infants develop kernicterus. Drillien (1964) has observed an increasing number of low-average, dull, retarded, and/or otherwise defective children as birth weight falls below two kilograms. When the birth weight was below 1360 grams, Drillien noted that less than one-third of these children were of low-average or better ability, that over one-third would require special educational treatment but could attend normal school, and that over one-third would require special schooling because of physical and/or mental handicap.

Drillien's study of 440 premature children tested at school age revealed that 17.5% exhibited some hearing defect. In 1% of these, the hearing impairment was felt to be of congenital onset; however, in the 72 children with birth weights below 1360 grams, the incidence of congenital onset was estimated to be 8%. A history of otitis media was elicited in 24% of the 440 children and a history of recurrent upper respiratory infection in 34%. No obvious cause for the hearing deficit was found in 42%. Drillien comments that premature infants are more likely to sustain cerebral damage as a result of birth injury than are full-term infants, and that mental retardation and neurological defect may result in some cases. He also reminds us that postnatal symptoms that are commonly attributed to birth injury are in many instances due directly to the immaturity of the baby or to an underlying developmental defect, and Drillien concludes that one cannot assume without other evidence that a prematurely born child showing subsequent mental or neurological defect and having a history of abnormal postnatal symptoms did, in fact, suffer from trauma at birth.

Anoxia

Anoxia, or oxygen deficiency, is also a significant perinatal cause of hearing loss with a reported incidence ranging from 0.9% (Shimizu, 1976) to 10% (Marcus, 1970). Anoxia has been cited as being present in 5 to 10% of all births, although to a varying degree.

Birth Injury

Birth injury, as a primary etiology for hearing impairment, is cited by incidence figures ranging from 0.3% (Shimizu, 1976) to 2.5% (Schein and Delk, 1974).

In summary, the perinatal factors appear to be less common than prenatal and postnatal etiologies of hearing impairment; nevertheless, they are often combined with prenatal and postnatal conditions to which the hearing impairment may be totally and erroneously attributed.

POSTNATAL ETIOLOGIES

Hearing loss of postnatal onset is reported by Shimizu (1976) to be the primary cause in 50% of hearing-impaired children under 19 years of age. In this group, the most common disorder was otitis media (including serous and infectious) with an incidence of 33.4%. Other infections were reported to cause hearing loss in 6.9%; of this latter group 2.6% were secondary to meningitis.

Deafness (i.e., profound hearing loss) was reported in the NCDP study conducted by the National Association of the Deaf (NAD), in 1971 to be of postnatal onset in 41% of those under 19 years of age. In this study, the most common etiology cited was meningitis (9.7%); with a second category of scarlet fever, measles and pertussis combined (13.1%); a third category of other illnesses (13.2%) and trauma (5.1%). Differences between these data reflect, in part, varying definitions and methods of sampling.

Otitis Media

Acute Infectious Otitis Media. Acute infectious otitis media continues to be a major clinical problem, especially in infants. It is often associated with nasopharyngitis with extension of infection to the nose, paranasal sinuses, and chest. Enlarged adenoid tissue, blocking the nasopharynx, and the short straight eustachian tube of the child contribute to the spread of infection in the middle ear. While the incidence of otitis media has decreased since the advent of antibiotics, the condition remains a major source of hearing impairment in children.

Serous Otitis Media. This subacute or chronic, usually painless, condition is characterized by the presence of sterile fluid in the middle ear and by an associated hearing impairment of conductive type. It is common in children from 2 to 8 years old who exhibit enlarged tonsils and adenoids and who give a history of frequent upper respiratory infections. In about one-third of cases, there is a positive allergy history. In some, the condition appears to be an aftermath of an attack of acute otitis media, particularly after antibiotic therapy. It is especially common (50-65%) in children who have cleft palates or other palatal abnormalities.

Serous otitis media is thought to arise as a result of inadequate aeration of the middle ear via the eustachian tube. The process appears to be one of resorption of gases within the middle ear—leading to retraction of the tympanic membrane—followed by secretion of a transudate (Juhn et al., 1973) that later becomes mucoid or exudative in consistency, especially when the disorder is of long duration. In many instances, the condition tends to persist despite attempts to control apparent predisposing factors.

Incidence of Otitis Media. Eagles et al. (1967), in a survey of elementary school children, found an overall incidence of hearing impairment secondary to otitis media and/or tympanic membrane perforation of 33 to 39% in several studies—an incidence similar to the 33.4% reported by Shimizu (1976) from a large medical center.

Table 1-5 shows the frequency and incidence of hearing loss for otoscopically abnormal school children. Adhesive and serous otitis media account for 87.2% of all diagnoses. The incidence of hearing impairment for at least one ear is 38.3%. Conditions showing the highest incidence of hearing loss per diagnosis include acute, serous and adhesive otitis media.

In summary, the majority of hearing impairments of postnatal onset originate in the middle ear and are primarily of the conductive type. Such conditions may be transient, as with acute otitis media, or prolonged, as with serous otitis. Some require surgery for amelioration or correction. Most of the predisposing conditions are infectious or allergic. One congenital malformation, cleft palate, is associated with serous or suppurative otitis media in about 45% of those afflicted. The incidence of hearing impairment is reported in a range from 25 to 90%, with an average figure of 60%. In 1972, cleft palate was reported in the history obtained from deaf respondents in 0.4% of those between the ages of one and 64 years of age in the United States.

Complications of Otitis Media. Certain complications of otitis media can produce hearing impairment by mechanisms other than tympanic membrane retraction or fluid in the middle ear. Complications of serous otitis media include adhesive otitis media, tympanosclerosis, retraction-pocket cholesteatoma, and rarely, granulation tissue growth. Scarring of the tympanic membrane, unless extensive, rarely produces a hearing loss of significance. However, if the scar binds the tympanic membrane, or if it limits motion of the ossicles—as in advanced adhesive otitis media—the conductive loss may be significant and difficult to correct.

Complications of infectious otitis media may include tympanic membrane perforation, necrotizing otitis media, cholesteatoma, mastoiditis (including petrous bone infection), labyrinthitis, meningitis, subdural or brain abscess, and sensorineural hearing loss. Tympanic membrane perforation and necrotizing otitis media are less common since the advent of antibiotic therapy. At times, however, and particularly when the infection is caused by a virulent streptococcus or staphylococcus organism, destruction of a major part of the tympanic membrane and/or ossicles may be extensive.

Cholesteatoma denotes an abnormal presence of skin in the middle ear or mastoid. Primary cholesteatoma, arising from embryonal epithelial cell remnants within the middle ear or mastoid bone, is rare. Secondary or acquired cholesteatoma generally arises in one of two ways: from epithelial growth within a

TABLE 1-5. Relationship of Otoscopically Abnormal Children To Diagnosis and Significant Hearing Impairment

Diagnosis	Number	Frequency of Diagnosis by %	Incidence of Hearing Loss by %
Adhesive otitis media	249	70.7%	70.6%
Serous otitis media	58	16.5%	93.5%
Beginning or subsiding otitis media	23	6.5%	39.1%
Tympanic membrane perforation	21	6.0%	44.4%
Acute otitis media	1	0.3%	100.0%
Totals:	352	100.0%	38.3%*

Source: Adapted from Eagles et al., 1967.

*Overall incidence of hearing loss for poorer ear.

retraction pocket of the tympanic membrane (particularly in the attic area from the pars flaccida) or by growth of auditory canal epithelium into the middle ear through a perforation of the tympanic membrane. Expansion of the cholesteatoma may limit motion of the membrane and/or ossicles or may destroy the membrane and/or ossicles, or may erode the bony walls of the cochlea, the labyrinth, the lateral sinus, or the middle cranial or posterior cranial fossae. In such circumstances, secondary infection, which is often present as a result of tympanic membrane perforation, can easily extend to these structures to produce labyrinthitis, lateral sinus infection and thrombosis, meningitis, subdural abscess, and brain abscess. Meningitis, which will be discussed next, can arise from infectious otitis media through the diploic blood vessels in the absence of mastoiditis, cholesteatoma, or any significant bony destruction. Miningitis sometimes develops as an extension of middle ear infections through anomalous defects of the stapes, otic capsule, or temporal bone. Since the advent of antibiotic agents, however, the incidence of otitic meningitis has dropped to about 1% of the prepenicillin rate.

Sensorineural hearing impairment may occur as a sequel to infectious otitis media from damage to the cochlea by infection, inflammation, or toxic reaction. This effect may be enhanced by noise trauma or by the use of ototoxic agents to combat the infection. Konigsmark and Gorlin (1976) have also described instances where a hereditary sensitivity towards ototoxic agents may be a factor.

Meningitis

Meningitis, the second most common cause of hearing impairment of postnatal onset, ranks considerably below otitis media. However, it is the leading postnatal cause of hearing loss among school-age deaf children. Meningitis may be aseptic or exudative (i.e., suppurative). The latter type is most frequently associated with hearing loss. Fifty percent of meningitis is reported in children under 5 years old, predominantly under 2½ years. Mortality rates have decreased from about 13% in 1969 to the present 6 to 8%, except for newborns whose mortality rates are still slightly greater than 50%. Sequellae are not uncommon; 25 to 38% show multiple handicaps; 9.8% have more than one severe handicap beside hearing impairment. In many of the children the infection occurred between the ages of 1 and 4 years. In addition to hearing loss, complications most frequently reported are aphasia, mental retardation, emotional disturbances, and cerebral palsy. Impairment of hearing may occur from ototoxicity when the therapy includes ototoxic agents, such as the aminoglycosides.

Meningitis due to Hemophilus influenza is by far the most common type and accounts for 45 to 50% of pediatric infections under 15 years of age and for 80% of infants under two years. Hearing loss has been reported in 1 out of every 27 cases by Barrett.[2] Long term follow-up of 56 cases has shown 29% with residual handicaps and 14% with possible minimal residual impairments (Sproles et al., 1969).

Pneumococcal meningitis ranks second to influenza. Incidence figures range from 20 to 25% of all meningitis in children below 15 years of age to 10% of all meningitis in those below 3 years of age. Pneumococcal meningitis is reported to infect the frontal lobes more often than do other types.

Meningococcal meningitis ranks in incidence about equal to or slightly below pneumococcal infection and is reported to cause 15 to 25% of all meningitis. About 45% of cases occur in children below 15 years of age; of these, one-fourth occur in children below age 5 and about one-seventh occur in those under 1 year of age. The pathological process of meningococcal infection is a purulent inflammation of the arachnoid and pia mater (layers of the meninges), especially over the parietal and occipital lobes and the cerebellum, with secondary damage to the optic, auditory, and facial nerves and the development of hydrocephalus. Such damage is more likely when the infection occurs under 3 years of age. The mortality for treated meningococcal meningitis is now 1 to 2%, unless widespread infection or meningococcemia has developed, in which instance the mortality ranges from 20 to 50%.

Streptococcal meningitis is less common and staphylococcal meningitis, the least common of the exudative types. The latter is most common in children under 6 months of age. Infant mortality is 45 to 50% during the first week of life and drops to 10 to 15% after this period. Streptococcal and staphylococcal meningitis in older children frequently result from other deafness-producing conditions such as otitis media and mastoiditis.

Of the aseptic types, tuberculous meningitis and labyrinthitis remain promi-

[2] Personal communication from Dr. F. Barrett, Baylor College of Medicine, Houston, Texas, 1976.

nent causes of hearing impairment and carry a high probability of other neuro-logical sequellae including: hemiplegia, paraplegia, ocular palsy, epilepsy, and optic atrophy.

The overall incidence of profound hearing loss from meningitis has ranged, in various public health surveys, from 18% in 1920 (Best, 1943) to 10% in 1970 (Marcus, 1970) to 9.7% in 1971 (Schein and Delk, 1974). The persistence of meningitis as an etiological cause may be attributable to several factors in-cluding: bacterial and viral resistance to chemotherapeutic agents, better survival rates for severely infected children, and secondary damage to the auditory sys-tem by ototoxic agents.

Other Infections and Disorders

There appears to be less consensus regarding the relative incidence of some of the less common and poorly defined disorders producing hearing loss. In part, this state of affairs can be attributed to the manner in which statistics are gathered and tabulated. The National Census of the Deaf Population in the NAD survey of 1971 lists relative causes for deafness (as defined earlier in this chap-ter) as follows:

Meningitis	9.7%
Scarlet fever	6.2%
Measles	4.3%
Pertussis	2.6%
Fall	3.0%
Other injury	2.0%
Other illnesses	13.2%

The reviewer should remember that many individuals interviewed in this study acquired their hearing loss before the development of anit-inflammatory and antimicrobial agents.

In a survey of children under age 19 with hearing impairment, Shimizu (1976) found the following incidence of hearing loss during the period of 1965–74:

Meningitis (all types)	2.6%
Mumps	2.3%
Trauma	1.2%
Pneumonia	0.9%
Viral infections (unspecified)	0.4%
Simulated hearing loss	0.4%
Measles	0.3%

And, in decreasing frequency:

Ototoxic agents

Acoustic trauma

Meniere-like disease

Encephalitis

Neoplasm

Unexplained high fever

Influenza

Varicella (chickenpox)

Anoxia from respiratory failure.

Prelingual Impairment

An examination of the data for prelingual impairment is useful because it gives some indication of those children who may be expected to have difficulty with language and speech development because of their early hearing loss. In most studies, prelingual hearing impairment or deafness is defined as occurring before age 3. The NAD survey indicates that almost 75% of those who became deaf before the age of 19 had lost their hearing in the prelingual period; more than 50% had lost their hearing during the first year of life. Only about 11.5% became deaf when 6 years old or older.

The experience of Shimizu with 1408 children with prelingual hearing loss indicated that approximately 60% were of unknown etiology. Those with known factors were distributed as shown in Table 1-6. Both the NAD survey and the Shimizu study agree that, despite differences in criteria and the difficulty in assigning the period of onset in many instances, most severe hearing impairments of children are present before birth or occur during the first twelve months of life.

TABLE 1-6. Distribution of Hearing Loss of Known Onset

Period of Onset	Percent Distribution
Prenatal (prenatal & hereditary factors predominating)	68%
Perinatal (premature birth, hyper-bilirubinemia, & anoxia predominating)	24%
Postnatal	8%

Source: Adapted from Shimizu, 1976.

SUMMARY

Approximately 66 of 1,000 persons in the United States have a significant hearing impairment. Of these, about 33 report significant hearing difficulties in both ears, and 8 or 9 are deaf. Of the deaf individuals, 2 date their hearing loss prior to 19 years of age and 1, before the age of 3.

One-third of persons under age 19 report no demonstrable cause for their hearing impairment; slightly less than one-third are of prenatal or perinatal onset, and slightly more than one-third, postnatal.

The most common prenatal factors appear to be heredity, maternal rubella, and ear deformity. The common perinatal factors include prematurity, low birth weight, hyperbilirubinemia, anoxia, and infection. The most common postnatal factors are otitis media, meningitis, other types of bacteriological and/or viral infections, and trauma. A review of the relative incidence and a brief outline of the pathology of the most common causes of hearing impairment have been outlined.

RESEARCH NEEDS

What is particularly needed is research directed towards prevention, diagnosis, and study of the course of disease, and management of certain disorders which cause hearing impairment. Continuing periodic surveys of incidence and prevalence are also needed.

Prospective studies, particularly of hereditable causes and of prenatal and neonatal infections, should be performed because of the frequency with which these conditions are associated with hearing loss. The quintet of prematurity, low birth weight, hyperbilirubinemia, anoxia, and sepsis deserve concentrated inquiry because these factors are so often found, in various combinations, to lead to hearing impairment during the prenatal, perinatal, and postnatal periods of life.

Otitis media, meningitis, and head trauma together account for over 80% of postnatal hearing loss. The control and prevention of otitis media, in particular, must be supported by active research.

Prevention of these handicapping conditions requires scientific inquiry of the highest quality and priority.

REFERENCES

Alford, B.R., "Rubella—la bête noire de la médecine," *Laryngoscope,* 78 (1968), 1626–1659.

Best, H., *Deafness and the Deaf in the United States.* New York: Macmillan Co., 1943.

Bordley, J.E., and B.R. Alford, "The Pathology of Rubella Deafness," *International Audiology*, 9 (1970), 58–67.

Brookhouser, P.E., and J.E. Bordley, "Congenital Rubella Deafness," *Archives of Otolaryngology*, 98 (1973), 252–257.

Catlin, F.I., "The Public Health Aspects of Deafness," *The Nervous System*, edited by D.B. Tower, Vol. 3: Human Communication and Its Disorders. New York: Raven Press, 1975.

Crosse, V.M., "The Incidence of Kernicterus (Not Due to Haemolytic Disease) Among Premature Babies," *Kernicterus: Report Based on a Symposium Held at the IX International Congress of Paediatrics*, ed. A. Sass-Kortsak, pp. 4–9. Toronto: University of Toronto Press, 1961.

Dahle, A.J., F.P. McCollister, B.A. Hamner, D.W. Reynolds, and S. Stagno, "Subclinical Congenital Cytomegalovirus Infection and Hearing Impairment," *Journal of Speech and Hearing Disorders*, 39 (1974), 320–329.

Drillien, C.M., *The Growth and Development of the Prematurely Born Infant.* Edinburgh and London: E&S Livingstone, Ltd., 1964.

Dublin, W.B., *Fundamentals of Sensorineural Auditory Pathology.* Springfield, Ill.: Charles C. Thomas, 1976.

Eagles, E.L., S.M. Wishik, and L.G. Doerfler, *Hearing Sensitivity and Ear Disease in Children: A Prospective Study.* St. Louis, Mo.: The Laryngoscope Press, 1967.

Fraser, G.R., "Profound Childhood Deafness," *Journal of Medical Genetics*, 1 (1964), 118–151.

Fulton, R.T., and L.L. Lloyd, "Hearing Impairment in a Population of Children with Down's Syndrome, *American Journal of Mental Deficiency*, 73 (1968), 298–302.

Glousky, L., "Audiological Assessment of a Mongoloid Population," *Training School Bulletin (Vineland)*, 63 (1966), 27–36.

Grewar, D.A.I., "Experiences with Kernicterus in Premature Infants," in *Kernicterus, Report Based on a Symposium Held at the IX International Congress of Paediatrics*, edited by A. Sass-Kortsak, pp. 13–19. Toronto: University of Toronto Press, 1961.

Hanshaw, J.B., "Congential Cytomegalovirus Infections," Editorial, *New England Journal of Medicine*, 288 (1973), 1406–1407.

Hardy, J.B., "Fetal Consequences of Maternal Viral Infections in Pregnancy," *Archives of Otolaryngology*, 98 (1973), 218–227.

Hayes, K., D.M. Danks, H. Givas, and I. Jack, "Cytomegalovirus in Human Milk," *New England Journal of Medicine*, 287 (1972), 177–178.

Hyman, C.B., J. Keaster, V. Hanson, I. Harris, R. Sedgwick, H. Wursten, and A.N. Wright, "CNS Abnormalities after Neonatal Hemolytic Disease or Hyperbilirubinemia," *American Journal of Diseases of Children*, 117 (1969), 395–405.

Juhn, S.K., J.S. Huft, and M.M.Paparella, "Lactate Dehydrogenase Activity and Isoenzyme Patterns in Middle Ear Effusions," *Annals of Otology, Rhinology and Laryngology*, 82 (1973), 192–195.

Konigsmark, B.W., and R.J. Gorlin, *Genetic and Metabolic Deafness*, Philadelphia, Pa.: W.B. Saunders Co., 1976.

Lindsay, J.R., "Profound Childhood Deafness, Inner Ear Pathology," *Annals of Otology, Rhinology and Laryngology*, 82 (1973), Supplement 5.

Marcus, R.E., "Reduced Incidence of Congenital and Prelingual Deafness," *Archives of Otolaryngology*, 92 (1970), 343–347.

Masland, R.L., Forward in Niswander KR, Gordon, Editorial Committee: *The Collaborative Perinatal Study of the National Institute of Neurological Diseases and Stroke: I. The Women and their Pregnancies*. Philadelphia, Pa.: W.B. Saunders Co., 1972.

McCracken, J.S., "Rubella in the Newborn," *British Medical Journal*, 2 (1963), 420–422.

Montgomery, R., L. Youngblood, and D.N. Medearis, Jr., "Recovery of Cytomegalovirus from the Cervix in Pregnancy," *Pediatrics*, 49 (1972), 524–531.

Reynolds, D.W., S. Stagno, T.S. Hosty, M. Tiller, and C.A. Alford, "Maternal Cytomegalovirus Excretion and Perinatal Infection," *New England Journal of Medicine*, 289 (1973), 1–5.

Schein, J.D., and M.T. Delk, *The Deaf Population of the United States*. Silver Spring, Md.: National Association of the Deaf, 1974.

Sells, C.J., R.L. Carpenter, and C.G. Ray, "Sequelae of Central Nervous System Enterovirus Infection," *New England Journal of Medicine*, 298 (1974), 1–4.

Shimizu, H., "Medical Assessment of Deafness." From an unpublished paper, 1976.

Skinner, C.W., "The Rubella Problem," *American Journal of Diseases of Children*, 101 (1961), 78–86.

Sproles, E.T., J. Azerrad, M.S.W. Williamson, and R.E. Merrill, "Meningitis due to Hemophilus Influenza: Long-term Sequelae," *Journal of Pediatrics*, 75 (1969), 782–788.

Stern, H., S.D. Elek, J.C. Booth, and D.G. Fleck, "Microbial causes of Mental Retardation," *Lancet*, 2 (1969), 443–448.

Strauss, M., and G.L. Davis, "Viral Disease of the Labyrinth: Review of the Literature and Discussion of the Role of the Cytomegalovirus in Congenital Deafness," *Annals of Otology, Rhinology and Laryngology*, 82 (1973), 577–583.

Zuelzer, W.W., and A.K. Brown, "Mechanisms and Significance of Hyperbilirubinemia in the Newborn with Reference to Kernicterus," *Kernicterus and its Importance in Cerebral Palsy*. Springfield, Ill.: Charles C. Thomas, 1961, 4–12.

SUGGESTED READINGS

Incidence of Hearing Loss

Eagles, E.L., S.M. Wishik, and L.G. Doerfler, *Hearing Sensitivity and Ear Disease in Children: A Prospective Study.* St. Louis, Mo.: The Laryngoscope Press, 1967.

Schein, J.D., and M.T. Delk, *The Deaf Population of the United States.* Silver Springs, Md.: National Association of the Deaf, 1974.

Etiology of Hearing Impairment

Bordley, J., "The Effect of Viral Infection on Hearing," *Archives of Otolaryngology,* 98 (1973), 217.

Drillien, C.M., *The Growth and Development of the Prematurely Born Infant.* Edinburgh and London: E & S Livingstone, Ltd., 1964.

Fraser, G., *The Causes of Profound Deafness in Childhood.* Baltimore, Md.: Johns Hopkins University Press, 1976.

Konigsmark, B.W. and R.J. Gorlin, *Genetic and Metabolic Deafness.* Philadelphia, Pa.: W.B. Saunders Co., 1976.

Pathology

Dublin, W.A., *Fundamentals of Sensorineural Auditory Pathology.* Springfield, Ill.: Charles C. Thomas, 1976.

Schuknecht, H., *Pathology of the Ear.* Cambridge, Mass.: Harvard University Press, 1974.

Miscellaneous

Tower, D.B., ed., *Human Communication and Its Disorders,* Vol. 3, The Nervous System. New York: Raven Press, 1975.

CHAPTER TWO

Effects of Early Hearing Impairment on Normal Language Development

STEPHEN P. QUIGLEY

INTRODUCTION

Although this chapter is intended as a general introduction to the effects of hearing impairment on language development, an important secondary purpose is to influence audiologists and those who design their training programs to become involved in the problems of profoundly hearing-impaired (deaf) people. In the foreseeable future the audiologist is likely to become a key person in the education of deaf children. He is likely to be the first informed person to diagnose and prescribe for the deaf child. His prescription should include more than recommendations for amplification devices and aural training, which have definite but limited value for many deaf children. The audiologist, to be fully effective, must have extensive knowledge of the specialized educational programs and techniques for teaching deaf children, and of the intellectual, emotional, social, occupational, and other consequences of early profound hearing impairment. He should be at least reasonably fluent in manual communication, so that he can communicate with deaf parents and other deaf individuals in the form most deaf people in the United States use and understand. This requires that audiologists and those who train them abandon their present narrow conception of language as involving only spoken language and its derivatives and of communication as involving only oral communication.

CHAPTER OBJECTIVES

The objectives of this chapter are: first, to present a brief summary of "normal" language development; second, to show some effects of hearing impairment on language development, with separate sections about hard-of-hearing and deaf individuals; and third, to detail some major research needs in the area. The effects of hearing impairment on various aspects of language development—morphology (word structure), syntax (sentence structure), and semantics (meaning)—will be described. Phonology, while of major importance in the education of hearing-impaired children, is not treated here because of its extensive coverage in other chapters of this book and in the recent book by Ling (1976).

Studies cited in the chapter were chosen as illustrative of the thesis that hearing impairment has a profound effect on all aspects of language development and that degree of hearing impairment is related to degree of language deficit. The studies are not meant to represent exhaustive reviews of the literature.

HEARING IMPAIRMENT

Before proceeding, a definition of hearing impairment is required. If we consider hearing impairment as a generic term, covering all degrees of disability, then it is fair to say that clinicians have tended to include in the term two subcategories—hard-of-hearing individuals and deaf individuals. Attempts to subdivide within these subcategories, on the ground that they are too broad to be clinically or educationally useful, have had little effect on research or on clinical or educational practices. We therefore use the two broad categories in this chapter.

Let us first point out some of the present problems of definition. Table 2-1 shows the classification of hearing threshold levels used by the Department of Public Health in the State of Illinois, a classification adapted from one presented by Davis (1965). In past practice, and usually in present practice as well, individuals with hearing-threshold levels within the first three categories have been referred to as hard-of-hearing; those within the final one, as deaf. Those falling within the fourth one are considered "educationally deaf." One great research need is to determine the validity of the reported educational effects, including the effects on language, that degrees of hearing impairment impose on those within the various categories in such classifications. It is obvious to any clinical observer that a child with a hearing threshold level of 70dB (ISO) has greater language and educational problems than a similar child with a level of 30dB (ISO). But what of the difference between 50dB and 60dB? Most such classifications are based on clinical "experience" or "intuition." They require verification by research. Although they represent an improvement over the two broad categories of "hard-of-hearing" and "deaf," they have had little impact on research or educational practice.

If, because of lack of research verification and use of finer gradations of hearing impairment, we must classify the research literature into two broad categories—"hard-of-hearing" and "deaf"—we at least must try to differentiate between the two terms. Our definition of "deafness," although a rough one, is, we believe, a useful one. While hearing impairment, as measured by pure-tone audiometry and represented on an audiogram, can be considered as a continuum, somewhere along that continuum is a point where an individual ceases to be linked to the world of language and communication primarily by his ears and instead becomes linked to it primarily by his eyes. The problem then is no longer a

TABLE 2-1. Relationship of Degree of Handicap to Educational Needs

Degree of Handicap	Effect of Hearing Loss on the Understanding of Language and Speech	Educational Needs and Programs
Slight 16 to 29dB (ASA) or 27 to 40dB (ISO)	May have difficulty hearing faint or distant speech. Will not usually experience difficulty in school situations.	May benefit from a hearing aid as loss approaches 30dB (ASA) or 40dB (ISO). Attention to vocabulary development. Needs favorable seating and lighting. May need lip-reading instruction. May need speech correction.
Mild 30 to 44dB (ASA) or 41 to 55dB (ISO)	Understands conversational speech at a distance of 3–5 feet (face-to-face). May miss as much as 50% of class discussions if voices are faint or not in line of vision. May exhibit limited vocabulary and speech anomalies.	Child should be referred to special education for educational follow-up if such service is available. Individual hearing aid by evaluation and training in its use. Favorable seating and possible special class placement, especially for primary children. Attention to vocabulary and reading. May need lip-reading instruction. Speech conservation and correction, if indicated.
Marked 45 to 59dB (ASA) or 56 to 70dB (ISO)	Conversation must be loud to be understood. Will have increasing difficulty with school situations requiring participation in group discussions. Is likely to have defective speech. Is likely to be deficient in language usage and comprehension. Will have evidence of limited vocabulary.	Will need resource teacher or special class. Special help in language skills, vocabulary development, usage, reading, writing, grammar, etc. Individual hearing aid by evaluation and auditory training. Lip-reading instruction. Speech conservation and speech correction. Attention to auditory and visual situations at all times.

Severe 60 to 79dB (ASA) or 71 to 90dB (ISO)	May hear loud voices about one foot from the ear. May be able to identify environmental sounds. May be able to discriminate vowels but not all consonants. Speech and language defective and likely to deteriorate. Speech and language will not develop spontaneously if loss is present before one year of age.	Will need full-time special program for deaf children, with emphasis on all language skills, concept development, lip reading, and speech. Program needs specialized supervision and comprehensive supporting services. Individual hearing aid by evaluation. Auditory training on individual and group aids. Part-time in regular classes only as profitable.
Extreme 80dB or more (ASA) or 91dB or more (ISO)	May hear some loud sounds but is aware of vibrations more than tonal pattern. Relies on vision rather than hearing as primary avenue for communication. Speech and language defective and likely to deteriorate. Speech and language will not develop spontaneously if loss is present before one year.	Will need full-time special program for deaf children with emphasis on all language skills, concept development, lip reading, and speech. Program needs specialized supervision and comprehensive supporting services. Continuous appraisal of needs in regard to oral and manual communication. Auditory training on group and individual aid. Part-time in regular classes only for carefully selected children.

Source: R.J. Bernero and H. Bothwell, "Relationship of Hearing Impairment to Educational Needs," Illinois Department of Public Health and Office of the Superintendent of Public Instruction, 1966.

39

difference in degree, but becomes a difference in kind. That point is where "hard-of-hearingness" becomes "deafness"; it seems to occur at about 90dB (ISO). In terms of the classification in Table 2-1, most persons in the fifth category, as well as many in the fourth category, would be considered deaf. Many other qualifying factors, such as intelligence and socioeconomic status of the family, can enter into the determination, but these two rough categories will serve for our discussion of how hearing impairment affects language development.

NORMAL LANGUAGE DEVELOPMENT

McCarthy (1954) provided an extensive review of early research on language acquisition and various factors that influence it. The early studies, primarily descriptive, provided information on the first "sounds" the child makes, the first words he uses and at what age he uses them, and the growth of his vocabulary. The studies of articulation and sentence structure reported regarded the child's "errors" (articulation errors and incomplete and ungrammatical utterances) as a problem rather than a source of information. The research, in retrospect, seems atheoretical; because little effort was made to formulate and test hypotheses, no clear picture of the language development process emerges (Quigley et al., 1976).

In contrast, during the years since McCarthy's review, researchers have proposed a number of theories to explain a relatively small amount of data. Researchers are now focusing on the "how" of language acquisition, not just the "when." The major theoretical formulations and the developmental process of language acquisition they attempt to explain will be described briefly as a standard against which to compare the research findings on how hearing impairment affects language development. I will concentrate primarily on studies based on the theories of transformational-generative grammar, theories that have been the major force influencing language research during the past 20 years. Traditional studies are summarized by McCarthy (1954), and summaries of studies based on the formulations of structural linguistics are available in Harrell (1957) and Loban (1963).

Recent Theories

Recent theories of language acquisition can be loosely grouped into three categories: behaviorist, nativist, and cognitive. The behaviorist theories of language acquisition have their roots in the traditional psychology of learning. Skinner (1957) has presented perhaps the most comprehensive of the behaviorist theories. Language is described as a network of associations, a large number of stimulus and response connections. It is acquired through operant conditioning and reinforcement and is extended to new situations through response generalization. For the behavior theorists, language universals are those laws of learning that have long existed in psychology and that are believed to explain all learning. Structural linguistics is closely associated with behaviorism.

The behaviorist theories have been attacked by N. Chomsky (1957) and Weksel (1965), among others. The basic criticisms are that reinforcement and generalization are inadequate to explain the data, that language is too variable for the child to learn the appropriate connections, that language is essentially creative, and that the language user has available an infinite number of possible utterances which are produced by a finite number of grammatical rules. These writers argue that if the child learned language in a stimulus-response fashion, he could never acquire all of the sentences that he is, in fact, capable of producing.

An alternative to the behaviorist approaches comes from linguistic traditions, especially the ideas of N. Chomsky and later transformationalists. Proponents of this nativist theory place heavy emphasis on an innate biological propensity for language that they claim exists in every individual. Lenneberg (1967) proposed that language develops as a maturational process of the neurological structures. McNeill (1966) emphasized the nature of exposure to language, and theorized that speech sounds are distinguishable from other sounds in the environment, that linguistic input can be organized into categories, and that the developing linguistic system undergoes constant re-evaluation. The transformationalists claim that there are language universals common to all men and language.

The primary criticism of the nativist theories has been that there is little physiological evidence to support the biological-neurological organization proposed by proponents of the theories. The language-acquisition device they describe is hypothetical, without support of known biological data.

The third position falls between the two extremes of the pure behaviorist, for whom everything is learned, and the pure nativist, for whom everything is innate. This theoretical view may best be described as "cognitive." Slobin (1966a & 1966b), Fodor (1966), and Bever (1970) are recent proponents of this position; Piaget may be viewed as an early proponent. The cognitive theorists emphasize the interaction between a biological predisposition to use language and the environment. The development of the cognitive ability to deal with the world, the limitations of the memory in short-term and long-term retention, and the mechanisms for processing information place limits on the rate of language acquisition. Language functions as a means of communicating information and depends on the general cognitive development of the child for its development. This position is compatible with transformational grammar and has been espoused by many transformationalists.

Studies Based on Generative Grammar

Linguistics posits three levels of language—sound, shape, and sense, or more technically, phonology, morphology (including syntax), and semiology. Studies have indicated that most of a language's phonology is mastered by the typical child by the age of 4. While articulation "errors" still occur with older children, most of the sounds are under at least passive control (Moores, in press). The shape of a language refers to its grammar (morphology plus syntax), with syntax referring to word order and morphology to word forms. Although many psycholinguists consider the child to have mastered the grammar of his language by about age 5, some studies (C. Chomsky, 1969; Hunt, 1965; O'Donnell, Griffin, and Norris, 1967) indicate that some grammatical structures continue to develop at much later ages. Semiology refers to the meaning and vocabulary of language and, according to Joos (1964), most of the words people know are learned by the age of 20 years.

Thus, for the normal child acquisition of the phonological component of language is relatively complete at 4 or 5 years of age, the syntactic component at about the same age, and the semantic component by the age of 20. As will be seen, for the hearing-impaired child the situation is much different.

THE HARD-OF-HEARING CHILD

To assess the effects of a very slight (less than 15dB) to marked (70dB) hearing impairment on language performance and comprehension, Quigley and Thomure (1968) identified, as an experimental group, public school students who had been diagnosed as having a hearing impairment, but for whom special educational provisions had not been made. The subjects of the study ranged in age from 7 to 17 years. Each subject received an audiometric evaluation consisting of individual pure-tone air- and bone-conduction testing, and a language evaluation consisting of the word meaning, paragraph meaning, and language subtests of the *Stanford Achievement Test*. Table 2-2 shows the differential effects of hearing impairment across a less-than-15dB to 70dB (ISO) range on language comprehension.

Two significant items may be readily noted from study of Table 2-2. First, for every subtest in the hearing-level category, actual performance was lower than expected performance. Second, there were steady increases in the gaps between expected and actual performance on each subtest through the various hearing-threshold categories, with the exception of the last category where only the language subtest maintained the increase. Of particular interest in Table 2-2 is the language retardation in the first two categories of hearing-threshold level (less than 15dB and 15-26dB ISO). These data indicate that the effects of a slight hearing impairment on language development should not be minimized or dismissed. Additionally, the overall data support the hypothesis that children classified as hard-of-hearing do not form a homogeneous group, at least in language performance.

TABLE 2-2. Differences Between Expected Performance and Actual Performance of the Subjects on Various Subtests of the *Stanford Achievement Test*

Hearing Threshold Level (Better ear)	Number of Subjects	IQ	Word Meaning	Paragraph Meaning	Language	Subtest Average
Less than 15 dB	59	105.14	-1.04	-0.47	-0.78	-0.73
15-26dB	37	100.81	-1.40	-0.86	-1.16	-1.11
27-40dB	6	103.50	-3.48	-1.78	-1.95	-2.31
41-55dB	9	97.89	-3.84	-2.54	-2.93	-3.08
56-70dB	5	92.40	-2.78	-2.20	-3.52	-2.87
Total Group	116	102.56	-1.66	-0.90	-1.30	-1.25

Source: S.P. Quigley and F.E. Thomure, *Some Effects of Hearing Impairment Upon School Performance.* Springfield, Ill.: Office of the Superintendent of Public Instruction, 1968.

Expected Grade Placement in School (N = 116) M, 6.90; sd, 2.63

Actual Grade Placement in School   (N = 116) M, 5.78; sd, 2.61

Syntactic Development

Children with moderate degrees of impairment are likely to make language errors as a result of their deficient hearing. If such a child says, "My father work in the garden," it could be because he has not heard the "s" or the "ed" ending of the verb "work." Errors of agreement between subject and verb, and in verb tenses, are quite common (Streng, 1958).

Presnell (1973) found such verb-form difficulties in a sample of severely hard-of-hearing children. Her subjects ranged in age from 5 years to 13 years 3 months, and in hearing impairment from 50dB to greater than 93dB (ISO). All subjects had been identified as hearing-impaired before the age of 2 and none was known to have any additional problems that might interfere with language acquisition. The Northwestern Syntax Screening Test (NSST) was administered to each subject individually, and results were compared to the norms for the test. No hearing-impaired child scored above the norm on any of the syntactic forms.

Wilcox and Tobin (1974) found that certain verb constructions were difficult for children whose impairments were less severe than those of the Presnell study. These children were enrolled in special public-school classes for hard-of-hearing children. The mean age for the group was 10 years 4 months with a range of 8 years 10 months to 11 years 8 months. The mean IQ was 106 with a range of 87 to 147. The normal-hearing subjects were from the same grade level and age ranges and all had IQ scores within the normal range. The hard-of-hearing children all had congenital hearing impairments. Unaided pure-tone averages for the speech range were from 47 to 88dB with a mean of 61dB

(ISO). Although all of the hard-of-hearing children wore hearing aids at home and at school, their aided hearing threshold levels were not reported. The verb constructions used in the study, all in third person singular, were: present tense auxiliary (be + ing), auxiliary (have + en), auxiliary (will), passive and negative passive. Analysis of the data indicated that the linguistic performance of the hard-of-hearing children was significantly inferior to that of the normal-hearing children for all verb constructions tested.

Goetzinger (1962) and Harrison (1964) have shown that children with hearing impairments of less than 35dB (ASA) experience difficulty in language development. Goetzinger's work is especially interesting in that he collected his data longitudinally from cases he saw in his audiological clinic. All children when first seen were about 6 to 7 years old. He found that children with a 30 to 35dB impairment in the better ear were also retarded in language development by about one year.

Semantic Development

Young and McConnell (1957) studied the vocabulary level of 20 children with a mean hearing-threshold level of 51 dB (range: 32–75 dB) at 500 to 2000 Hz (ASA) enrolled in regular classes to determine if it differed significantly from that of 20 comparable children with normal hearing. Using verbal and visual presentation of the Ammons Full-Range Picture Vocabulary Test, they found a statistically significant difference between the two groups in favor of the children with normal hearing. Nor was the difference just a group difference, since no hard-of-hearing child received a higher score on the vocabulary test than did his matched control subject. In another study investigating semantic development in hearing-impaired children to assess the effects of hearing impairment on their social use of language, Lewis (1968) found a direct relationship: As hearing decreased, language performance decreased.

Effects of Early Intervention

Since basic language development for typical children with normal hearing takes place during the first few years of life, there has long been interest in attempting to improve the language development of hearing-impaired children through intensive early intervention. One study of such intervention is discussed here; another, in the following section of this chapter.

McConnell and Horton (1970) designed a study patterned after the home training program of the John Tracy Clinic. It involved: (1) a home setting for parent training; (2) intensive and continuing hearing evaluation of the children; (3) providing hearing aids for the children; (4) informing the parents of the nature and effects of hearing impairment; and (5) instructing the parents in how the home setting could be used to develop language and communication. During the three-year project 94 children participated; extensive data are given on these children, their families, and the results achieved. However, a number of uncontrollable factors resulted in lack of continuity of attendance for many children, and the data presented are based on 28 children who had attended continuously for 27.8 months.

Table 2-3 gives background data on the children and their parents. Of particular interest are the data on the hearing levels of the children. The initial unaided Speech Awareness Level for the group has a mean of 71.6dB with a range of 40 to 100dB. While the project was designed to deal with very young deaf children, the hearing level is not as severe as that usually associated with the term "deaf." This is even more apparent in the initial aided Speech Awareness Level, where the group mean was 48.6dB with a range of 20 to 100dB. These data raise questions concerning the degree and type of hearing impairment, as do the data for the final aided examination, where the mean was 27.1dB and range 8 to 65dB. This point is being emphasized to caution against overgeneralization of the results of the study to children with more severe degrees of hearing impairment.

Table 2-4 shows the results in language development that were obtained with the 28 children. Using the Communicative Evaluation Chart (Anderson, Miles, and Matheny, 1963) to measure langauge age, one sees the children progressed 20.8 months during the 27.8 months of instruction at home and in the demonstration home setting—very notable progress indeed.

These few data are sufficient to indicate that very early intervention in a cooperative program between professionals and families can improve language and communication development. As stated earlier, caution should be exercised in generalizing to children with more severe degrees of hearing impairment.

TABLE 2-3. Summary Description of 28 Children with Respect to Parental Occupational Classification, Amount of Home Program Instruction, and Hearing Level for Speech

	Mean	*Stand. Dev.*	*Range*
Parent's occupational classification	3.9	1.8	1–7
Number home visits	21.2	12.8	7–57
Number hours instruction	27.2	16.1	7–68.5 hr.
Hearing Level			
Speech awareness level, 1st exam unaided	71.6dB	15.2dB	40–100dB
Speech awareness level, 1st exam aided	48.6dB	21.3dB	20–100dB
Speech awareness level, last exam, aided	27.1dB	17.2dB	8–65dB

Source: F. McConnell and K.B. Horton, "A Home Teaching Program for Parents of Very Young Deaf Children," Vanderbilt University School of Medicine, Project No. 6-1187, Grant No. OEG 32-52-0450-6007. U.S. Office of Education, Final Report, January, 1970.

TABLE 2-4. Pre- and Postinstruction Comparisons for 28 Children on Chronological, Language, and Performance Age

	Mean	Standard Deviation	Range	Difference
Chronological age				
Preinstruction	27.5 months	8.2	10-40 months	27.8 months
Postinstruction	55.3 months	8.6	34-69 months	
Language age				
Preinstruction	8.4 months	2.3	4.7-13.8 months	20.8 months
Postinstruction	29.2 months	13.0	12.7-57.0 months	
Performance age				
Preinstruction	23.2 months	—	9.2-30.8 months	24.7 months
Postinstruction	47.9 months	—	26.6-60.0 months	

Source: F. McConnell and K.B. Horton, "A Home Teaching Program for Parents of Very Young Deaf Children," Vanderbilt University School of Medicine, Project No. 6-1187, Grant No. OEG 32-52-0450-6007. U.S. Office of Education, Final Report, January, 1970.

THE DEAF CHILD

Morphology

Before examining language development in deaf children, let us examine a now-classic study of morphology in hearing children. Berko (1958) reasoned that if a child could supply correct plural forms for words he had never heard before, then it could be assumed that he was using a general rule for forming plurals, not memorizing the plural forms of a large number of words. Berko conducted studies using nonsense words such as "wug" and "gutch" to test her hypothesis. Items were, for example: "There is a wug. Now there is another one. Now there are two of them. There are two ____."

The child was expected to complete the sentence with the plural form "wugs." Using similar techniques, Berko investigated the ability of preschoolers and first-graders to supply noun plurals and possessives, past tenses of verbs, simple third person singular markings, present progressive, and regular comparison of adjectives—all inflectional morphemes—as well as such derived forms as diminutives, adjectives, agentive nouns, and some compound nouns. She found that children could perform these tasks quite successfully and there was a developmental order among the various inflected and derived morphemes studied.

Studies of deaf children's acquisition of morphology indicate that although the sequence is generally the same as for hearing children, it is greatly delayed. Cooper (1967), working with deaf children and using an approach similar to that used by Berko, found that noun plurals and possessives were usually learned earlier than verb tense markers; that the progressive marking for verbs occurred before the past, which in turn was learned before the third person singular, simple present; that superlative adjective forms were easier than comparatives; and that inflected morphemes were easier than derived ones. In an extensive study of samples of deaf children's written language, Taylor (1969) found that verb problems were more severe than noun problems and that plural forms of nouns exhibited more errors than possessive forms.

While these studies indicate that the order of difficulty of morphological forms for deaf children is generally similar to their order of acquisition by hearing children, caution should be exercised in accepting order of difficulty as being the same as order of acquisition. Studies of language acquisition by hearing children generally are conducted on the spoken language of very young children; studies on deaf children are conducted on the written language of older children. Whereas very young hearing children can be assumed to be learning language in a more or less "natural" fashion, the deaf children studied usually have been exposed to direct and formal intervention in their language acquisition process by teachers and other professionals.

Syntax

In this section on syntax, we also consider general measures of reading comprehension, which are heavily influenced by the deaf child's syntactic ability.

Reading Ability. Furth (1966) reported on a comprehensive survey of the reading abilities of 4,624 deaf subjects between the ages of 10½ and 16½ years conducted by Wrightstone, Aronow, and Moskowitz in 1963. The scores of the deaf subjects were compared with the norms established for hearing children on the *Metropolitan Elementary Reading Test,* Test 2. It was found that the mean score for silent reading achievement rose from a grade equivalence of 2.7 around age 11 to 3.5 around age 16. Furthermore, only 12% of the 1,075 subjects between the ages of 15½ and 16½ years and 10% of the 1,035 subjects between 14½ and 15½ years of age reached a grade equivalence of 4.9 or higher. The grade equivalences cited by Furth have been supported in other studies (Goetzinger and Rousey, 1959; Myklebust, 1960), including a large national study by DiFrancesca (1972), who reported the results of approximately 17,000 *Stanford Achievement Tests* given to deaf students between the ages of 6 and 21 years. Analysis of the paragraph meaning subtest indicated that the highest average grade-equivalent score was 4.36 at age 19. The average reading growth for the students was 0.2 grade level for each year of schooling.

Studies published early in this century by Pintner and Paterson (1916) and Pintner (1918) provide evidence that deaf students in schools at that time performed no better than those reported on by Furth and DiFrancesca. The earlier studies used scores on the *Trabue Language Completion Tests* as their dependent variable. Pintner and Paterson reported that the reading abilities of the majority of the deaf children were between grades 2 and 4 and that only 6.4% reached scores above the fourth-grade level. These findings were based on test results from 570 deaf students in two residential schools. When Pintner administered two scales of the *Trabue Language Completion Test* to 1,720 deaf students in four residential schools, he found that the medians for fourth-grade hearing children were higher than any of the medians at any of the four schools for deaf children (Moores, in press).

The Cloze Procedure. The studies cited thus far all indicate that deaf students' abilities to read written English are poor and that their growth in this area is slow. Each of these studies used tests standardized for hearing students. Moores (1967), however, reported that reading scores achieved by deaf students on such standardized tests, even though very low, provide inflated estimates of reading ability; grammatical and semantic insufficiencies among the deaf subjects that are not reflected in the reading test scores lower their reading ability still further. To demonstrate this, Moores matched an experimental group of 37 deaf students with a control group of 37 hearing students on reading scores on the *Stanford Achievement Test*. The experimental group had a mean grade reading level of 4.77, and the control group had a mean grade level score of 4.84. Moores selected three passages of approximately 250 words each from a fourth-, a sixth-, and an eighth-grade reading test. From these passages every fifth word was deleted and the subjects were asked to supply the missing word. The technique, known as the "cloze procedure," has been demonstrated by Taylor (1953, 1954, and 1956) to be a reliable tool for measuring reading ability.

When the subjects had supplied words for each of the blanks in the passages, three scores were given. If the subjects supplied the exact word deleted from the text, they were given a correct score for verbatim reproduction. If the exact word was not supplied, but the subjects responded by filling in a word from the same grammatical class, a correct score for form-class reproduction was given. The third score was the percentage of verbatim responses given for the correct form-class responses.

A significant difference between groups at each level was found for verbatim reproduction, supporting the assumption that standardized reading tests give inflated estimates of deaf subjects' abilities to comprehend written English. Significant differences were also found for the form-class reproduction at the fourth- and sixth-grade levels, indicating inadequately developed grammatical relations in English for the deaf subjects. Significant differences at all three reading levels for the verbatim given form-class reproduction indicated semantic insufficiencies in the form of redundant, stereotyped modes of expression and limited vocabulary on the part of the deaf subjects in spite of the fact that they were supposedly equal in reading ability to the hearing subjects.

Studies of Specific Syntactic Structures. If, as the above studies indicate, standardized reading tests do not adequately measure the ability of deaf children, it would seem appropriate to define more precisely what comprehension problems deaf children might encounter in reading. Schmitt (1968) provided one of the first investigations into comprehension and production of specific syntactic structures. These types of investigations were furthered by Power (1971), Power and Quigley (1973), and Quigley et al. (1976).

Schmitt (1968) developed materials that included pictures in a multiple-choice format to assess the comprehension and production of simple sentences that varied in transformations and verb tenses. Deaf subjects at ages 8, 11, 14, and 17 years were compared with a control group of hearing children at ages 8 and 11 years. The three transformations studied were the negative, passive, and passive negative; the three tenses were past, present progressive, and future. Schmitt found no differences in verb tense difficulties across all the tasks. The most difficult transformation was found to be the passive followed by the passive-negative, declarative, and negative. He also found that comprehension tasks were easier than production tasks.

Power and Quigley (1973) extended Schmitt's work by investigating deaf children's comprehension and production of nonreversible, reversible, and agent-deleted passive sentences. Ten boys and ten girls between the ages of 9 and 10, 11 and 12, 13 and 14, 15 and 16, and 17 and 18 years were presented with comprehension, production, and recognition tasks. A criterion of 75% correct responses was established. The percentage of deaf subjects between the ages of 17 and 18 years achieving the criterion on each of the tasks is shown in Table 2-5. For the deaf subjects, the most difficult task was production, with comprehension and recognition following in decreasing order of difficulty. A similar study by Turner and Rommetveit (1967) indicated that approximately 95% of hearing children comprehend and produce the passive structure by age 8.

The research by Quigley et al. (1976) expanded the study of specific syntactic structures to include aspects of relativization, conjunction, complementation, pronominalization, question formation, negation, and the verb system. The

TABLE 2-5. Percentage of Children at the Age of 17–18 Years Reaching Criterion of 75% of Sentences Correct

Task	Age 17–18
Comprehension	
Nonreversible sentences	65%
Reversible sentences	60
Agent-deleted sentences	35
Production	40
Recognition	70

Source: D.J. Power, "Deaf Children's Acquisition of the Passive Voice." Unpublished doctoral dissertation, University of Illinois, 1971.

Test of Syntactic Ability (TSA), which consists of 22 subtests, was developed to assess the comprehension and production of those structures.

The TSA was administered to 450 prelingually deaf students between the ages of 10 and 18. At each age level, 25 boys and 25 girls were randomly selected from 16 educational programs with 100 or more students; the programs were also randomly selected after they had been stratified by geographical region of the United States and type of program (day or residential). Four major questions motivated this study and a fifth question was added later:

1. How well established are the syntactic rules of English in the language of deaf students at age levels from 10 to 18 years?
2. Are there developmental stages for these rules and, if so, how do the stages compare with those for hearing individuals?
3. Is there an order in which the various syntactic structures are acquired by deaf individuals, and is this order similar to the order in which the structures are acquired by hearing individuals?
4. Do deaf individuals acquire the same syntactic rules as hearing individuals, but at a retarded rate, or do they acquire some rules that never operate in the grammar of hearing persons? (Quigley et al., 1976, p. 2)

The fifth question which developed during the investigation was:

5. How does deaf children's understanding of various syntactic structures compare to the occurrence of those structures in their reading materials? (p. 184)

Table 2-6 gives summary data on questions 1, 2, and 5. The structures are listed in the table by their order of difficulty for the deaf subjects, from the easiest to the most difficult. Although the orders of difficulty are not identical between the deaf and hearing subjects, it is of interest that the three easiest structures for the deaf students were also the easiest for the hearing sample. In like manner, pronominalization, the verb system, complementation, and relativization were most difficult for both samples. The only major difference in order of difficulty appeared with the disjunction and alternation subtest.

Table 2-6 also illustrates the extent to which the syntactic rules of English are established in the language of deaf children. Among deaf students most of the structures were not well established even among the 18-year-olds, whereas among the hearing subjects virtually all of the structures had been mastered by the age of 10. The disparity between the deaf subjects' knowledge of specific syntactic structures and their appearance in the textbook series *Reading for Meaning* (McKee et al., 1966) is also depicted in Table 2-7. As an example 18-year-old deaf students had a mean score of 63% correct on the Complementation subtest. This structure first appeared in the second primer of the reading series 4 times per 100 sentences; at the sixth-grade level it had increased to 32

TABLE 2-6. Summary of Performance on Syntactic Structures and Their Frequency of Occurrence Per 100 Sentences in the *Reading for Meaning* Series

Structure	Deaf Students				Hearing Students	Frequency of Occurrence	
	Average Across Ages	Age 10	Age 18	Increase	Average Across Ages	Level at Which Structure First Appeared	Frequency in 6th Grade Text
Negation							
be	79%	60%	86%	26%	92%	1st Primer–13	9
do	71	53	82	28	93		
have	74	57	78	21	86		
Modals	78	58	87	29	90		
Means	76	57	83	26	90		
Conjunction							
Conjunction	72%	56%	86%	30%	92%	1st Primer–11	36
Deletion	74	59	86	27	94		
Means	73	57	86	29	92		
Question Formation							
WH questions:							
Comprehension	66%	44%	80%	36%	98%	2nd Primer–5	6
Yes/no questions:							
Comprehension	74	48	90	42	99	1st Primer–5	3
Tag questions	57	46	63	17	98		
Means	66	46	78	32	98		
Pronominalization							
Personal pronouns	67%	51%	88%	37%	78%		
Backward pronominalization	70	49	85	36	94	4th grade–1	0 (4/1000)
Possessive adjectives	65	42	82	40	98	1st grade–4	27

(continued)

TABLE 2-6. (Continued)

Structure	Deaf Students				Hearing Students	Frequency of Occurrence	
	Average Across Ages	Age 10	Age 18	Increase	Average Across Ages	Level at Which Structure First Appeared	Frequency in 6th Grade Text
Possessive pronouns	48	34	64	30	99	3rd Primer-1	0 (3/1000)
Reflexivization	50	21	73	52	80	2nd grade-1	2
Means	60	39	78	39	90		
Verbs							
Verb auxiliaries	54%	52%	71%	19%	81%	1st grade-1	18
Tense sequencing	63	54	72	18	78		
Means	58	53	71	18	79		
Complementation							
Infinitives and gerunds	55%	50%	63%	13%	88%	2nd Primer-4	32
Relativization							
Processing	68%	59%	76%	17%	78%	3rd Primer-2	12
Embedding	53	51	59	8	84		
Relative Pronoun referents	42	27	56	29	82		
Means	54	46	63	18	82		
Disjunction & alternation	36%	22%	59%	37%	84%	1st grade-1	7

Source: Cited in B. Jones (1976), as adapted from Quigley et al. (1976).

times per 100 sentences. It would appear, therefore, that at age 18 deaf students would experience difficulty in comprehending approximately one-third of the sentences in the sixth-grade text merely on the basis of this one structure. Similar results were obtained for the other structures.

Studies on language acquisition among hearing children have indicated that children acquire specific syntactic structures through developmental stages. This has been shown by Klima and Bellugi-Klima (1966) and Bellugi (1971) for question formation and by Bellugi (1967) for negation. Question three asked if deaf children go through similar stages. The data from the TSA could not provide a direct answer to this question, since it measures degrees of syntactic difficulty rather than the acquisition process for specific structures in the language of children. Also, since the subjects for the study ranged in age from 10 to 18 years, one could not reasonably expect the data to answer definitive questions concerning the language acquisition process. The authors did, however, offer a tentative conclusion that syntactic structures for deaf children develop in a manner similar to those of hearing children, but at a slower rate. They were able to reach this conclusion on the basis of comparison from psycholinguistic literature on hearing children and data from the TSA. They did, however, find exceptions; this was the concern of question 4.

Table 2-7 presents syntactic structures that appeared consistently in the comprehension and production of many of the deaf subjects, but not among the hearing sample. One might reasonably assume, because of their being both consistent and persistent, that these structures are rule ordered. The extent to which deaf subjects acquire syntactic structures different from those of hearing subjects would be expected to affect their abilities to comprehend written English.

The studies cited present a depressing picture of the syntactic problems in the language of deaf children, but as the following samples of written language from "typical" deaf children show, the picture is a realistic one.

The man pull many her fish. He see one large fish. The boy saw many, many her fish and turtle. The man saw two red fish. He will see not out more and fish. The boy is sorry. (10-year-old female, performance IQ of 97, born deaf, better ear average of 99dB, ASA.)

The girl help to dog eat. The children had talk. The family went to trip. The boy saw to dog. A boy was happy to met dog. A dog want to in car. Our family leave to on trip. Our family arrived to rest in park. The two boy played to ball or with the dog. Some Children was hungry. A woman cooked to the hamburg. A girl want to eat. (14-year-old male, performance IQ of 118, born deaf, better ear average of 99dB ASA.)

Mrs. Gloria made some sandwich and other some any food and drink. A little girl got a sandwich. She give a dog eat a cheese and ham in sandwich. She brother Bill tooked I gave basketball for bring park. and father got a bat and ball. A Family arrived father is car. He drive car It is on. Happen Bill saw a dog walked on the sidewalk. He told father, He said stop. He say what. "I saw may a

TABLE 2-7. Some Distinct Syntactic Constructions in the Language of Deaf Students

Structural Environment in Which Construction Occurs	Description of Construction	Example Sentences
Verb system	Verb deletion	The cat under the table.
	Be or have deletion	John sick. The girl a ball.
	Be-have confusion	Jim have sick.
	Incorrect pairing of auxiliary with verb markers	Tom has pushing the wagon.
	By deletion (passive voice)	The boy was pushed the girl.
Negation	Negative outside the sentence.	Beth made candy no.
Conjunction	Marking only first verb	Beth threw the ball and Jean catch it.
	Conjunction deletion	Joe bought ate the apple.
Complemention	Extra for	For to play baseball is fun.
	Extra to in POSS-ing complement	John goes to fishing.
	Infinitive in place of gerund	John goes to fish.
	Incorrectly inflected infinitive	Bill liked to played baseball.
	Unmarked infinitive without to	Jim wanted go.
Relativization	NP's where whose is required	I helped the boy's mother was sick.
	Copying of referent	John saw the boy who the boy kicked the ball.
Question formation	Copying	Who a boy gave you a ball?
	Failure to apply subject-auxiliary inversion	Who the baby did love?
	Incorrect inversion	Who TV watched
Question formation, Negation	Overgeneralization of contraction rule	I amn't tired. Bill willn't go.
Relativization, Conjunction	Object-object deletion	John chased the girl and he scared. (John chased the girl. He scared the girl.)
	Object-subject deletion	The dog chased the girl had on a red dress. (The dog chased the girl. The girl had on a red dress.)
All types of sentences	Forced subject-verb-object pattern	The boy pushed the girl. (The boy was pushed by the girl.)

Source: Cited in B. Jones (1976), as adapted from Quigley et al. (1976).

dog. Open a door. Bill jumped on the side walk. He love him dog. He laught them Now We went to trip for park. About 1:30 oclock. Mrs. Gloria cooked hamburger and other sandwich. Father son Bill played baseball. A dog running to Bill because a dog get a ball. but we have good time for park. (18-year-old male, performance IQ of 99, born deaf, better ear average of 99dB ASA.)

Semantics

It has usually been held that it is easier to teach vocabulary than connected language to deaf children. While this might be true, it does not seem that deaf children's vocabularies are superior to their understanding of syntax, at least as far as standardized test results are concerned. Studies have consistently shown that scores on vocabulary subtests of achievement batteries are not usually higher than those on subtests with such labels as "paragraph meaning," and they have sometimes been reported to be lower (Cooper and Rosenstein, 1966; O'Neill, 1973). These findings are supported by a large-scale study of deaf students using the *Stanford Achievement Test* (DiFrancesca, 1972). It was reported that "vocabulary scores" were below those for "word meaning" and "paragraph meaning," even at the oldest ages studied. Studies by Goetzinger and Rousey (1959) and by Myklebust (1960) confirm these vocabulary findings and show that the average deaf student, by the time he leaves school, has a vocabulary equivalent to that of the average nine-year-old hearing child.

Two studies in the early sixties (Kates, Kates, and Michael, 1962; Jurmaa, 1973), designed to investigate the relationship of language to thinking in deaf children, indicated the semantic problems of deaf children on various semantic measures. Kates, Kates, and Michael tested deaf adolescents and adults and found that whenever the task was changed from object- to word-sorting, categorization performance seriously declined. This large gap did not exist for the hearing subjects. Jurmaa (1973) administered five vocabulary tests to deaf children and adolescents, ages 12 to 17. The tasks consisted of naming pictures, naming as many words as possible beginning with *k* and *s,* giving the opposites to simple words, choosing words in the same category, and testing combined general knowledge and vocabulary. As expected, the deaf subjects were significantly inferior to the matched controls on all measures.

Koplin et al. (1967) also observed a performance gap between deaf and hearing children on semantic measures. They administered a word association task to 266 deaf students between the ages of 11 and 21 years and to 325 matched hearing controls. The control group made fewer idiosyncratic responses (a response to a stimulus word given by only one subject) than the deaf group and performed significantly better on a contrast (opposites) test. While the superordinate reponses (the stimulus word is a member of a larger class which is given a response: eagle[s]-bird[r]; cabbage[s]-vegetable[r]) and paradigmatic responses (words similar in meaning used as a substitute for the stimulus word) of the hearing group were more mature, the difference between the deaf group and the hearing group did not reach significance. The investigators concluded that the gap was quantitative and did not represent a developmental difference.

Rosenstein and MacGinitie (1969) confirmed these results and also found that the responses among the deaf children of their study were quite similar. In addition, the performance of the deaf subjects did not improve with age. Related studies by Silverman and Rosenstein (Rosenstein and MacGinitie, 1969) indicated that deaf children used more associations in defining words than did hearing children, but with these associations they constructed less adequate definitions. A further study found that deaf subjects were less able to identify synonyms than were hearing controls.

Nunnally and Blanton (1966) also found that deaf children produced fewer paradigmatic responses at any given age than hearing children. If the extent of this responding is a true reflection of the level of semantic development of deaf children, then apparently they are deprived of sufficient linguistic experiences and tend to perform at a less mature level than hearing children.

Effects of Early Intervention

The studies cited lead one to question whether deaf subjects provided with optimum opportunities to learn standard English would have better comprehension skills. This question led Brasel and Quigley (1977) to investigate whether early intervention could enhance the acquisition of English among deaf children and, if so, which types of intervention would be most successful. Four groups of deaf subjects between the ages of 10 years and 18 years 11 months were selected and given the TSA and the language and reading subtests of the Stanford Achievement Test. A total of 72 subjects (18 for each group) participated in the study. The four groups were dichotomized according to whether the parents were hearing or deaf. Those with deaf parents were then assigned to one of two groups: those whose parents used manual English; those whose parents used some form of Ameslan (American Sign Language) with their deaf children during infancy and early childhood. The subjects with hearing parents were also divided into two groups: those whose parents provided them during the early childhood years with an intensive oral education at home and in preschool; those who provided an average oral education for their children.

The results for the TSA are shown in Table 2–8. It can be seen that the manual English group had the highest means for all structures; they were followed by the average manual, the intensive oral, and average oral groups. These findings suggest that the development of a standard English language base early in life would lead to better English skills and that visual presentation through manual English might be the most effective method of developing such a language base. The findings for the TSA were supported by identical findings for the four groups on the subtests of the Stanford Achievement Test.

TABLE 2-8. Test of Syntactic Ability, Mean Percentage Scores, Ranges and Standard Deviations, by Group and Structure (N = 72)

Group	Relativization	Question Formation	Negation	Conjunction	Verb Usage	Pronominalization
ME						
Mean %	80.87	89.8	91.9	87.5	82.2	89.9
Range %	40.8–95.2	59.2–99.3	82.9–100.0	36.3–98.8	65.8–94.7	66.7–99.3
SD %	11.94	11.36	4.86	15.80	8.86	9.54
IO						
Mean %	66.3	76.0	84.9	73.1	69.4	71.2
Range %	47.6–92.4	34.5–99.3	53.4–97.3	26.3–100.0	42.1–89.5	23.3–98.0
SD %	13.29	19.74	12.30	21.23	14.34	23.07
AM						
Mean %	66.4	81.3	86.7	76.5	74.5	78.7
Range %	47.6–90.3	52.1–94.4	47.3–97.3	37.5–96.3	50.0–90.8	40.7–96.0
SD %	13.56	15.31	12.41	16.79	11.39	19.07
AO						
Mean %	58.1	64.0	79.4	67.6	66.8	64.6
Range %	43.6–75.8	28.2–94.4	43.8–95.2	30.0–93.8	51.3–85.5	32.7–97.3
SD %	8.53	18.63	15.29	15.84	10.71	19.31
Total						
Mean %	67.89	77.78	85.72	76.20	73.20	76.08
Range %	43.6–95.2	28.2–99.3	43.8–100.0	26.3–100.0	42.1–94.7	23.3–99.3
SD %	11.12	13.63	10.32	16.6	10.83	15.42

Source: K.E. Brasel, and S.P. Quigley, "Influence of Certain Language and Communication Environments in Early Childhood on the Development of Language in Deaf Individuals." Journal of Speech and Hearing Research, 20, (1977), 96–107.

SUMMARY

Early hearing impairment has definite effects on language development and the effects seem closely related to degree of impairment. As shown by Quigley and Thomure (1968), Goetzinger (1962), Harrison (1964), and others, even very mild impairments of hearing (less than 30dB) are often related to language and other educational deficits. This relation of hearing impairment and language deficit is evident in all aspects of language—phonological, morphological, syntactic, and semantic.

While the relationship between degree of impairment and severity of language deficit seems to be continuous at the mild and moderate levels of impairment, at some point (perhaps at about 80 or 90dB, ISO) the child passes from having language problems to having no language at all, unless intensive and specialized educational procedures are employed. This point, which is influenced by several factors, can be considered the demarcation line between hard-of-hearing and deaf, terms which still have some educational value despite the present antipathy of educators for such labels. At this point and beyond, the child is linked to the world of communication primarily by his eyes rather than by his ears.

The language problems of children with mild and moderate degrees of hearing impairment have not been investigated sufficiently to specify the probable type and extent of the problem at a particular level of impairment. Research, however, has increased considerably in the past decade, and there now are at least a few studies in each of the several aspects of language. Expansion of the research and clinical studies should result in definitive statements about the phonological, morphological, syntactic, and semantic effects of different degrees of impairment; such statements will be not only informative, but also clinically and educationally useful.

With profound degrees of impairment (deafness), the situation is different. Although many fewer children fall into this category, effects of the impairment have been more thoroughly investigated, and the clinical, educational, and rehabilitation services provided are much more extensive than those for hard-of-hearing children. Studies by Cooper (1967) and Taylor (1969) in morphology; Power and Quigley (1973) and Quigley et al. (1976) in syntax; and Koplin et al. (1967) in semantics illustrate the considerable number of investigations that are beginning to provide a body of clinically and educationally useful knowledge about the language of deaf children. Of particular interest are recent findings in morphology and syntax that show that the considerable "deviations" of the language productions of deaf children from standard English are not random occurrences, but occur in many instances with such consistency that the "deviations" must be considered rule-ordered (Taylor, 1969; Quigley et al., 1976). These findings open up new possibilities for diagnosis and remediation of the language problems.

RESEARCH AND TRAINING NEEDS

Just as this chapter could contain only samplings of the research literature, so this section can list only a sampling of the major research and training needs:

1. The indications that hearing impairments even as mild as 20dB can result in language and educational deficiencies should be thoroughly investigated. Research and other endeavors in hearing impairment during the past 15 to 20 years have concentrated mostly on individuals with profound degrees of impairment (deaf persons), while the much larger population of hard-of-hearing children has been relatively neglected.

2. Related to this is the need to determine the specific problems in each aspect of language—phonology, morphology, syntax, and semantics—at varying degrees of hearing impairment. In other words, do the various classifications of hearing-threshold levels have educational and clinical validity and value?

3. A determination is needed of whether there is a point (or range) on the hearing-threshold scale beyond which there is a shift from degree of problem to kind of problem, as is believed to exist between the language problems of hard-of-hearing children and those of deaf children.

4. Dodd (1976) and Quigley et al. (1976) have presented evidence indicating that deaf children exhibit phonological and syntactic "deviations" from standard English usage persistent and consistent enough to indicate they are rule-ordered and not random happenings. This type of investigation should be expanded with deaf persons and extended to other degrees of hearing impairment.

5. Diagnostic language tests and individualized remedial programs and materials based on the tests are needed. Much of the work with language problems of hearing-impaired children involves clinical teaching, which requires specific diagnostic and remedial techniques, not the more general educational approaches common to classroom teaching.

6. The first five listed needs deal primarily with expanding knowledge of the extent and nature of the language effects of hearing impairment. An investigation of the effectiveness of various types of formal and informal intervention programs in alleviating language problems is a major need. Of particular concern here we mention the use of oral and manual methods of communication, alone or in combination, with deaf children. An increasing number of investigations in this area have been conducted during the past 20 years, but much more is needed.

7. The audiologist can play a vital role in the education of deaf children, but to do so he requires much more extensive training in the specific educational programs and techniques for deaf children, in manual communication (the lan-

guage of signs and fingerspelling), and in the intellectual, emotional, social, occupational, and other consequences of early profound hearing impairment.

8. One final listing also deals with training. We see a need for the training of educational or clinical specialists to teach those schoolchildren who now seem to "fall between the cracks." These are children whose hearing problems are too severe for the limited availability and the limited training of itinerant speech and hearing specialists, but not severe enough for the highly specialized, very intensive, and often segregated programs provided for deaf children.

REFERENCES

Anderson, R.M., M. Miles, and P.A. Matheny, *Communicative Evaluation Chart from Infancy to Five Years.* Cambridge, Mass.: Educators Publishing Service, Inc., 1963.

Bellugi, U., "The Acquisition of Legation." Unpublished doctoral dissertation, Harvard University, 1967.

Bellugi, U., "Simplification in Children's Language" in *Language Acquisition: Models and Methods,* edited by R. Huxley and E. Ingram. New York: Academic Press, 1971.

Berko, J., "The Child's Learning of English Morphology," *Word,* 14 (1958), 150–177.

Bernero, R.J., and H. Bothwell, *Relationship of Hearing Impairment to Educational Needs.* Springfield, Ill.: Illinois Department of Public Health and Office of Superintendent of Public Instruction, 1966.

Bever, T.G., "The Cognitive Basis for Linguistic Structures," in *Cognition and the Development of Language,* edited by J.R. Hayes. New York: John Wiley & Sons, Inc., 1970.

Brasel, K.E., and S.P. Quigley, "Influence of Certain Language and Communication Environments in Early Childhood on the Development of Language in Deaf Individuals," *Journal of Speech and Hearing Research,* 20, (1977), 96–107.

Chomsky, C., *The Acquisition of Syntax in Children from 5 to 10.* Cambridge, Mass.: M.I.T. Press, 1969.

Chomsky, N., *Syntactic structures.* The Hague: Mouton, 1957.

Cooper, R.L., "The Ability of Deaf and Hearing Children to Apply Morphological Rules," *Journal of Speech and Hearing Research,* 10 (1967), 77–86.

Cooper, R.L., and J. Rosenstein, "Language Acquisition of Deaf Children." *Volta Review,* 68, (1966), 58–67.

Davis, H., "Guide for the Classification and Evaluation of Hearing Handicap in Relation to the International Audiometric Zero," *Transactions of the American Academy of Ophthalmology and Otolaryngology,* July–August 1965, 740–751.

DiFrancesca, S., *Academic Achievement Test Results of a National Testing Program for Hearing Impaired Students, United States, Spring, 1971.* Washington, D.C.: Gallaudet College, Office of Demographic Studies, 1972.

Dodd, B., "The Phonological Systems of Deaf Children," *Journal of Speech and Hearing Disorders,* 41 (1976), 185–198.

Fodor, A., "How to Learn to Talk: Some Simple Ways," in *The Genesis of Language: A Psycholinguistic Approach,* edited by F. Smith and G.A. Miller. Cambridge, Mass.: M.I.T. Press, 1966.

Furth, H.G., "A Comparison of Reading Test Norms of Deaf and Hearing Children," *American Annals of the Deaf,* 3 (1966), 461–462.

Goetzinger, C.P., "Effects of Small Perceptive Losses on Language and on Speech Discrimination," *Volta Review,* 64 (1962), 408–414.

Goetzinger, C.P., and **C.L. Rousey**, "Educational Achievement of Deaf Children," *American Annals of the Deaf,* 104 (1959), 221–231.

Harrell, L.E., Jr., "A Comparison of Oral and Written Language in School Age Children, *Monographs of the Society for Research in Child Development,* 22, (1957).

Harrison, C.W., "A Study of Small Perceptive Hearing Losses in School Age Children," paper presented at the Annual Convention of the American Speech and Hearing Association, San Francisco, November 1964.

Hunt, K.W., *Grammatical Structures Written at Three Grade Levels.* Champaign, Ill.: National Council of Teachers of English, 1965.

Jones, B., "The Abilities of Deaf Students to Comprehend and Produce Written English: A Review of the Literature." Mimeographed. Urbana, Ill.: University of Illinois, 1976.

Joos, M., "Language and the School Child," *Harvard Educational Review,* 34 (1964): 203–210.

Jurmaa, J., "On the Ability Structure of the Deaf," in *The Handicapped Child,* edited by R. Dinnage. London: Longman Group Limited and the National Children's Bureau, 1973.

Kates, S.L., W.W. Kates, and **J. Michael**, "Cognitive Processes in Deaf and Hearing Adolescents and Adults," *Psychological Monographs: General and Applied,* 76 (1962), 1–34.

Klima, E., and **U. Bellugi-Klima**, "Syntactic Regularities in the Speech of Children," in *Psycholinguistic Papers,* edited by J. Lyons and R.J. Wales. Chicago, Ill.: Aldine, 1966.

Koplin, J., P. Odom, R. Blanton, and **J. Nunnally**, "Word Association Test Performance of Deaf Subjects," *Journal of Speech and Hearing Research,* 10 (1967), 126–132.

Lenneberg, E.H., *Biological Foundation of Language.* New York: John Wiley and Sons, 1967.

Lewis, M., *Language and Personality in Deaf Children.* London: Cambridge University, 1968.

Ling, D., *Speech and the Hearing Impaired Child: Theory and Practice.* Washington, D.C.: A.G. Bell Association for the Deaf, 1976.

Loban, W., *The Language of Elementary School Children.* Champaign, Ill.: National Council of Teachers of English, 1963.

McCarthy, D., "Language Development in Children," in *Manual of Child Psychology,* edited by L. Carmichael. New York: John Wiley and Sons, 1954.

McConnell, F., and K.B. Horton, *A Home Teaching Program for Parents of Very Young Deaf Children.* Vanderbilt University School of Medicine, Project No. 6-1187, Grant No. OEG 32-52-0450-6007. U.S. Office of Education, Final Report, January, 1970.

McKee, P., M.L. Harrison, A. McCowen, E. Lehr, and W.K. Durr, *Reading for Meaning* (4th ed.). Boston: Houghton Mifflin Co., 1966.

McNeill, D., "Developmental Psycholinguistics," in *The Genesis of Language,* edited by F. Smith and G.A. Miller. Cambridge, Mass.: M.I.T. Press, 1966.

Moores, D.F. "Applications of 'Cloze' Procedures to the Assessment of Psycholinguistic Abilities of the Deaf." Unpublished doctoral dissertation, University of Illinois, 1967.

Moores, D.F., *Educating the Deaf.* Boston: Houghton Mifflin Co. (in press).

Myklebust, H.R., *The Psychology of Deafness.* New York: Grune & Stratton, 1960.

Nunnally, J.C., and R.L. Blanton, "Patterns of Word Association in the Deaf," *Psychological Reports,* 18 (1966): 87–92.

O'Donnell, R.C., W.J. Griffin, and R.C. Norris, *Syntax of Kindergarten and Elementary School Children: A Transformational Analysis.* Champaign, Ill.: National Council of Teachers of English, 1967.

O'Neill, M.A., "The Receptive Language Competence of Deaf Children in the Use of the Base Structure Rules of Transformational-generative Grammar." Unpublished doctoral dissertation, University of Pittsburgh, 1973.

Pintner, R., and D.G. Paterson, "A Measure of the Language Ability of Deaf Children," *Volta Review,* 20 (1918), 755–764.

Pitner, R., and D.G. Paterson, "A Measure of the Language Ability of Deaf Children, *Psychological Review,* 23 (1916), 413–436.

Power, D.J., "Deaf Children's Acquisition of the Passive Voice." Unpublished doctoral dissertation, University of Illinois, 1971.

Power, D.J., and S.P. Quigley, "Deaf Children's Acquisition of the Passive Voice," *Journal of Speech and Hearing Research,* 16 (1973), 5–11.

Presnell, L., "Hearing Impaired Children's Comprehension and Production of Syntax in Oral Language," *Journal of Speech and Hearing Research,* 16 (1973), 12–21.

Quigley, S.P., and F.E. Thomure, *Some Effects of Hearing Impairment upon School Performance.* Springfield, Ill.: Illinois Office of Education, 1968.

Quigley, S.P., R.B. Wilbur, D.J. Power, D.S. Montanelli, and M.W. Steinkamp, *Syntactic Structures in the Language of Deaf Children.* Urbana, Ill.: Institute for Child Behavior and Development, 1976.

Rosenstein, J., and W.H. Macginitie, *Verbal Behavior of the Deaf Child: Studies of Word Meanings and Associations.* New York: Teachers College, 1969.

Schmitt, P., "Deaf Children's Comprehension and Production of Sentence Transformations and Verb Tenses." Unpublished doctoral dissertation, University of Illinois, 1968.

Skinner, B.F., *Verbal Behavior.* New York: Appleton-Century-Crofts, 1957.

Slobin, D.I., "Comments on Developmental Psycholinguistics," in *The Genesis of Language; A Psycholinguistic Approach,* edited by F. Smith and G.A. Miller. Cambridge, Mass.: M.I.T. Press, 1966a.

Slobin, D.I., "Grammatical Transformations and Sentence Comprehension in Childhood and Adulthood," *Journal of Verbal Learning and Verbal Behavior,* 5 (1966b), 219–227.

Streng, A., *Hearing Therapy for Children.* New York: Grune and Stratton, 1958.

Taylor, L., "A Language Analysis of the Writing of Deaf Children." Unpublished doctoral dissertation, Florida State University, 1969.

Taylor, W.L., "'Cloze Procedure': A New Tool for Measuring Readability," *Journalism Quarterly,* 30 (1953), 415–533.

Taylor, W.L., "Application of Cloze and Entropy Measures to the Study of Contextual Constraints in Samples of Continuous Prose." Unpublished doctoral dissertation, University of Illinois, 1954.

Taylor, W.L., "Recent Developments in the Use of 'Cloze Procedure,'" *Journalism Quarterly,* 33 (1956), 42–48.

Turner, E.A., and R. Rommetveit, "The Acquisition of Sentence Voice and Reversibility," *Child Development,* 38 (1967), 649–660.

Weksel, W., Review of *The Acquisition of Language,* edited by U. Bellugi and R. Brown, *Language,* 41 (1965), 692–709.

Wilcox, J., and H. Tobin, "Linguistic Performance of Hard-of-hearing and Normal-hearing Children," *Journal of Speech and Hearing Research,* 17 (1974), 286–293.

Wrightstone, J. W., M.S. Aronow, and S. Moskowitz, "Developing Reading Test Norms for Deaf Children," *American Annals of the Deaf,* 108 (1963), 311–316.

Young C., and F. McConnell, "Retardation of Vocabulary Development in Hard-of-Hearing Children," *Exceptional Children,* 33 (1957), 268–270.

CHAPTER THREE

Psychological Aspects
of Hearing Loss in Children

CORNELIUS P. GOETZINGER

INTRODUCTION

Interest in the harmful effects of hearing impairment upon the psychological and educational growth of children arose around the turn of the century. Several investigators compared deaf and hearing children on a number of mental and physical tests. In 1912, Pintner and Paterson (1915) attempted to administer the Binet Test (an individual, verbal test of intelligence) to deaf children and as a result concluded that the test was not suitable for the deaf. They subsequently developed both an individual performance scale and a group nonverbal test of intelligence that were suited to use with the deaf.

With the advent of the pure-tone audiometer in the early 1920s (Bunch, 1943), research was directed toward the effects of degree of deafness on the psychological and educational progress of children. In addition, researchers studied the effect of age at onset of deafness and whether the disability was congenital or adventitious. More recently, how etiology relates to heredity and "in utero" factors has been examined to obtain a better understanding of the effects of deafness.

CHAPTER OBJECTIVES

The purposes of this chapter are: first, to review a number of the variables which contribute to differences in the effects of hearing impairment upon the educational and psychological development of children; second, to present the research associated with the impact of hearing impairment upon the educational, psychological, and motor abilities of children; third, to consider learning in hearing-impaired children; fourth, to discuss multiple-handicapped hearing-impaired children; fifth, to consider psychological tests for the hearing-impaired; sixth, to present case histories of hearing-impaired children for illustration.

BACKGROUND OF PROBLEM

Degree of Hearing Impairment

The degree of hearing impairment refers to the loss in sensitivity in hearing that exceeds the accepted normal limits of hearing. Table 3-1 shows the normal range of hearing as well as the hearing levels that define the various classifications of hearing loss. As is apparent, hearing losses, in the better ear, of between 25 and 40dB are classified as slight, between 40 and 55dB as mild, between 55 and 70dB as marked, between 70 and 90dB as severe, and above 90dB as profound. The table also outlines the relationship of hearing loss to the understanding of speech, to psychological problems, to the need for a hearing aid, and to the percent of children within each classification as determined in the Pittsburgh study (Eagles, Hardy, and Catlin, 1968).

Age at Onset of Hearing Impairment

Children who are either congenitally deaf or become deaf before the acquisition of language are more retarded educationally than children who lose their hearing after language has been established. The early research of Pintner and Paterson (1917), Reamer (1921), and Day, Fusfeld, and Pintner (1928) showed that the age range from 4 to 6 years was critical. Thus, children who lose their hearing after language has been established benefit because of their early hearing.

It should be noted that age 3 rather than from 4 to 6 years is now regarded as being critical, primarily because of early diagnosis, parent-infant programs, and preschools for hearing-impaired children. Recently, it has been shown that slight congenital and/or prelingual hearing impairment may have a retarding effect on language development (Goetzinger, 1962). Interestingly, research in linguistics indicates that one's native language is mastered fundamentally by ages 3 to 4½ years (McNeill, 1965). It is clear, therefore, that age at onset of deafness is an important psychological variable.

Type and Etiology of Hearing Impairment

Generally, the handicapping effects of hearing impairment are related to the type of deafness. For example, auditory discrimination, or the ability to understand speech clearly, is usually good to excellent (80-100% on PB words) in conductive hearing loss, regardless of degree of deafness. Conversely, in sensorineural deafness, auditory discrimination may range from good to a total inability to understand the spoken word. In short, sensorineural hearing loss is usually accompanied by distortion of the speech sounds to greater or lesser extent. Furthermore, it may be more pronounced in VIIIth nerve lesions than in cochlear hair cell lesions. Thus, a child with a 60dB sensorineural hearing loss is

TABLE 3-1. Classification of Hearing Handicap for the Better Ear Relative to the Speech Frequencies (500–2000 Hz).

ANSI dB	Handi-cap	Speech Discrimination*	Psychological Implications	Hearing Aid Need†	Pittsburgh, Pa. Study of 4064 Subjects for C.A. 5–10 Years.‡
0	None	Excellent	None	None (CROS with unilateral cases at times)	Number in class was 3996 (98.3% of total).
25	Slight	Difficulty with faint speech	Children may show a slight verbal deficit.	Increased use with better "all-in-ear" aids	Number in class was 36 (0.9%).
40	Mild	Trouble frequently with normal speech at one meter (SPL of 65–70dB.)	Psychological problems are measurable in children. The beginning of social inadequacy in adults	Hearing aids needed, particularly with children	Number in class was 19 [21 §] (0.5%).
55	Marked	Frequent difficulty with loud speech	In general, children are retarded educationally if they do not receive special help. Emotional and social problems are frequent. Psychological problems are measurable in adults.	Generally the area of greatest satisfaction from an aid	Number in class was 9 (0.2%).
70	Severe	Might understand shouted or amplified speech, but this will depend on other factors such as type of impairment, etc.	Congenitally and prelingually deaf children usually show marked educational retardation. Emotional and social problems may obtain in children & adults.	Generally good results, but benefits depend on auditory discrimination, etc.	Number given as 2 (0.05%). It includes the extreme class.

(continued)

TABLE 3-1. *(Continued)*

ANSI dB	Handi- cap	Speech Discrimination*	Psychological Implications	Hearing Aid Need†	Pittsburgh, Pa. Study of 4064 Subjects for C.A. 5–10 Years.‡
90	Extreme	Generally, no under-standing of speech, even amplified	Congenitally and prelingually deaf may show severe educational re-tardation and emotional under-development. Deafened adults may have personal and social problems.	Help from aid depends on objectives. Lip-reading & voice quality are helped often.	
	Total				

*Adapted from Davis and Silverman (1960) and Eagles, Hardy, and Catlin (1968).

†Adapted from the lectures of Dr. Raymond Carhart.

‡The Pittsburgh study provides an estimate of the percentages of children in the public schools who fall within the various hearing impairment classifica-tions. Adapted from Eagles, Hardy, and Catlin (1968).

§The number should probably be 21. There is an error in the authors' table.

usually more handicapped than one with a 60dB conductive hearing loss. When the lesion involves the VIIIth nerve and the cochlea, as may occur in meningitic deafness, there is often poorer auditory discrimination than is found generally in cochlear impairment.

As noted previously, age at onset of hearing impairment can have a deleterious impact on the acquisition of language and on later educational achievement. In addition, the effect of congenital deafness on the child can depend on whether the etiology is endogenous (that is, hereditary transmission through the genes associated with dominant, recessive, or sex-linked characteristics) or is exogenous (deafness related to conditions that arise "in utero," such as maternal rubella and Rh incompatibility). Research within the past 15 years has produced evidence of the importance of these variables with reference to psychological and educational growth in children.

PSYCHOLOGICAL CONSIDERATIONS OF HEARING IMPAIRMENT

Children in the Regular Schools

The early investigators selected for study such variables as intelligence, school achievement, emotional adjustment, and motor ability in their comparisons of normal and hearing-impaired children. The latter consisted of children in schools for the deaf—those with severe and profound deafness. The devices then available for measuring degree of hearing loss were crude, consisting of such tests as tuning forks, the watch tick, whispered and spoken voice, and an audiometer that generated, usually, one impure tone (Bunch, 1943). Obviously, the tests were not sufficiently sensitive to allow studies of degrees of hearing loss and their effects upon behavior; therefore, if any behavioral differences did exist between normal and hearing-impaired persons, they were more likely to be apparent in comparisons between those with normal hearing and the profoundly deaf. Thus, the early researchers compared the normal-hearing with the deaf, rather than with the hard-of-hearing.

It may be said that the deaf are defined presently as those whose hearing disability precludes successful processing of linguistic information through audition, with or without a hearing aid. For them vision rather than hearing is the primary avenue of language acquisition and communication. The hard-of-hearing are those who, generally with the use of a hearing aid, have sufficient residual hearing to enable successful processing of linguistic information through audition (Report, Ad Hoc Committee, 1975). For the hard-of-hearing, the auditory channel, with the help of a hearing aid, is primary for the acquisition of language and for communication; in contrast, the deaf cannot acquire language through the ear alone, with or without a hearing aid.

Intelligence. Soon after the development of the Western Electric 2-A pure-tone audiometer in the 1920s, Waldman, Wade, and Aretz (1930) compared normal and hard-of-hearing children on group verbal intelligence tests and found the latter to be slightly retarded. About the same time Madden (1931) administered mental tests to normal and hard-of-hearing children and reported that the latter group evinced retardation.

In a comprehensive investigation Pintner and Lev (1939) compared more than 1100 normal and hard-of-hearing children in grades five through eight on the Pintner IQ Test (a group verbal test). The subjects with hearing losses were within the 10 to 40dB range by today's ISO and ANSI standards; they were found to be retarded by five IQ points. Pintner and Lev further divided their hard-of-hearing subjects into two groups, the one with 10 to 25dB hearing levels and the other with 25 to 40dB hearing levels. The former were not significantly different in IQ from the normal-hearing subjects. The latter, however, were retarded eight IQ points; hearing losses between 25 and 40dB induced a retardation in verbal skills that was reflected in the verbal IQ test. Pintner and Lev concluded that the difference, though significant, was not large and indicated that their hard-of-hearing subjects were within the normal range of intelligence. When they tested smaller samples of the same two groups with the Pintner Non-Language Mental Test, they did not find a significant difference. Consequently, they recommended the use of nonlanguage tests for assessing the mental ability of hearing-impaired children.

Educational Achievement. The impact of hearing loss on a child's academic accomplishment in school has long been of concern to educators and psychologists. Comparisons between normal and hearing-impaired children in the public schools have relied on incidence of grade repetition (Caplin, 1937) and scores of standardized educational tests (Pintner, Eisenson, and Stanton, 1946). In general, the results indicated that the hearing-impaired children repeated more grades and were somewhat retarded in educational achievement. However, many of the large-scale investigations were conducted before 1941.

Henry (1947) studied hearing loss in relation to reading attainment. His subjects were given air-conduction hearing tests and the results classified into low-, middle-, and high-frequency losses. No information was provided concerning degree, type, and age at onset of hearing loss. The results indicated that low-tone hearing losses did not differentiate the poorest from the best readers. Significant differences in threshold between the poorest and best readers were found for children with middle- and high-frequency losses.

In England, Fisher (1966) studied vocabulary and basic school subjects in 83 children with hearing impairment in the public schools. Their mean hearing level was 38dB with a range of 20 to 64dB (this, the British standard, which is similar to ANSI). Their mean of 38dB falls within the slight hearing loss classification as shown in Table 3-1. Their mean chronological age (C.A.) was 10.1

years. Fisher reported that they were substantially retarded in vocabulary and in basic school subjects, although their intelligence as measured with Raven's Progressive Matrices, a nonverbal test, was normal.

The impact of slight to mild hearing loss, usually congenital, upon language development in children has received little attention from researchers. Goetzinger (1962), after longitudinal observation of children with sensorineural hearing losses of 20 to 45dB (ANSI) in the better ear, tentatively concluded that such losses induce a language lag of 12 to 18 months at age 3 when intelligence is normal and frequently cause a speech deficit. Children between 2 and 4 years of age with slight to mild sensorineural hearing losses are often misdiagnosed as being aphasic, retarded, emotionally disturbed, or learning disabled.

Goetzinger, Harrison, and Baer (1964) compared 20 normal children to 20 children with sensorineural deafness on auditory and educational tests. The mean hearing losses in the better and poorer ears of the experimental subjects were 36.7 and 47.6dB respectively. Data available from the school files on reading achievement for the two groups did not permit a statistical comparison. Mean percentiles that were reported suggested a reading lag in the children with sensorineural deafness.

Recently, Ling (1975) commented on the deleterious effects of chronic conductive hearing loss upon the educational progress of children. He noted that educational retardation has been demonstrated for reading, arithmetic, and language.

As hearing loss increases, the impact upon educational achievement is more pronounced. Young and McConnell (1957) compared normal and hearing-impaired children matched for age, sex, grade, and socio-economic status in intelligence using the standard (1938) Raven's Progressive Matrices, and in vocabulary with Ammon's Full-Range Picture Vocabulary Test. The experimental subjects had a mean hearing loss of 61dB (ANSI) in the better ear. Although the groups did not differ in intelligence, the normal children showed a significant superiority over the hearing-impaired subjects in vocabulary.

Emotional Adjustment. In an early study Habbe (1936) administered a battery of adjustment- and behavior-rating scales to normal and hearing-impaired boys matched for age, school, grade, IQ, nationality, and socioeconomic level. The mean pure-tone hearing losses in the right and left ears of the experimental group were reported to be 27 and 29dB respectively. By today's ANSI standard these levels would be 37 and 39dB. The normal control subjects tended to show better adjustment than the hard-of-hearing on five of the six scores derived from the tests, but none of the differences was statistically significant. The hearing-impaired group tended to be more introverted and submissive than the normal group.

Pintner (1942) compared normal and hearing-impaired children in a number of areas of adjustment. The two groups did not differ significantly in ascendentsubmissive behavior; however, subjects with hearing losses greater than 40dB (ANSI) did show a tendency to aggressive behavior and less emotional stability. Pintner concluded that the hearing-impaired children were inclined to be introverted and were not as well adjusted as the normal children.

Several smaller studies of normal and hearing-impaired children have been conducted during the past 20 years on personal and social adjustment (Reynolds, 1955; Goetzinger, Harrison, and Baer, 1964; Fisher, 1966), ability to handle frustration (Kahn, 1957), and acceptance-rejection by classmates (Elser, 1959). In general, hearing-impaired children with 40dB or greater hearing levels in their better ears tend to be less well adjusted than children with normal hearing (Goetzinger, Harrison, and Baer, 1964; Fisher, 1966). Furthermore, the hearing-impaired children were not as well accepted by their classmates (Elser, 1959). Kahn's study indicated that his hearing-impaired subjects handled their frustrations more constructively than the control subjects.

Children in Special Schools

Children with hearing losses of 70dB or greater in the better ear are classified as educationally deaf according to Eagles, Hardy, and Catlin (1968). These children are educated predominantly in special residential and day schools for the deaf, although some may be found in special classes in the regular school systems.

In recent years, there has been a movement to mainstream, or integrate, selected deaf children (Northcott, 1973; Bitter, Johnson, and Bringhurst, 1974; Katz, Mathis and Merrill, 1974; Craig and Salem, 1975) into the regular public-school classroom. Obviously, such an undertaking requires large-scale cooperation of the administration, the classroom teachers, the children with normal hearing, the special tutors, and the parents of both the hearing and deaf children. Just how widespread mainstreaming of the deaf child is likely to become is contingent on many factors, most of which are treated extensively in other chapters of this book.

Intelligence. The initiation of psychological study of the deaf in this country is mainly attributable to Pintner and Paterson (1915). They showed that the Goddard revision of the Binet Test, an individual verbal test of intelligence, was not suitable for use with deaf children. Pintner developed an individual performance scale of intelligence (Pintner and Paterson, 1923) and also a group nonverbal test (Pintner, 1929) before 1920. Neither of these tests was dependent upon language, and both could be used with the deaf. Research with the Digit-Symbol and Symbol-Digit tests before 1920 and with the Pintner Non-Language Mental Test later found deaf children to be from two to three years retarded in intelligence (Pintner, 1915; Pintner and Paterson, 1916; Reamer, 1921; Day, Fusfeld, and Pintner, 1928). Only the study by Newlee (1919) reported deaf children to be normal in intelligence. The results of her study of 85 deaf children in the Chicago Public School System with the Digit-Symbol and Symbol-Digit Tests were criticized because of the small number in her sample and her selection of subjects.

Drever and Collins (1936), using their own performance scale of intelligence, found the deaf to be equal to or better than the subjects with normal hearing. These results did not agree with Pintner and his associates, who had used non-verbal group tests, and subsequently gave rise to a number of studies comparing the two types of tests.

In general, the deaf scored as retarded on some nonverbal tests (MacKane, 1933; Oleron, 1950; Levine and Iscoe, 1955; Goetzinger, Wills, and Dekker, 1967), but not on the Chicago Non-Verbal Test (Johnson, 1947 and 1948; Goetzinger, Wills, and Dekker, 1967). Similarly, deaf children obtain IQs within normal limits on performance scales of intelligence (MacKane, 1933; Burchard and Myklebust, 1942; Goetzinger and Rousey, 1957). It appeared, therefore, that the group nonverbal tests were more abstract than the performance scales and that the retarded language development of the deaf contributed to their inferior showing on these tests.

However, Furth (1964) in about 1958 initiated studies which demonstrated eventually that the inferior results of deaf children on many nonverbal cognitive tasks were not observed in deaf adults. He attributed the poor performance of children on these tasks to an experiential deficit rather than to retardation, since retardation, as a permanent condition, would also be noted in adults. He further maintained that the retarded language of the deaf did not negatively affect their performance. Furth concluded, in agreement with the later position of Oleron (Levine, 1963), that language is not as significant in problem solving and relational language as was formerly thought.

In 1960 my colleagues and I (Goetzinger, Wills, and Dekker, 1967) began a series of studies using the Standard Raven's Progressive Matrices (1938). Earlier Oleron (1950) and Levine and Iscoe (1955) had reported that deaf children were about two years retarded in mental development as measured with this test. Although our investigation did reveal the expected two-year retardation for children whose average age was 13½ years, the deficit was not apparent in a study of older children at the same school whose average age was 18½ years. In the earlier studies, paragraph meaning and vocabulary subtests of the Stanford Achievement Test had also been administered and correlated to give indirect measures of language ability of the subjects. The results showed that the correlations between the mental tests and either the paragraph meaning or vocabulary tests were significant but low. In addition, the older children were less than 6 months advanced over the younger children on the two educational tests, even though they had been in school five years longer. Furthermore, individual performance IQs on both groups had indicated no difference in intelligence. The findings were interpreted as indicating only a weak relationship between language ability and the nonverbal test scores. The results, therefore, supported Furth's conclusions.

During the past two or three decades, considerable research effort has been focused on the perceptual and conceptual abilities of deaf children. Results on tests of visual perception have been controversial. Myklebust and Brutten (1953) reported that deaf children were inferior to those with normal hearing in visual foreground-background differentiation, but subsequent studies have not confirmed their results (Embrey, 1955; Larr, 1956).

The research appears to be in accord that deaf children are inferior in verbal conceptualization to their hearing peers. Templin (1950) found that deaf children's explanations of physical causality were similar to those of much younger children with normal hearing. Other investigators reporting on different aspects of verbal conceptualization have also found the deaf to be inferior (Heider and Heider, 1940, 1941; Larr, 1956; Myklebust, 1960; Rosenstein, 1960, 1964). Conversely, the deaf perform as well as the hearing on nonverbal tests of conceptualization. Differences that occur are related to experiential deficit.

Because of the discrepancy between verbal and nonverbal conceptualization of the deaf, inferiority in abstract concepts would be expected if exposure to the concept is contingent upon language. Blake, Ainsworth, and Williams (1967) examined inductive and deductive reasoning in deaf and hearing subjects, and found the deaf to be inferior in the recognition and use of concepts. They attributed the differences to the poorer language facility of their deaf subjects.

Language is not now considered as important for the deaf in nonverbal cognitive reasoning and conceptualization as once thought. However, the acquisition and extension of knowledge and conceptualization at higher levels are limited unless a verbal language is developed. It appears reasonable to maintain that a rich and comprehensive written language is not likely to evolve without a verbal language (an example would be the congenitally deaf). Furthermore, without a written language for the storage and retrieval of information, the higher levels of conceptualization are not likely to be attainable. One of the most important characteristics of advanced cultures is a written language. From this line of thought, it follows that the congenitally and prelingually deaf cannot reach their full potential for mental growth until they have developed a basic verbal language—one that is sufficiently complete so that they are able to learn to read and bridge the hearing gap through the written or printed language without the language weakness usually encountered. In short, their problems associated with learning to read and deciphering the written word are basically related to language deficiency, not to the problems of word recognition as such, so commonly found with normal children. This aspect of the problem will be discussed more fully in the learning section of this chapter.

Educational Achievement. The educational achievement of deaf children has been investigated ever since the advent of standardized achievement tests. Pintner and Paterson (1917); Reamer (1921); Day, Fusfeld, and Pintner (1928) reported that deaf children were from 4 to 6 years retarded in educational achievement. Later, Pugh (1946), Miller (1958), Goetzinger and Rousey (1959), and Boatner (1965) found educational retardation of deaf children to be about the same as in the Pintner era. Myklebust (1960) reported progressive retardation with age for deaf children using the Columbia Vocabulary Test. At age 16, the deaf were more than 6 years retarded.

The Babbidge (1965) report emphasized again the limited educational achievement of the deaf. Also, Gentile and Di Francesca (1969) provided evidence of the severe educational retardation of hearing-impaired children. The most recent demographic survey of academic achievement of hearing-impaired students conducted by Gallaudet College found a paragraph meaning subtest grade level of 4.36 years at age 19 (Report of Advisory Council, 1975). These findings seem to suggest that during the last 50 years there has not been marked success in raising the educational achievement level (as measured by standardized test results) of severely and profoundly hearing-impaired children.

Emotional Adjustment. Studies of the personality and emotional adjustment of deaf children were conducted by Brunschwig (1936); Bradway (1937); Springer (1938); Kirk (1938); Heider and Heider (1940, 1941); Burchard and Myklebust (1942b); Avery (1948); McAndrew (1948); Levine (1956); Bindon (1957); Myklebust (1960); Goetzinger, Ortiz, Bellerose, and Buchan (1966), and Vegely and Elliott (1968). The researchers used personality tests of the paper-and-pencil type, projective techniques such as the Rorschach and MAPS (Make-A-Picture Story), inventories, drawings, and so forth. In general, the research has indicated that deaf children are not as well adjusted as those with normal hearing. Also, there is a higher incidence of immaturity among the deaf, and they tend to be more egocentric, rigid, and neurotic.

Motor Ability and Locomotion. Motor ability and locomotion are generally regarded as primary aspects of development and maturation. Locomotion, which is reflected by the age at which a child begins to walk, is used often as supportive evidence in the diagnosis of mental retardation. However, there is no clear-cut relationship between motor and mental abilities even at early ages, but rather there is much overlapping of functions (Bayley, 1935; Gesell and Amatruda, 1948). Yet, as Myklebust (1946, 1949, 1954) has stressed, motor evaluation is important in the differential diagnosis of aphasia, deafness, autism, and mental retardation in children.

Motor tests for clinical use were developed by Bayley (1935), Oseretsky (Doll, 1946), Heath (1942, 1943, 1944), and others. Heath devised a railwalking test to measure gross locomotor ability and published norms for children and adults. Goetzinger, Ortiz, Rousey, and Dirks (1961) re-evaluated the Heath test for male and female children for the age range of 8 to 16 years inclusive and obtained excellent agreement with Heath's norms. Recently, Cunningham and Goetzinger (1972) published normative data on children, 8 to 18 years, for the Floor Ataxia Test Battery.

Heath (1944) stressed that both motor and sensory pathways are involved in a test of equilibrium as measured through railwalking. The sensory pathways indicate to an individual that he is off balance. The motor pathways enable him to regain balance. A poor performance is often difficult to attribute to either sensory or motor disability, or to central coordinating mechanisms such as of the cerebellum. In conjunction with the vestibular apparatus consisting of the semicircular canals, the utricle, and the saccule, vision and the kinesthetic sense also contribute to equilibrium. Myklebust (1946), and Scanlon and Goetzinger (1969) have provided evidence of the inferiority of deaf children on the Heath railwalking test. Scanlon and Goetzinger (1969) also reported poorer performance for the deaf on the Fukuda vestibular tests. However, there was large variability among deaf subjects in both studies, a finding which would be expected because of the differences in etiology and in degree of hearing loss. For example, the meningitic deaf show severe locomotor disturbance on the Heath railwalking test because of destruction of the semicircular canals, the utricle, and saccule. In Scheibe's deafness, which is characterized by normal semicircular canals and utricles, but anomalous development of the cochlea and saccule, one would expect normal locomotor performance on the Heath railwalking test (Omerod, 1960; Whetnall and Fry, 1964; Lindsay, 1967; Schuknecht, 1967). Moreover, Sandberg and Terkildsen (1965) studied subjects in a school for the deaf and reported a higher incidence of abnormal calorics[1] (which would account for poor Heath test scores) for subjects with greater than 90dB hearing loss through the speech range (500–2000 Hz) as compared to those with less than 90dB loss. It is clear, therefore, that tests of locomotion, balance, and so forth have a place in the diagnosis, treatment, and education of hearing-impaired children.

Learning in Hearing Impaired Children—Auditory, Visual, and Combined Modalities

Effects of Slight, Mild, Marked, and Severe Hearing Impairment. In 1967 Gaeth reported the results of a number of studies he had conducted during the preceding decade on learning in hearing-impaired children. Using a paired-associates paradigm, he investigated the effectiveness of unimodal and bimodal methods of

---

[1]Calorics refer to tests which are performed by irrigating the ears first with cool water, then with warm water under controlled conditions to determine the functionality of the vestibular system. The normal reaction is an eye jerk referred to as a nystagmus. The absence of nystagmus as well as other atypical manifestations in the nystagmus are indicative of abnormality.

presenting material for learning. His three methods were auditory, visual, and auditory-visual combinations. His visual stimuli were printed words and nonsense syllables. He did not use lip movements as in lipreading.

Gaeth compared normal with hearing-impaired children of differing degrees of hearing loss, namely 26 to 40dB, 41 to 55dB, 56 to 70dB, and 71 to 85dB in the better ear. He found no significant differences for his normal hearing subjects among the three methods of learning. His hearing-impaired subjects within the 26 to 40dB (slight), 41 to 55dB (mild), and 56 to 70dB (marked) classifications of hearing loss did not differ significantly in performance on the visual and audio-visual methods. In short, the three groups with hearing loss performed as well under the visual as under the audio-visual method. However, they performed significantly better under the audio-visual method than under the purely auditory approach. When children with the 71 to 85dB hearing loss classification were compared using the three methods of learning, the visual method was superior to the audio-visual as well as to the auditory.

Gaeth checked his results by repeating the experiments and also by using new material, hypothesizing that the bimodal presentation is critical when either normal or hearing-impaired children are learning new words and concepts. For these new studies he used nonverbal and nonmeaningful symbols, nonsense syllables, simple meaningful words, and nonmeaningful sounds. As a result of his experiments, he concluded that the child learns originally through either one or the other modality (visual or auditory) but not through both simultaneously. Furthermore, the child selects the channel from which he receives the more meaningful information.

Profound Hearing Impairment. Gaeth felt that when deaf children show benefit from a bimodal presentation, as in the combination of lipreading and hearing with a hearing aid, it is attributable to the integration of rapidly alternating unimodal stimulation, and not to the integration of the simultaneous bimodal presentation.

There is ample support in the research literature for Gaeth's comment on the superiority of a bimodal method (auditory-visual) over the visual when the latter modality is lipreading (Heider, 1943; Numbers and Hudgins, 1948; Hudgins, 1951; Prall, 1957; Purcell and Costello, 1970; Sanders, 1971). However, the obvious divergence in results between Gaeth's findings of no significant difference between the audio-visual and the visual methods and those researchers who found the audio-visual to be superior is due simply to the stimuli used for the visual modality. Briefly, Gaeth used either words, nonsense syllables, or nonsense symbols, all of which were in printed form; the other investigators, in contrast, employed speech or lip movements. Because printed forms are visual stimuli that may be repeated over and over again without any changes in stimulus properties, they provide a precise and accurate method for thought transmission. Lip or speech movements are comparatively imprecise and highly ambiguous because of variations in the formation of words and sounds from speaker to speaker. Furthermore, homophenous words—words like *man-pan* that look the same on the lips—add to the receiver's confusion in reading lips.

Gaeth's subjects using the audio-visual method concentrated on the printed words to the exclusion of the distorted auditory signals. Conversely, the subjects of Number and Hudgins; Hudgins, Prall, Purcell, and Costello; and Sanders were exposed to the relatively distorted visual (i.e., lip movements) and auditory (discrimination very poor) signals simultaneously, and thus received cues from each modality. Hence, the bimodal representation is usually superior to the unimodal, whether visual or auditory.

Whether or not the bimodal is superior to the unimodal reception for the severely hearing-impaired when lip movement (speechreading) and hearing, instead of the printed word and hearing, are the stimuli is contingent upon speechreading and auditory discrimination abilities, as well as the balance between the abilities. For example, for the past 20 or more years in our clinic at Kansas University Medical Center (KUMC), tests of speechreading and auditory discrimination—separate as well as combined—are frequently conducted in conjunction with hearing aid evaluations. Scores of, say, 20% each for lipreading and auditory discrimination frequently increase to between 60 and 70% under the bimodal condition (Goetzinger, 1963). However, the imbalance at which a difference in scores between modalities (as 70% auditory and 20% lipreading or vice versa) results in an absence of improvement when there is bimodal stimulation has not been determined completely, although O'Neill (1954) has reported data along these lines.

It will be recalled that in Gaeth's study bimodal reception was not superior to unimodal visual reception, and in some instances bimodal was poorer. Actually, in Gaeth's experiments, it would appear that the visual modality was so far superior to the auditory, particularly for the deaf, that the subjects ignored the auditory and concentrated on the visual.

Related is a study conducted at the National Technical Institute for the Deaf (NTID) comparing the relative efficacy of lipreading, sign language, and printed material in conveying information to deaf students (Struckless, 1971, reporting on the research of Robert Gates, 1970). Gates selected 140 deaf subjects in the beginning class at NTID and randomly assigned them to 7 groups of 20 each. Criteria for selection were the absence of any serious visual defects and at least an eighth-grade reading ability. Each group received the same 2,000-word test passage under seven different presentation conditions using videotape and a split-screen technique. A 39-item multiple-choice test was developed to test their comprehension. The seven presentations were: (1) unvocalized speech, or lipreading; (2) manual communication only; (3) printed graphic or reading symbols alone; (4) lipreading and symbols combined; (5) lipreading and reading combined; (6) symbols and reading combined; (7) lipreading, symbols, and reading combined.

Several of the findings are important to the current discussion. Lipreading (L.R.) and manual communication resulted in low mean scores (mean = 13.5; 15.05). Combining the two did not increase understanding (mean = 13.7). However, there was a significant increase in the score (mean = 26.05) when the printed word (reading) was the medium. In addition, the score remained virtually the same for combinations which included reading (Reading + L.R. mean = 25.65; Reading and signs mean = 23.95). When reading was combined with lipreading and signs, the mean score of 25.65 was essentially the same as from reading alone (mean = 26.05).

In this study, the manual method was not any more effective than lipreading. In addition, combining the two did not improve the scores. However, presenting the material through reading significantly improved the score over either lipreading or signs alone, and over combinations of all three. Also, the score significantly improved when reading was combined either with signs or lipreading or with both (reading, signs, and lipreading).

These results suggest that the printed word is superior both to lipreading and signs for conveying information. Also, when three different methods of presenting information visually are used simultaneously, the method that is inherently the clearest is selected. In this case it was reading. The data of Gates suggest that the person cannot process more than one visual method at a time. For example, combining signs and lipreading did not improve reception over either one alone.

Carson and Goetzinger (1976) completed a study that was designed to explore whether or not combined audio-visual methods of presenting material for learning by deaf children are superior either to auditory or visual presentations alone. The study involved comparisons among seven different conditions of auditory-visual learning of nonsense syllables by deaf children within the age range of 8 to 10 years inclusive; 35 children were assigned randomly to the learning conditions forming 7 groups of 5 subjects each. The learning conditions were: (1) lipreading; (2) signs; (3) auditory; (4) lipreading and auditory; (5) lipreading and signs; (6) signs and auditory; (7) lipreading, signs, and auditory. Each group participated in a test session consisting of 10 trials. A trial consisted of the presentation of 6 nonsense syllables. In the sign conditions 6 nonsense signs were paired with the nonsense syllables.

A female teacher was videotaped speaking and giving the sign for each nonsense syllable. The 6 videotaped presentations were randomized 10 times to accommodate the 10 trials. Provisions were made to present lipreading, signs, and the auditory conditions singly and in the appropriate combinations. The closed-circuit TV system and studio at the school were used for the experiment. Statistical analyses were based upon 300 responses for each group and consisted of comparisons of differences among groups.

The results indicated that the lipreading-auditory condition was superior to signs alone, auditory alone, and the signs-auditory conditions. The lipreading-signs-auditory condition was significantly superior to auditory alone and to the signs-auditory conditions. No other differences among conditions were significant. The lipreading-signs-auditory condition, as implied, was not significantly different from the lipreading-auditory condition. Since the former condition is essentially the same as "Total Communication" (Kent, 1971; Katz, Mathis, and Merrill, 1974), the results appear to raise some questions about the reported superiority of this method of teaching the deaf (Meadow, 1968; Vernon and Koh, 1970). Total Communication utilizes not only bimodal but also bivisual stimuli; therefore, it requires the simultaneous processing of two distinctly different visual signals (lip movements and hand signs) in conjunction with the auditory stimuli.

A surprising finding of the study was the lack of significant difference between the auditory-lipreading and the signs-lipreading conditions. It will be recalled that the former is bimodal (hearing and vision) and that the latter is unimodal but bivisual (both signs and lipreading are processed through the visual system). In my view, the organism is capable of summating bimodal stimuli—for example, lip movements and vocalizations—because they occur simultaneously. Obviously, one or the other may become dominant if there is a large difference between the effectiveness of the channels.

Conversely, bivisual stimuli or signals would be difficult to encode simultaneously, since either one or the other would compete for the system. Of course, switching back and forth between visual modes could be a possibility. However, Gates' data provided no evidence of the superiority of the combined lipreading-manual condition over either one alone for connected discourse. Therefore, the finding of a non-significant difference between the auditory-lipreading and the signs-lipreading conditions in the Carson-Goetzinger study is not in agreement with the Gates result and, furthermore, does not support the postulations presented above.

The explanation might be found in the difference of stimulus materials used in the two studies. Gates employed a story, which is connected discourse, whereas the Carson-Goetzinger investigation used a task involving the perception only of a nonsense syllable and a nonsense sign at any given time. In the latter instance, a type of simultaneous perception might be possible; however, simultaneous visual perception and processing does not seem reasonable when sentences, or connected discourse, are used. There is, of course, the possibility that the organism could switch back and forth between stimulus conditions (namely, between lipreading and signs combined with finger spelling). Yet, in view of the manner in which signs and/or finger spelling are executed, it does not appear to me that switching would be effective—first, because of the length of the eye-sweep required to move from the lips to the hands and vice versa; second, because of the poor synchronization between the lips and the hands. Although in Total Communication the receiver has the option of selecting the modality of his choice, it nevertheless does not seem logical that he could improve reception by simultaneous perception or processing, or in fact, that it is possible within the confines of this discussion. More than likely, he will choose the condition under which he has been schooled. The options should be: (1) the lipreading-auditory condition; (2) lipreading alone; (3) signs and finger spelling. They should not be either the combination of signs and finger spelling with the auditory, or lipreading in conjunction with the signs–finger spelling for the reasons which were previously advanced.

A number of studies during the past 10 to 15 years purport to show that deaf children, brought up in a manual communication environment, show greater educational achievement than those from an oral background. Stuckless and Birch (1966), Meadow (1968), and Vernon and Koh (1970) compared deaf children of deaf parents with deaf children of hearing parents and reported superiority of the former over the latter in most educational areas. Furthermore, Klopping (1972) and Moores, Weiss, and Goodwin (1973) reported success with Total Communication. However, the majority of these studies were descriptive; the need for experimental investigation in this area is critical.

One possibility for increasing the reception of severely hearing-impaired individuals may be through the use of Cornett's Cued Speech (Cornett, 1967) in conjunction with the bimodal auditory-visual condition. The cues consist of 12 hand positions executed around the face which give additional information. Cued speech does not constitute the addition of a second visual method as, for example, the sign language or a combination of signs and finger spelling used along with speechreading and auditory amplification as in Total Communication. The cues are just that and nothing more. Because they are executed essentially at the lips, they are incorporated into the ongoing lip movement to assist in the comprehension of obscure motion. Therefore, the cues could be expected to enhance rather than deter understanding and language development because of their location and moderate use.

Ling and Clark (1975) and Clark and Ling (1976) recently published the results of two studies of cued speech with deaf children. The first studied 12 subjects within the age range of 7 to 11 years; the second, 8 subjects within the 8- to 11-year range. In both studies their deaf subjects obtained significantly higher scores with cues than without cues in identifying words, phrases, and sentences both with and without the use of hearing aids. Nevertheless, there were no significant differences in the scores between cuing with hearing aids and cuing without hearing aids. In other words, cuing did not improve reception when the children put on their hearing aids. Clark and Ling remarked that this finding was unexpected, particularly as the children were ". . . consistent and avid users of powerful, individual, radio-frequency aids" (Clark and Ling, 1976, p. 32).

Earlier, Erber (1972a) reported that profoundly deaf children with greater than 90dB hearing losses in the better ear were only slightly more accurate in categorizing the test consonants by place of articulation under bimodal auditory-visual (lipreading) stimulation than under unimodal visual (lipreading) stimulation alone. In another study, Erber (1972b), testing word-recognition performances using vision alone and vision plus hearing, compared six profoundly deaf children (greater than 95dB ISO) to six children ranging from 10 to 15 years of age and six adults from 23 to 31 years of age. The scores for the deaf subjects, regardless of the acoustical signal, were 7 to 11% higher for the bimodal than for the unimodal visual stimuli. Those with normal hearing also showed a 6 to 8% improvement in the bimodal condition.

In the experiments of Ling and Clark (1975) and Clark and Ling (1976), the cues significantly enhanced the scores of their subjects when used with speechreading. This finding appears to support my hypothesis that the second visual input (speechreading plus the cues) can be processed when it is minimal and if it occurs close to the primary movement (near the lips in this case). The failure of Clark and Ling to find improvement with the addition of auditory stimulation may simply be related to the profound deafness of their subjects, and hence, to a large diminution in auditory cues.

The question of how deaf children process a combined audio-visual signal has theoretical as well as utilitarian implications. Gaeth (1967) concluded that the improvement from a bimodal presentation consisting of speechreading and auditory amplification with a hearing aid results from the integration of rapidly alternating visual and auditory stimuli rather than from the simultaneous integration of the two.

However, one may speculate that there could be simultaneous processing in bimodal reception, at least in the instance of vocalized speech. Furthermore, there appears to be some evidence for this position from clinical observation. For example, we have for years utilized monosyllabic words (CID PBs) in our clinic to evaluate auditory discrimination as well as lipreading ability (Goetzinger, 1963). It is not uncommon to have patients with scores of 24% in each modality improve dramatically under the bimodal (audio-visual) condition. It is difficult to explain such improvement in any way other than simultaneous processing of the audio-visual stimuli. One would be forced to conclude that the organism switches back and forth rapidly during a single PB word! This position is not to say that the organism may not resort to the modus operandi of Gaeth, which would be feasible in encoding sentences, but in my opinion, it does not explain improvement in PB word scores.

Habilitation of Hearing-Impaired Children

Slight, Mild, and Marked Hearing Impairment. According to the data of Eagles, Hardy, and Catlin (1968), shown in Table 3-1, more than half of the children with hearing impairment within the age range of 5 to 10 years fell within the slight hearing loss classification of 25 to 40dB (ANSI). As discussed earlier, Pintner and Lev (1939) found an 8-point deficit in verbal intelligence in children

within this range of hearing loss. In the absence of any serious specific disabilities, children with slight hearing losses are educated exclusively in the conventional classrooms. They do, however, require additional help relative to the use
of hearing aids, placement in the classroom, speechreading, language work, and
emotional support. It is very important to their emotional well-being that the
teacher as well as the parents have an understanding of the educational and
psychological implications of hearing impairment, and furthermore, that the
children in the classroom be made aware of the hearing impairment; otherwise,
problems may develop over partially heard greetings, instructions, and so forth.

Sensorineural hearing loss of about 40dB in the better ear induces a language retardation of a year to a year and a half when it exists from birth (Goetzinger, 1962). Furthermore, emotional problems are measurable when hearing
loss in the better ear is 40dB or greater (Pintner, 1942; Goetzinger, Harrison,
and Baer, 1962; Fisher, 1966). It will be recalled from the Eagles, Hardy, and
Catlin (1968) study that 0.5% (or about a third of the hearing-impaired children)
fell within the mild loss classification of 40 to 55dB. Such children require
hearing aids and their use should be begun as soon after diagnosis as possible.
Because early diagnosis of slight and mild hearing losses is becoming more
common in hearing and speech centers, procedures can be instituted to overcome the language retardation. Early remediation will help to alleviate many of
the problems such as language lag, speech defects, and emotional adjustment
encountered after the child enters school.

Early remediation of itself is not likely to be a panacea or cure-all for hearing
impairment. Continuous help, particularly through the elementary grades, is
likely to be required. In the earlier years, the home will be involved as closely as
the school. I cannot overemphasize the need for such continuing help. As one
who has helped evaluate candidates for enrollment at the Kansas School for the
Deaf during the past 25 years, I have observed that the number of children with
mild hearing losses who have been referred to the school because of failure in the
conventional classrooms has been incredible. Simply put, placing such children
in the regular classroom is not enough. These children must be given understanding and special help. When appropriate steps are taken to provide them with
additional help and with suitable hearing aids, there is no logical reason why
they should not succeed in the regular class, provided their intelligence and
adjustment are reasonably normal. Since children with mild hearing losses represent the largest segment currently in the public schools, special effort should be
made to analyze their problems so as to develop more efficient techniques for
their educational and psychological progress.

Table 3-1 shows that about 0.2% of the cases, or about two children per
1,000, had marked hearing loss of 55 to 70dB in the better ear. These children
unquestionably need auditory amplification. They are frequently found to be
retarded in educational achievement (Young and McConnell, 1957) and to have

more social and emotional problems. These children very often require additional help in the classroom and at home. In many instances, special classes for the hearing-impaired will be required for children with this degree of hearing loss.

Severe and Profound Hearing Impairment. By referring to Table 3-1 again it may be seen that only 2 of 4064 children in the sample had hearing loss in the better ear of 70dB or greater. These children are generally classified as educationally deaf. For the majority of these children, the visual channel is the primary means of acquiring language. Thus, the child who is either born deaf or suffers deafness before the acquisition of language is severely circumscribed in acquiring language through hearing alone. Hearing is an omnidirectional sense, and is peculiarly constituted for perceiving at distances. The child with normal hearing is continuously saturated with spoken language from the moment of birth, much of it in the form of incidental language. The severely and profoundly deaf child is isolated almost totally from incidental language. His language experiences are mainly visual and are almost nil unless the speaker is in his direct line of vision. Therefore, the need is great to expose this child to language during the formative years and to provide him with the best possible means of acquiring incidental language.

The use of auditory amplification as soon as possible after the diagnosis of deafness is the only means of supplementing the meager incidental contacts with language for the congenitally and prelingually deaf child. Obviously, the question of benefit from auditory amplification arises with children whose deafness exceeds the 90dB hearing level and who are profoundly deaf. Since many children with greater than 90dB hearing losses apparently do profit from auditory amplification (Northcott, 1975; Kennedy et al., 1976), there is a critical need to study and define the variables which contribute to success and failure. Clinical observation suggests that children with severe and profound deafness who respond to sound at low frequencies by bone conduction, as differentiated from vibro-tactile sensation, develop better voice quality with auditory amplification than those who cannot perceive sound by bone conduction.

Perhaps children who are born with intact VIIIth cranial nerves, even though with defective cochleas, might profit from early auditory stimulation. For example, assuming that Scheibe's deafness accounts for a substantial number of children in schools for the deaf in the United States, as it does in England (Whetnall and Fry, 1964), the presumption of a functioning VIIIth cranial nerve may be reasonable. In fact, Schuknecht (1967) states that the spiral ganglion is usually normal in Scheibe's deafness and, furthermore, that it may remain so until late in life. (Scheibe's deafness is of genetic origin. There is aplasia involving the cochlea and saccule of the inner ear. However, the bony labyrinth is fully developed. The utricle and semicircular canals are histologically and functionally normal.) With the incredible recent advances in radiological techniques, it is possible that in the not too distant future a contrast technique could be developed that would permit a differentiation between a functional and nonfunctional auditory portion of the VIIIth cranial nerve in Scheibe's type deafness and in other severe and profound hearing impairments.

The vast majority of congenitally deaf children are now educated either in residential or day schools for the deaf; however, within the last decade or so there has been a movement to integrate deaf children into conventional public school classes for hearing children. Mainstreaming, to use the current educational lingo, is acquiring ever-increasing support from educators of children with atypical physical and mental development. The tempo appears to be increasing with regard to the hearing-impaired, judging by articles in the literature as well as papers at national and international conventions. This topic is discussed in greater detail elsewhere in this book.

However, successful adjustment of deaf children to conventional public school classes will depend on several psychological factors. Several adjustment patterns may develop as a result of impaired hearing. First, new psychological situations are a potential source of poor adjustment. Since audition is a tool of behavior, its loss predisposes the individual more frequently to new psychological situations. Furthermore, the loss of hearing imposes on the person overlapping psychological roles. Meyerson (1963) has presented three general patterns of adjustment in terms of these psychological concepts.

In adjustment pattern one, the individual essentially retreats to the circumscribed world of the disability. The hard-of-hearing withdraw from the vastly larger life-space of those with normal hearing into the sheltered and protected atmosphere of societies and clubs for the hearing-impaired. The deaf may stay within the safe and secure confines of deaf society. These people either reject or are rejected by the world of the hearing. Meyerson remarks that this particular pattern of adjustment is condemned by all but those who practice it. He further maintains that withdrawal is not necessarily a maladjustive reaction; in many cases it is appropriate. Although it decreases the variety of satisfactions and gratifications which can accrue from the overlapping normal life-space, demands upon the individual are fewer, more easily anticipated, and easier to carry out. Hence, the problem of overlapping roles is solved.

In adjustment pattern two, the person aspires to the world of the hearing and rejects the world of the hearing-impaired. This particular pattern is frequently lauded by hearing persons, who view the handicapped individual as having spunk.

At times the barrier between the two worlds can be penetrated successfully by the handicapped person because of a particular skill, because of wealth, or because of social position. But penetration of the barrier does not necessarily mean acceptance. Hostility may be prevalent. He who adopts pattern two must develop a high tolerance for frustration. Indeed, tension and conflict are certain. He is not likely to have the emotional support of other hearing-impaired friends. Although he may make a more or less effective adjustment to the hearing society, he will, nevertheless, be more or less disorganized and maladjusted as a person. Adjustment pattern three is an acceptance of both worlds by the individual. He realizes there are benefits to be derived from each one. He does not consider himself to be inferior because of his hearing disability, although he recognizes that some skills are dependent upon hearing. His emphasis is upon what he can do and reasonably expect to accomplish, rather than upon limitations imposed by the hearing problem. He stresses the positive rather than the negative aspects of his life situation (Meyerson, 1963).

Educators of hearing-impaired children would do well to acquaint themselves with the advice of Meyerson. Children grow up to be adults who must interact with a hearing world. Acceptance rather than denial of the effects of hearing impairment contributes unquestionably to a more fulfilling and rewarding life.

Multiple-Handicapped Children

Hardy (1969) recently discussed the problem of children with multiple handicaps caused by prenatal rubella. As a result of the rubella epidemic of late 1963 and early 1964, an estimated 20,000 to 30,000 children in the United States were born with handicaps. The triad of congenital heart disease, cataracts, and deafness has long been associated with rubella.

Vernon (1967a) evaluated psychologically, educationally, and physically 129 rubella-handicapped children who were referred for admission to a school for the deaf from 1954 to 1964. He found 53% of them to have multiple handicaps. Educationally, they scored below other groups of deaf children, even when IQ was taken into consideration. Their poor educational achievement was ascribed to a high incidence of aphasia, reported to be 21.9%. Emotional problems were reported to be frequent. In comparison to four other groups (deafness caused by heredity, Rh factor, premature birth, and meningitis) the children with rubella-caused hearing loss had the highest incidence of psychological maladjustment.

Vernon (1967b) also studied 114 post-meningitic deaf children. Their mean age at onset of deafness was 20 months. Although 38% of this group had multiple handicaps, only 8.6% had more than one handicap in addition to deafness. Aphasia, emotional disturbance, mental retardation, and spasticity were the most common secondary handicaps. These children achieved educationally at two-thirds the rate of deaf children of deaf parents.

In the same sample of children Vernon (1967c) isolated 46 with definitely established Rh-factor deafness. Of this group, 71.1% were multiple handicapped. In addition, 51.5% of the total group were cerebral palsied and 22.8% aphasic. These children achieved at a rate that was 5/7 that of the hereditarily deaf.

Vernon (1967d) studied the premature deaf for whom there was no other cause of deafness. About 9.7% of these children were dismissed from school as ineducable. Another 10% had been denied admission because of a lack of potential. They progressed academically at a rate that was 2/3 that of the hereditarily deaf.

These studies therefore found the hereditarily deaf to be educationally, intellectually, and emotionally superior to those whose deafness was due to rubella, meningitis, Rh factor, and prematurity. They also had fewer secondary handicaps.

Jensema (1974) reported a study of 43,946 children enrolled in special educational programs for the hearing-impaired during the 1972/73 school year. Of these, 7,739 were reported to have suffered hearing loss as a result of rubella. Jensema found these children to have greater hearing loss than those with deafness from other causes. In addition, they had a higher frequency of additional handicaps, including visual, behavioral, and heart-related problems. Jensema postulated that a higher proportion of those with rubella-caused deafness are enrolled in full-time special education programs because of their greater hearing loss and additional handicaps.

Hereditary Deafness

Konigsmark (1969) reviewed recently causes of hereditary deafness. However, studies of the psychological effects of hereditary—in contrast to congenital—deafness are meager. Owsley (1962) studied intelligence and school achievement of children with Waardenburg's syndrome in schools for the deaf. The syndrome is characterized by unilateral or bilateral congenital deafness, a white forelock of hair, lateral displacement of the inner canthi of the eyes and of the interior lacrimal puntae producing a broad, nasal root, heterochromia of the iris, and confluence of the eyebrows with hypertrichosis of the medial ends. Owsley's findings indicated that his subjects had normal intelligence. Their educational achievement was the same as that of other congenitally deaf children.

Psychological Tests with Hearing-Impaired Children

Individual performance scales and group nonverbal tests of intelligence are widely used to evaluate children with hearing impairment. Only one of the performance scales and none of the nonverbal tests have been standardized on deaf subjects. Other than the Hiskey-Nebraska Scale of Learning, I am not acquainted with any other individual scale of intelligence for which norms were derived using hearing-impaired subjects. As a consequence, most psychologists use gestures interspersed with a few signs, if they know any, for directions.

The Hiskey-Nebraska Scale was standardized on both normal-hearing and deaf subjects. In general, the norms for the deaf are slightly lower than for the normal-hearing subjects.

That verbal versus nonverbal directions have a significant effect on performance outcome is well known. Graham and Shapiro (1953) in a well-controlled study showed that the standard verbal directions, as compared to pantomime, in the administration of the Wechsler Intelligence Scale for Children (WISC) to hearing subjects resulted in a five-point difference in IQ with the verbal directions giving the higher rating. They also administered the Performance Scale to a group of deaf subjects and obtained a mean IQ of 95, which was the same as the normal-hearing subjects who had been given the pantomime directions. Therefore, they recommended that psychologists add five points to the Performance Scale IQ when it is used with deaf subjects. This recommendation by Graham and Shapiro has proven to be remarkably appropriate over the years.

A group nonverbal test, the Chicago Non-Verbal Examination, has been standardized on hearing subjects using verbal and nonverbal directions (see appendix). Because the type of directions, either verbal or nonverbal, influences the test results, two sets of norms were derived. Verbal directions result in higher scores for normal-hearing subjects.

Since there are no standardized directions for administering the Wechsler tests, Goetzinger and Proud (1975) published directions for administering the WISC and Wechsler Adult Intelligence Scale (WAIS) to hearing-impaired subjects. Practice material is also included to aid in clarifying the pantomime directions. These directions may serve as interim procedures until such time as standardized directions are available.

A list of mental and adjustment tests that may be used with hearing-impaired subjects is given in the appendix. The age ranges of the tests as published by the developers are also provided. In some instances, the lower level of the test range is not suitable for deaf children. For example, I do not advise giving the WISC Performance Scale below age 8 in most cases. Also the Standard Raven's Progressive Matrices (1938) should not be used for intermediate-grade deaf children, since they more than likely will show a two-year retardation. The test is reserved for deaf subjects 18 years old and above (Goetzinger, Wills, and Dekker, 1967).

The following case histories illustrate the use of verbal and performance tests with hearing-impaired children to demonstrate the effects of hearing impairment upon language acquisition. There are, of course, a number of tests available today to measure verbal language level in children. However, with hearing-impaired children, individual verbal tests of intelligence are essentially measures of language acquisition and/or language level. Such tests provide an indirect index of the effect of hearing impairment upon verbal acquisition when the results are compared with the performance scale. Hence, for hearing-impaired children, the difference between verbal and performance scales gives quantitative information for habilitative and rehabilitative educational emphasis.

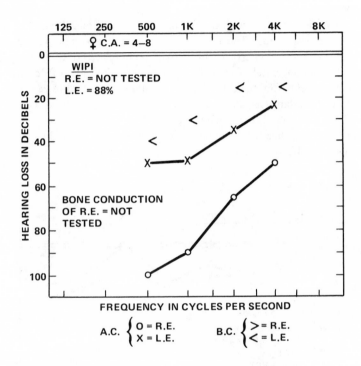

A.C. { O = R.E. / X = L.E. } B.C. { > = R.E. / < = L.E. }

Female   C.A.=4 years 8 months   WPPSI*Verbal Scale=94
WPPSI Performance Scale=105

This little girl weighed 4 pounds 5 ounces at birth, which was at full term and without problems. A neurologist made a diagnosis of epilepsy at an early age. A recent EEG and skull X-ray were normal. She has strabismus and is currently under the care of an ophthalmologist. As may be seen, a recent audiogram revealed a bilateral hearing loss by air conduction of 43dB and 85dB respectively in the left and right ears. The bone-conduction average for the left ear was 28dB, thus indicating a mixed hearing loss. Bone-conduction testing of the right ear was not conducted. Auditory

*See Appendix to this chapter for a listing of tests that can be used with hearing-impaired children and adults, used in these case studies.

discrimination on the left ear was 88% using the Word Intelligibility by Picture Identification (WIPI) Test (Ross and Lerman, 1971). The right ear was not tested. Tympanometry showed bilateral tympanograms which peaked at -150 MM H^2O pressure. The child was treated for otitis media by an otologist.

Her ability as measured with the Wechsler Pre-School and Primary Scale of Intelligence was normal. The 11-point differential between her verbal and performance results (94 vs. 105) is more than likely related to the hearing loss, which was congenital. The average bone-conduction loss of 28dB (her basic hearing level before the ear infection) would be expected to cause a 10-point deficit in language acquisition, which is reflected in the verbal results. This child attends her neighborhood preschool. Her teacher has been acquainted with her hearing problem so that appropriate classroom management can be initiated.

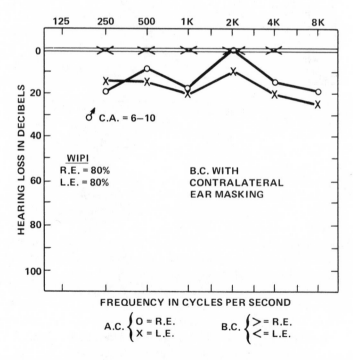

Male   C.A.=6 years, 10 months   WPPSI Verbal Scale=81
                                      WPPSI Performance Scale=82

This little boy had a history of recurrent middle-ear infections. As shown in the figure he had a bilateral conductive hearing impairment. Auditory discrimination as measured with the WIPI test was 80% in each ear. His verbal and performance WPPSI results were 81 and 82 respectively, which indicates that his conductive hearing impairment had not perceptibly affected his language development as indirectly measured by the verbal scale. Interestingly, his WIPI scores of 80% virtually reflect his verbal WPPSI score of 81. When auditory discrimination is reduced in children with slight conductive hearing loss, it is well to recommend that they be given a full-scale (performance and verbal) examination to determine whether the deficit is related to the hearing loss or is a basic inability. A discrepancy between the verbal and performance scale (if, for example, the Verbal had been 80 and the Performance 100 in this case) favoring the performance would suggest that hearing loss caused the deficit, but when both are reduced, as they are in this case (Verbal 81 and Performance 82) there is a very strong suggestion that deficiency in ability is the cause of the auditory discrimination problem. This child attends a class for slower learners and is progressing well.

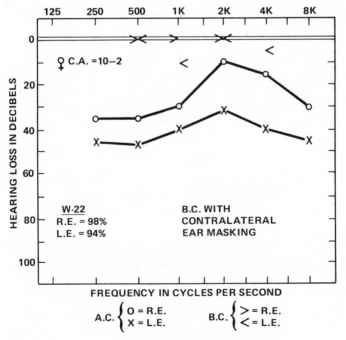

Female   C.A.=10 years 2 months   WISC Verbal Scale=101
                                     WISC Performance Scale=100

This child was seen for evaluation in May 1973. As may be seen in the figure, she had a bilateral conductive hearing loss which was diagnosed by her otologist as glue ear. Although she had suffered recurrent slight to mild hearing loss for a number of years, there had not been any deleterious effects on her verbal development as indirectly measured with the WISC. Her verbal and performance IQs of 101 and 100, respectively, were virtually identical. In our experience, slight to mild hearing losses even when existing from an early age rarely retard language development significantly, since auditory discrimination is always good, unless a central problem is present. Furthermore, such hearing losses are often amenable to surgical correction. The fluctuating nature of many middle-ear problems at times leads to emotional problems, particularly when the hearing loss approaches 35 to 40dB in the better ear. This is not to state that lesser hearing loss does not give rise to psychological problems. However, it is measurable with current tests at these levels (i.e., 35-40dB).

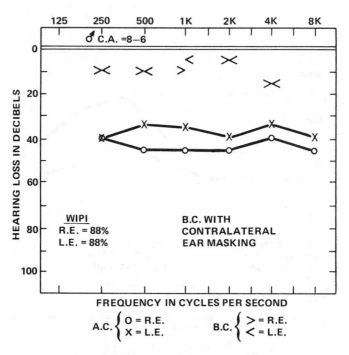

Male   C.A.=8 years 6 months   WISC Verbal Scale=57
                                 WISC Performance Scale=55

This young boy again illustrates a bilateral conductive hearing impairment. He suffered constant middle-ear infections with hearing loss. His psychological results using the WISC produced a verbal score of 57 and a performance score of 55. The child was retarded. However, despite his persistent conductive hearing loss and retardation as determined by the performance scale, his language acquisition and verbal ability as measured with the verbal scale are not out of line with his basic ability. These findings suggest that slight to mild conductive hearing impairment does not have any greater negative effect upon the retarded than upon normal children with respect to verbal and language acquisition as indirectly measured with verbal tests. Of course, several language tests are available; however, the verbal IQ tests are superior from the point of view of standardization and, in addition, offer an indirect measure of language, which may be compared to the performance results for increased efficiency of diagnosis and for habilitation or rehabilitation.

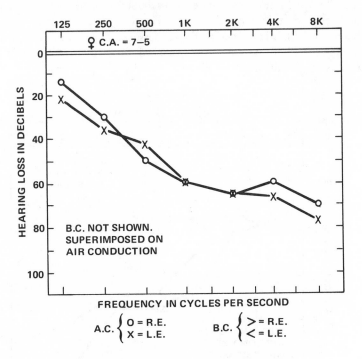

Female   C.A.=7 years 5 months   WISC Verbal Scale=62
WISC Performance Scale=101

This child's marked, bilateral sensorineural hearing impairment was caused by measles at 18 months of age as reported by the parents. Her WISC performance IQ was 110 in contrast to a verbal score of 62. The latter, of course, is not an IQ, but is an indirect index of her language and verbal acquisition at the time of the examination (February 13, 1974). In short, at a chronological age of 7 years 5 months, her mental age was about 8 years 3 months, and her verbal age, about 4 years 7 months.

This case points up the deleterious impact of prelingual sensorineural hearing loss upon the acquisition of language as indirectly measured with the WISC.

The child had been fitted with a hearing aid at 18 months of age when her deafness was diagnosed. She had attended kindergarten and the first two years of a regular public school in her home town. However, during her second year in school, she had experienced difficulty and the school administration, which had no provisions for special help, requested that she be transferred to a neighboring city with a program for hard-of-hearing children.

The reason for her difficulty in school is apparent in her verbal WISC of 62 or, as pointed out, in her verbal acquisition and facility level of 4 years 7 months. This child is not a candidate for a school for the deaf; yet, to plunge her into a conventional classroom without providing special help is tantamount to either ignorance or thoughtlessness. She was transferred to the neighboring school system with a special educational program and, at last report, was progressing rapidly both educationally and emotionally.

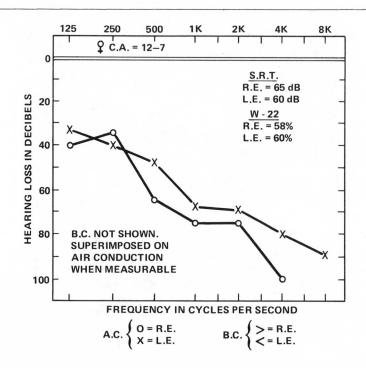

Female   C.A.=12 years 7 months   WISC Verbal Scale=74
WISC Performance Scale=107

This child was seen on numerous occasions in the KUMC Audiological Clinic. At age 4 years 3 months her audiograms indicated a bilateral sensorineural hearing loss of 45dB (ISO). At the time she scored at a 2-year-4-month level on the Mecham Verbal Language Development Scale—a finding that, in my experience, is consistent with the degree and type of hearing loss when intelligence is normal.

As is shown in the figure, her hearing loss on February 6, 1974, had progressed to 60 to 65dB. Auditory discrimination as measured with the W-22 recorded PB word test was 58 to 60%. She was given a psychological evaluation and obtained a WISC verbal score of 74 and a WISC performance IQ of 107. The latter was confirmed by a standard Raven's Progressive Matrices (1938) percentile rank of 50. This particular case illustrates the need for periodic checks of hearing sensitivity, as the lesion may be progressive. Had this child's hearing loss existed from birth, she would not have been likely to have obtained a WISC Verbal Score of 74 by age 12 years 7 months in the conventional educational system. Yet a score of 74 (mental age of 9 years 6 months), taken alone, indicates that she is still about three years retarded relative to a mental age of 13 years 4 months, in verbal acquisition as indirectly measured by the test. Hence, the impact of the hearing loss is indeed formidable.

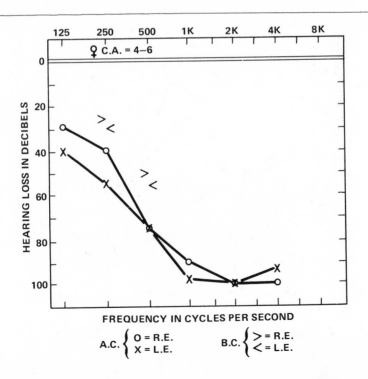

Female ˙ C.A.=4 years 6 months   Verbal Ability=a few words
Hiskey-Nebraska Scale=106

This little girl was congenitally deaf. As may be seen from her audiogram, she has a sharply sloping bilateral sensorineural hearing loss of 90dB and 93dB respectively for the right and left ears through the speech range of 500 to 2000 Hz. Her intelligence as measured with the Hiskey-Nebraska Scale at a chronological age of 4 years 6 months was 106, or normal. However, her verbal ability was limited to a few words and her understanding of spoken language with or without a hearing aid was essentially nil. This child had good voice quality because of her relatively good hearing in the low frequencies. Such children are not infrequently diagnosed as aphasic or emotionally disturbed. They respond to the low frequencies, at first consistently but later intermittently, which helps to increase the impression of aphasia, or emotional denial of hearing. Unfortunately, diagnoses are frequently made without having such essential information at hand as how well the child hears and sees.

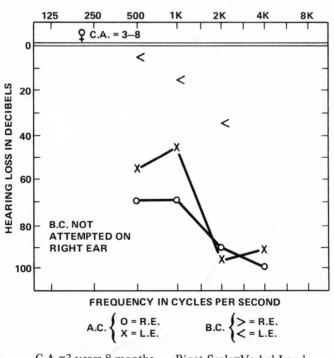

Female   C.A.=3 years 8 months   Binet Scale=Verbal Level
of 1½-2 yrs.
Leiter Performance Scale= 123

This figure shows the audiogram of a 3-year 8-month-old girl who has been seen in the Ear, Nose and Throat and Audiological Clinics on several occasions. The child has had middle-ear disease practically all of her life. Audiograms dating from age 2 years 11 months consistently show hearing loss similar to that in the figure. This child has normal voice quality, but her expressive and receptive language development is considerably retarded. The otologist did not elect to do corrective surgery at this time, as there was some question about authenticity of the bone-conduction responses and mental retardation. A Leiter Performance IQ of 123 was obtained at chronological age 3 years 8 months, indicating that the child had superior intelligence. A verbal test administered the same day revealed a verbal age of about 1½ to 2 years. As noted previously, the child's voice quality was normal. However, a hearing loss in excess of 55dB during the critical language development period will have a serious effect. In this child's case, the hearing impairment has persisted at least since age 2 years 11 months, the date of the earliest audiogram. However, according to the parents (who have three other normal-hearing children), the patient has never had normal hearing.

Since surgery is not presently contemplated and there were no medical contra-indications to the wearing of a hearing aid, the child was fitted with an air-conduction aid on the left ear. The child's responses after placing the aid on the left ear were dramatic. She will be brought back to the clinic in two months for follow-up otological, audiological, and psychological evaluation.

These case histories illustrate the need for persistent and complete evaluation with very young children in order to pinpoint the basic nature of the problem. They also point up the need for audiologists to understand the importance of type and degree of hearing loss upon language acquisition as well as the stages of language development in normal-hearing children. As I pointed out earlier in the chapter, linguists have shown that the normal-hearing child with normal ability has acquired basic language by age 3 to 4½ years. Hence, the audiologist and also the otologist should make every effort to channel speech to the hearing-impaired child during this very critical period, either through surgical correction or, if surgery is not possible, through a hearing aid.

SUMMARY

1. Children with hearing levels within the 0 to 25dB range do not show any measurable psychological deficiencies in either adjustment or intelligence as determined by research.

2. Children with hearing loss within the 25 to 40dB range (slight hearing

loss) in the better ear may show a significant retardation on group intelligence tests, but are still within normal limits. The reduction in IQ probably reflects a slight lag in verbal language development as a result of the slight loss.

3. Children with hearing impairment approaching 40dB in the better ear, particularly if congenital and sensorineural, may be retarded significantly in educational achievement as compared to normal-hearing children. They may also evince emotional and social maladjustment. These children need help to compensate for their problems.

4. Children who have sensorineural congenital or prelingual deafness of about 40dB seem to be retarded by a year to a year and a half in language development at age 3 years. These children are not infrequently misdiagnosed as aphasic or brain-injured.

5. Children who are born deaf are severely retarded on the average in educational achievement. However, intelligence as measured with performance scales is normal. Their retardation on some nonverbal group tests disappears with age and is a function of experiential deficit.

6. Deaf children compare well with hearing children in verbal reasoning when the language is within their understanding and facility. Their inferiority on many verbal tasks is associated with a lack of facility and breadth of language, not to an innate inferiority related to deafness.

7. Deafness in connection with rubella, meningitis, Rh factor, and prematurity is frequently accompanied by other handicaps.

8. Methods of teaching deaf children were discussed. Some theoretical implications of so-called "total communication" and of the "auditory-visual" approach (namely lipreading–auditory amplification) to language development in deaf children were presented. Although definitive research is still lacking, it was nevertheless concluded that the former is not superior to the latter. Furthermore, it was concluded that "cued speech," if used in conjunction with the lipreading–auditory amplification approach, may be the most effective method with deaf children, providing there is some residual perception of sound.

9. Some implications of the use of locomotor tests with hearing-impaired children were elucidated. It was shown that such tests have a place in the diagnosis, treatment, and education of hearing-impaired children.

10. A list of psychological tests which may be used with the hearing impaired appears in the appendix.

RESEARCH NEEDS

The need for experimental studies in how to most effectively communicate with the deaf has already been stressed. The child who is born deaf is in essence cut off from any incidental exposure to language. Vision, unlike hearing, is a unidirectional sense and as a medium for acquiring language, it is, in comparison to hearing, relatively inadequate. Cued speech in conjunction with speechreading and auditory stimulation appears to be the logical approach. Unfortunately, those involved in special education have long resisted cued speech. The Ling-Clark (1975) and Clark-Ling (1976) studies have shown cued speech in conjunction with lipreading to be effective, although the addition of the auditory modality failed to demonstrate additional gains in language reception.

If the deaf are to be educated to their potential, their receptive language competency must be brought to a level where they will be able to read on a par with their hearing peers. Therefore, efforts must be made to develop methods for establishing the basic language during the years from birth to age 6. Unless the deaf child has developed a receptive language comparable to his hearing peer by age 6, his probability of increased language growth through reading will be no better than it has been in the past. I am well acquainted with the early research of Helen Thompson in this area and suggest that prospective researchers review her study (Thompson, 1927).

Another area requiring definitive research is that of developing specific techniques to help the hearing-impaired with the transition from concrete to more abstract vocabulary and language concepts at about 12 years of age. One has only to peruse the recent data of Gentile and Di Francesca (1969) to verify the educational plateau with which every teacher of the deaf for the past half-century has been familiar. It is unlikely that research will find a magic formula; more probably, a technique such as that used by Winitz (1973) to teach German to college students will be modified to meet the needs of the deaf. Goetzinger and Proud (1975) have already suggested a basic outline for developing language at the beginning level.

Further research is needed on the use of powerful hearing aids and their effects on the hearing mechanism. Jerger and Lewis (1975) have recently reviewed the literature on this subject. Without doubt, powerful hearing aids can cause hearing deterioration. However, clinical observation over the years attests to the fact that there are legions of successful users, and at least one unpublished study failed to reveal statistically significant deterioration in hearing sensitivity for deaf children over a two-year period (Cosper, 1968). There is no question of the need for intense study in this particular area.

REFERENCES

American Annals of the Deaf, 121 (1976), 144.

Avery, C., "Social Competence of Pre-school Acoustically Handicapped Children," *Journal of Exceptional Children,* 15 (1948), 71–73.

Babbidge, H., *Education of the Deaf,* A Report to the Secretary of Health, Education and Welfare by His Advisory Committee on the Education of the

Deaf. Washington, D.C.: U.S. Department of Health, Education and Welfare, 1965.

Bayley, N., *The Development of Motor Abilities during the First Three Years.* Washington, D.C.: Society for Research in Child Development, National Research Council, 1, 1935.

Bindon, M., "Make-A-Picture-Story Test Findings for Rubella Deaf Children," *Journal of Abnormal and Social Psychology,* 55 (1957), 38–42.

Bitter, G.B., K.A. Johnson, and K.F. Bringhurst, *Facilitating the Integration of Hearing Impaired Children into Regular School Classrooms.* Project Need: University of Utah, 1974.

Blake, K.A., S.H. Ainsworth, and C.L. Williams, "Effects of Induction and Deduction on Deaf and Hearing Individuals' Attainment of First-Order Concepts," *American Annals of the Deaf,* 112 (1967), 606–613.

Boatner, E.B., "The Need for New Vocational-Technical Programs for the Deaf," *Report of the Proceedings of the 42nd Meeting of the Convention of American Instructors of the Deaf.* Washington, D.C.: U.S. Government Printing Office, No. 71 (1965), 201–206.

Bradway, K.P., "The Social Competence of Deaf Children," *American Annals of the Deaf,* 82 (1937), 122–140.

Broadbent, D.E., *Perception and Communication.* Don Mills, Ont.: Pergamon Press, 1964.

Brunschwig, L., *A Study of Some Personality Aspects of Deaf Children.* New York: Columbia University, Teachers College Contributions to Education, No. 687, 1936.

Bunch, C.C. *Clinical Audiometry.* St. Louis, Mo.: C.V. Mosby Company, 1943.

Burchard, E.M., and H.R. Myklebust, "A Comparison of Congenital and Adventitious Deafness with Respect to Its Effect on Intelligence, Personality and Social Maturity (Part I)," *American Annals of the Deaf,* 87 (1942a), 140–152.

Burchard, E.M., and H.R. Myklebust, "A Comparison of Congenital and Adventitious Deafness with Respect to Its Effect on Intelligence, Personality and Social Maturity (Part II: Social Maturity)," *American Annals of the Deaf,* 87 (1942b), 241–251.

Caplin, D., "A Special Report of Retardation of Children with Impaired Hearing in New York City Schools," *American Annals of the Deaf,* 82 (1937), 234–243.

Carson, P., and C.P. Goetzinger, "A Study of Learning in Deaf Children," *Journal of Auditory Research,* 15 (1975), 73–80.

Clark, B.R., and D. Ling, "The Effects of Using Cued Speech: A Follow-Up Study," *Volta Review,* 78 (1976), 23–34.

Cornett, R.O., "Cued Speech," *American Annals of the Deaf,* 112 (1967), 3–14.

Cosper, C.E., "A Study of the Effects of the Use of High-Powered Hearing Aids on the Auditory Thresholds of Deaf Children." Unpublished Master's thesis, University of Kansas Medical Center, 1968.

Craig, W.N., and J.M. Salem, "Partial Integration of Deaf with Hearing Students: Residential School Perspectives," *American Annals of the Deaf,* 120 (1975), 28–36.

Cunningham, D.R., and C.P. Goetzinger, "Floor Ataxia Test Battery," *Archives of Otolaryngology,* 96 (1972), 559–564.

Davis, H., and S.R. Silverman, *Hearing and Deafness.* New York: Holt, Rinehart and Winston, 2nd ed., 1960; 3rd ed., 1970.

Day, H.E., I. Fusfeld, and R. Pintner, *A Survey of American Schools for the Deaf.* Washington, D.C.: The National Research Council, 1928.

Doll, E.A., *The Oseretsky Test of Motor Proficiency.* Minneapolis, Minn.: Educational Test Bureau, 1946.

Drever, J., and M. Collins, *Performance Test of Intelligence.* London: Oliver and Boyd, 1936.

Eagles, E.L., W.G. Hardy, and F.I. Catlin, *Human Communication: The Public Health Aspects of Hearing, Language and Speech Disorders.* NINDB Monograph No. 7. Washington, D.C.: Public Health Service Publication No. 1745, U.S. Government Printing Office, 1968.

Elser, R.P., "The Social Position of Hearing Handicapped Children in the Regular Grades," *Exceptional Children,* 25 (1959), 305–309.

Embrey, R., "A Study of the Visual Perceptual Responses of Congenitally Deaf Children." Unpublished Master's thesis, University of Kansas, 1955.

Erber, N.P., "Auditory, Visual and Auditory-Visual Recognition of Consonants by Children with Normal and Impaired Hearing," *Journal of Speech and Hearing Research,* 15 (1972a), 413–422.

Erber, N.P., "Speech Envelope Cues as an Acoustic Aid to Lipreading for Profoundly Deaf Children," *Journal of the Acoustical Society of America,* 51 (1972b), 1224–1227.

Fisher, B., "The Social and Emotional Adjustment of Children with Impaired Hearing Attending Ordinary Classes," *British Journal of Educational Psychology,* 36 (1966), 319–321.

Furth, H.G., "Language and the Development of Thinking," *Report of the Proceedings of the International Congress on Education of the Deaf and of the 41st Meeting of the Convention of American Instructors of the Deaf.* Washington, D.C.: U.S. Government Printing Office, No. 106 (1964), 475–483.

Gaeth, J.H., "Learning with Visual and Audio-Visual Presentations," in *Deafness in Childhood,* edited by F. McConnell and P.H. Ward. Nashville: Vanderbilt University Press, 1967.

Gates, R.R., "The Differential Effectiveness of Various Modes of Presenting Verbal Information to Deaf Students through Modified Television Formats." Unpublished doctoral dissertation, University of Pittsburgh, 1970.

Gentile, A., and S. Di Francesca, *Academic Achievement Test Performance of Hearing Impaired Students.* Washington, D.C.: U.S. Office of Demographic Studies, Gallaudet College, 1969.

Gesell, A.L., and C.S. Amatruda, *Developmental Diagnosis.* New York: Paul B. Hoeber, 1948.

Goetzinger, C.P., "Effects of Small Perceptive Losses on Language and on Speech Discrimination," *Volta Review,* 64 (1962), 408–414.

Goetzinger, C.P., "Factors Associated with Counseling the Hearing Impaired Adult," *Journal of Rehabilitation of the Deaf,* 1 (1967), 32–48.

Goetzinger, C.P., "Management of Hearing Problems in Persons of Advanced Age," *Eye, Ear, Nose and Throat Monthly,* 42 (1963), 38–41.

Goetzinger, C.P., C. Harrison, and C.J. Baer, "Small Perceptive Hearing Loss: Its Effects in School-Age Children," *Volta Review,* 66 (1964), 124–131.

Goetzinger, C.P., J.D. Ortiz, B. Bellerose, and L.G. Buchan, "A Study of the S.O. Rorschach with Deaf and Hearing Adolescents," *American Annals of the Deaf,* 111 (1966), 510–522.

Goetzinger, C.P., J.D. Ortiz, C.L. Rousey, and D.D. Dirks, "A Re-evaluation of the Heath Railwalking Test," *Journal of Educational Research,* 54 (1961), 187–191.

Goetzinger, C.P., R.C. Wills, and L.C. Dekker, "Non-language I.Q. Tests Used with Deaf Pupils," *Volta Review,* 69 (1967), 500–506.

Goetzinger, C.P., and G.O. Proud, "The Impact of Hearing Impairment Upon the Psychological Development of Children," *Journal of Auditory Research,* 15 (1975), 1–60.

Goetzinger, C.P., and C.L. Rousey, "Educational Achievement of Deaf Children," *American Annals of the Deaf,* 104 (1959), 221–231.

Goetzinger, C.P., and C.L. Rousey, "A Study of the Wechsler Performance Scale (Form 2) and the Knox Cube Test with Deaf Adolescents," *American Annals of the Deaf,* 102 (1957), 388–398.

Graham, E., and E. Shapiro, "Use of the Performance Scale of the Wechsler Intelligence Scale for Children with the Deaf Child," *Journal of Consulting Psychology,* 17 (1953), 396–398.

Habbe, S., *Personality Adjustment of Adolescent Boys with Impaired Hearing.* New York: Columbia University, Teachers College Contributions to Education, No. 697, 1936.

Hardy, J., "Rubella and Its Aftermath," *Children,* U.S. Department of Health, Education and Welfare, 16 (1969), 91–93.

Heath, S.R., "Clinical Significance of Motor Defects with Military Implications," *American Journal of Psychology,* 57 (1944), 482–499.

Heath, S.R., "Railwalking Performance as Related to Mental Age and Etiological Type among the Mentally Retarded," *American Journal of Psychology,* 55 (1942), 240–247.

Heath, S.R., "The Military Use of the Railwalking Test as an Index of Locomotor Coordination," *Psychological Bulletin,* 40 (1943), 282–284.

Heider, F., "Acoustic Training Helps Deaf Children," *Volta Review*, 45 (1943), 135.

Heider, F., and G.M. Heider, "A Comparison of Sentence Structure of Deaf and Hearing Children," *Psychological Monographs*, 52 (1940), 42–103.

Heider, F., and G.M. Heider, "Studies in the Psychology of the Deaf," *Psychological Monographs*, 53 (1941), 1–158.

Henry, S., "Children's Audiograms in Relation to Reading Attainments," *Journal of Genetic Psychology*, 76 (1947), 49–63.

Hudgins, C.V., "Problems of Speech Comprehension in Deaf Children," *Nervous Child*, 9 (1951), 57–63.

Jensema, C., "Post-rubella Children in Special Education Programs for the Hearing Impaired," *Volta Review*, 76 (1974), 466–473.

Jerger, J.F., and N. Lewis, "Binaural Hearing Aids: Are They Dangerous for Children?" *Archives of Otolaryngology*, 101 (1975), 480–483.

Johnson, E.H., "The Ability of Pupils in a School for the Deaf to Understand Various Methods of Communication," *American Annals of the Deaf*, 93 (1948), 258–314.

Johnson, E.H., "The Effect of Academic Level on Scores from the Chicago Non-Verbal Examination for Primary Pupils," *American Annals of the Deaf*, 92 (1947), 227–233.

Kahn, H., "Responses of Hard of Hearing and Normal Hearing Children to Frustration," *Exceptional Children*, 24 (1957), 155–159.

Katz, L., S.L. Mathis, and E.C. Merrill, *The Deaf Child in the Public Schools: A Handbook for Parents of Deaf Children.* Danville, Ill.: Interstate Printers and Publishers, 1974.

Kennedy, P., W. Northcott, R. McCauley, and S.M. Williams, "Longitudinal Sociometric and Cross-Sectional Data on Mainstreaming Hearing Impaired Children: Implications for Preschool Programming," *Volta Review*, 78 (1976), 71–81.

Kent, M.S., "Total Communication at Maryland School for the Deaf," *The Maryland Bulletin*, 91 (1971), 69–86.

Kirk, S.A., "Behavior Problem Tendencies in Deaf and Hard of Hearing Children," *American Annals of the Deaf*, 83 (1938), 131–137.

Klopping, H., "Language Understanding of Deaf Students under Three Auditory-Visual Stimulus Conditions," *American Annals of the Deaf*, 117 (1972), 389–396.

Konigsmark, B.W., "Hereditary Deafness in Man," *The New England Journal of Medicine*, 281 (1969), 713–720; 774–778; 827–832.

Larr, A.L., "Perceptual and Conceptual Abilities of Residential School Deaf Children," *Journal of the International Council for Exceptional Children*, 23 (1956), 63–66.

Levine, B., and I. Iscoe, "The Progressive Matrices (1938), the Chicago Non-Verbal and the Wechsler-Bellevue on an Adolescent Deaf Population," *Journal of Clinical Psychology,* 11 (1955), 307–308.

Levine, E.S., "Studies in Psychological Evaluation of the Deaf," *Volta Review,* 65 (1963), 496–512.

Levine, E.S., *Youth in a Soundless World.* New York: New York University Press, 1956.

Lindsay, J.R., "Congenital Deafness of Inflammatory Origin," in *Deafness in Childhood,* edited by F. McConnell and P.H. Ward. Nashville, Tenn.: Vanderbilt University Press, 1967.

Ling, D., "Recent Developments Affecting the Education of Hearing Impaired Children," *Public Health Reviews,* 4 (1975), 117–152.

Ling, D., and B.R. Clark, "Cued Speech: An Evaluative Study," *American Annals of the Deaf,* 120 (1975), 480–488.

MacKane, K., *A Comparison of the Intelligence of Deaf and Hearing Children.* New York: Columbia University, Teachers College Contributions to Education, No. 585, 1933.

Madden, R., *The School Status of Hard of Hearing Children.* New York: Columbia University, Teachers College Contributions to Education, No. 499, 1931.

McAndrew, H., "Rigidity and Isolation: A Study of the Deaf and Blind," *Journal of Abnormal and Social Psychology,* 43 (1948), 476–494.

McNeill, D., "The Capacity for Language Acquisition," *Research on Behavioral Aspects of Deafness.* Proceedings of a National Research Conference on Behavioral Aspects of Deafness, U.S. Department of Health, Education and Welfare, Washington, D.C.: Vocational Rehabilitation Administration (1965), 11–28.

Meadow, K., "Early Manual Communication in Relation to the Deaf Child's Intellectual, Social and Communicative Functioning," *American Annals of the Deaf,* 113 (1968), 29–41.

Meyerson, L., "A Psychology of Impaired Hearing," in *Psychology of Exceptional Children and Youth,* edited by W.M. Cruickshank. Englewood Cliffs, N.J.: Prentice-Hall, 1963.

Miller, J.B., "Educational Achievement," *Volta Review,* 60 (1958), 302–304.

Moores, D., K. Weiss, and M. Goodwin, "Receptive Abilities of Deaf Children Across Five Modes of Communication," *Exceptional Children,* 44 (1973), 22–28.

Myklebust, H.R., *Auditory Disorders in Children.* New York: Grune and Stratton, 1954.

Myklebust, H.R., "Significance of Etiology in Motor Performances of Deaf Children with Special Reference to Meningitis," *American Journal of Psychology,* 59 (1946), 249–258.

Myklebust, H.R., *The Psychology of Deafness: Sensory Deprivation, Learning and Adjustment.* New York and London: Grune and Stratton, 1960.

Myklebust, H.R., "The Relationship Between Clinical Psychology and Audiology," *Journal of Speech and Hearing Disorders*, 14 (1949), 98–103.

Myklebust, H.R., and Brutten, M., "A Study of the Visual Perception of Deaf Children," *Acta Oto-Laryngologica*, Supplementum 105, Stockholm, Sweden, 1953.

Newlee, C.E., "A Report of Learning Tests with Deaf Children," *Volta Review*, 21 (1919), 216–223.

Northcott, W.H., *The Hearing Impaired Child in a Regular Classroom*. Washington, D.C.: A.G. Bell Association for the Deaf, 1973.

Northcott, W.H., "Normalization of the Preschool Child with Hearing Impairment," *Otolaryngologic Clinics of North America*, 8 (1975), 159–186.

Numbers, M.E., and C.V. Hudgins, "Speech Perception in Present Day Education of Deaf Children," *Volta Review*, 50 (1948), 449–456.

Oleron, P., "A Study of the Intelligence of the Deaf," *American Annals of the Deaf*, 95 (1950), 179–195.

Omerod, F.C., "Pathology of Congenital Deafness," *Journal of Laryngology and Otology*, 74 (1960), 919–950.

O'Neill, J., "Contribution of the Visual Components of Oral Symbols to Speech Comprehension," *Journal of Speech and Hearing Disorders*, 19 (1954), 429–439.

Owsley, P.J., "A Study of Intelligence and Achievement among Children Exhibiting Symptoms of the Waardenburg Syndrome," *Volta Review*, 64 (1962), 429–431.

Pintner, R., "A Class Study with Deaf Children," *Journal of Educational Psychology*, 6 (1915), 591–600.

Pintner, R., "Some Personality Traits of Hard of Hearing Children," *Journal of Genetic Psychology*, 60 (1942), 143–151.

Pintner, R., *The Pintner Non-Language Mental Test*, New York: Columbia University, 1929.

Pintner, R., J. Eisenson, and M. Stanton, *The Psychology of the Physically Handicapped*, New York: F.S. Crofts, 1946.

Pintner, R., and J. Lev, "The Intelligence of the Hard of Hearing School Child," *Journal of Genetic Psychology*, 55 (1939), 31–48.

Pintner, R., and D.G. Paterson, *Learning Tests with Deaf Children*. Psychological Monographs, XX, No. 88. Princeton, N.J.: The Psychological Review Com-

Pintner, R., and D.G. Paterson, *A Scale of Performance Tests*. New York: Appleton-Century-Crofts, 1923.

Pintner, R., and D.G. Paterson, *Learning Tests with Deaf Children*. Psychological Monographs, XX, No. 88. Princeton, N.J.: The Psychological Review Company, 1916.

Pintner, R., and D.G. Paterson, "The Binet Scale and the Deaf Child," *American Annals of the Deaf*, 60 (1915), 301–311.

Prall, J., Lipreading and Hearing Aids Combine for Better Comprehension," *Volta Review*, 59 (1957), 64–65.

Pugh, G.S., Summaries from Appraisals of Silent Reading Abilities of Acoustically Handicapped Children," *American Annals of the Deaf,* 91 (1946), 331–349.

Purcell, G., and **M.R. Costello**, "Multisensory Stimulation and Verbal Learning," *Bulletin of American Organization for the Hearing Impaired* (A.G. Bell Association for the Deaf), 1 (1970), 66–68.

Reamer, J.C., *Mental and Psychological Measurements of the Deaf.* Psychological Monographs, No. 132. Princeton, N.J.: The Psychological Review Company, 1921.

Report by the Advisory Council for the Deaf, "A Comprehensive Plan for the Education of Hearing Impaired Children and Youth in Massachusetts." Division of Special Education, Massachusetts Department of Education, 1975.

Report of the Ad Hoc Committee to Define Deaf and Hard of Hearing, *American Annals of the Deaf,* 120 (1975), 509–512.

Reynolds, L.B., "The School Adjustment of Children with Minimal Hearing Loss," *Journal of Speech and Hearing Disorders,* 20 (1955), 380–384.

Rosenstein, J., "Cognitive Abilities of Deaf Children," *Journal of Speech and Hearing Research,* 3 (1960), 108–119.

Rosenstein, J., "Concept Formation Problems," *Report of the Proceedings of the International Congress on Education of the Deaf and of the 41st Meeting of the Convention of American Instructors of the Deaf.* Washington, D.C.: U.S. Government Printing Office, No. 106 (1964), 518–523.

Ross, M., and **J. Lerman**, *Word Intelligibility by Picture Identification.* Pittsburgh, Pa.: Stanwix House, Inc. 1971.

Sandberg, L.E., and **K. Terkildsen**, "Caloric Tests in Deaf Children," *Archives of Otolaryngology,* 81 (1965), 350–354.

Sanders, D.A., *Aural Rehabilitation.* Englewood Cliffs, N.J.: Prentice-Hall, 1971.

Scanlon, S.L., and **C.P. Goetzinger**, "The Heath Rails and Fukuda Vestibular Tests with Deaf and Hearing Subjects," *Eye, Ear, Nose and Throat Monthly,* 48 (1969), 29–39.

Schuknecht, H.F., "Pathology of Sensorineural Deafness of Genetic Origin," in *Deafness in Childhood,* edited by F. McConnell and P.H. Ward. Nashville: Vanderbilt University Press, 1967.

Springer, N., "A Comparative Study of the Behavior Traits of Deaf and Hearing Children of New York City," *American Annals of the Deaf,* 83 (1938), 255–273.

Stuckless, E.R., "Assessing and Supporting Linguistic Development in Deaf Adolescents," Kansas University Medical Center Conference Handout, Post-Graduate Medicine, February, 1971, pp. 7–13.

Stuckless, E.R., and **J.W. Birch**, "The Influence of Early Manual Communication on the Linguistic Development of Deaf Children," *American Annals of the Deaf,* 111 (1966), 452–460; 499–504.

Templin, M., *The Development of Reasoning in Children with Normal and Defective Hearing.* Minneapolis: University of Minnesota Press, 1950.

Thompson, H., *An Experimental Study of the Beginning Reading of Deaf-Mutes.* New York: Columbia University, Teachers College Contributions to Education, No. 254 (1927).

Vegely, A.B., and L.L. Elliott, "Applicability of a Standardized Personality Test to a Hearing-Impaired Population," *American Annals of the Deaf,* 113 (1968), 858–868.

Vernon, M., "Characteristics Associated with Post-Rubella Children: Psychological, Educational and Physical," *Volta Review,* 69 (1967a), 176–185.

Vernon, M., "Meningitis and Deafness: The Problem, Its Physical, Audiological, Psychological and Educational Manifestations in Deaf Children," *Laryngoscope,* 77 (1967b), 1856–1874.

Vernon, M., "Rh Factor and Deafness: The Problem, its Psychological, Physical and Educational Manifestations," *Exceptional Children,* 33 (1967c), 5–12.

Vernon, M., "Prematurity and Deafness: The Magnitude and Nature of the Problem among Deaf Children," *Exceptional Children,* 34 (1967d), 289–298.

Vernon, M., and S.D. Koh, "Early Manual Communication and Deaf Children's Achievement," *American Annals of the Deaf,* 115 (1970), 527–536.

Waldman, J.L., F.A. Wade, and C.W. Aretz, *Hearing and the School Child.* Washington, D.C.: Volta Bureau, 1930.

Whetnall, E., and D.B. Fry, *The Deaf Child.* London: William Heinemann Medical Books, 1964.

Winitz, H., "Problem Solving and the Delaying of Speech as Strategies in the Teaching of Language," *Asha,* 15 (1973), 583–586.

Young, C., and F. McConnell, "Retardation of Vocabulary Development in Hard of Hearing Children," *Exceptional Children,* 23 (1957), 368–370.

Appendix

Publisher	*Individual Performance Scales of Intelligence*	*Range of Test by Age*
A	Leiter International Scale (Original Norms)	2–adult
A	Leiter International Scale (Grace Arthur Revised Scoring)	3–8
A	Merrill-Palmer Pre-School Performance Tests (19 subtests of nonverbal abilities)	Preschool through primary grades
B	Wechsler Pre-School and Primary Scale of Intelligence (WPPSI)	4–6½
B	Wechsler Intelligence Scale for Children (WISC)	5–15
B	WISC-R (Revised WISC)	5–15
B	Wechsler Adult Intelligence Scale (WAIS)	16–75+
B	Wechsler-Bellevue Intelligence Scale (Form 2 is the retest for the WAIS)	10–59
B	Arthur Point Scale of Performance (Revised Form 2)	5–15
C	Arthur Point Scale of Performance (Form 1, the original scale)	5–15
D	Hiskey-Nebraska Test of Learning Aptitude	3–16

	Group Nonverbal Tests of Intelligence	
B	Revised Army Beta Test	16–59
A–B	Raven's Progressive Matrices (Colored, 1947)	5–11
A–B	Raven's Progressive Matrices (Standard, 1938)	8–65
A–B	Raven's Progressive Matrices (1947 & 1962)	For above average adolescents and adults
B	Chicago Non-Verbal Examination	8–adult
E	Science Research Associates, Inc. (SRA Non-Verbal Form)	Adult

Publisher	Personality and Emotional Adjustment Tests (Must be used with caution with deaf)	Type of Test and Age Range
B	Make a Picture Story (MAPS Test)	Projective Children & adults
B	Thematic Apperception Test (TAT)	Projective Adolescents & adults
B	Rorschach Test	Projective Adolescents & adults
F	Psychological Evaluation of Children's Human Figure Drawings (Elizabeth Koppitz). Also Developmental Norms	5–12
G	California Personality Tests	Kindergarten–adult
A	The Hand Test (E.E. Wagner) Used experimentally by C.P.Goetzinger	Projective Adolescents & adults
A	Buttons: A Projective Test for Pre-Adolescents and Adolescents (Esther Rothman & Pearl Berkowitz). Used Experimentally by C.P.Goetzinger	(See Title)
H	Group Personality Projective Test (GPPT) (R.N. Cassell and T.C. Kahn) Used experimentally by C.P.Goetzinger	Projective Adolescents & adults

Other Tests

B	Benton Revised Visual Retention Test (A. Benton) (Visual Memory Test)	8–adult
F	Bender Gestalt (Elizabeth Koppitz)	5–12

PUBLISHERS

A	Western Psychological Services, 12031 Wilshire Boulevard, Los Angeles, California 90025
B	The Psychological Corporation, 304 East 45th Street, New York, New York 10017
C	C.H. Stoelting Co., 424 North Homan Avenue, Chicago, Illinois 60624
D	Union College Press, Lincoln, Nebraska

E   Science Research Associates (SRA) Inc.,
259 East Erie Street, Chicago, Illinois 60611

F   Grune & Stratton, Inc., 381 Park Avenue South,
New York, New York 10016

G   California Test Bureau, 5916 Hollywood Boulevard,
Los Angeles, California 90028

H   Psychological Test Specialists, Box 1441, Missoula, Montana 59801

Diagnosis

The adult hearing-impaired patient usually comes to the audiologist through his own motivation to learn of the nature of his auditory disorder so that he can take steps to lessen its effects. As a rule, the pediatric patient is an unwilling or unwitting participant in such measures. It is generally agreed that the assessment of hearing disorders in children is, if not more difficult than, at least different from evaluation of disorders among adults. With adults, evaluation begins from the audiologist's point of view. With children, the examiner must be sensitive enough to select a method which taps the child's interests.

Because of their age or the nature of their handicap, many children do not cooperate during behavioral measurements of hearing. Dr. Berlin's subject in Chapter 4 is the use of objective tests that have been developed to determine hearing sensitivity. The term "objective" in this context means that the patient offers no subjective response to a stimulus.

A large number of even very young children can be persuaded to cooperate during voluntary hearing tests. Dr. Hodgson in Chapter 5 focuses on procedures for the very young child. In Chapter 6, on pure-tone tests, Dr. Fulton admonishes the reader to adhere to the rigors of scientific control in the auditory assessment of young children. Upon reading this chapter, the practicing audiologist may be given pause to reflect on his own approaches and the degree to which pure-tone audiometry is an art versus a science. The values and methods of speech audiometry with children are discussed by me in Chapter 7.

In Chapter 8, on differential diagnosis, Drs. Wood and Cole look at auditory disorders from the viewpoint of the language pathologist. Rather than attempting to familiarize the reader with specific tests of language dysfunction, they illustrate behaviors suggestive of processing difficulties, which may be regarded as auditory disorders.

CHAPTER FOUR

Electrophysiological Indices of Auditory Function

CHARLES I. BERLIN

113

INTRODUCTION

There is no single behavioral or physiological test of "hearing" in the broad sense of understanding complex signals like speech or Morse code. However, some procedures emerging from laboratory practice can give us powerful insights into physiological function of parts of the auditory system. Although we can make inferences about children's auditory limitations from these procedures, we should *not* hope for results analogous to the all-too-familiar pure-tone air conduction, bone conduction, speech reception threshold, and discrimination scores. Some may consider this a major drawback; others more broadly oriented may consider it a relief from an artificial constraint. Insisting on physiological homologues to the traditional audiometric battery is about as productive as calling Cugnot's 1769 steam carriage a "failure" because it did not resemble a horse, or insisting the Wright brothers' plane was of little use because it did not resemble the wing-flapping bird.

CHAPTER OBJECTIVES

This chapter will consider three *direct* procedures for assessing children's auditory function:

1. Electrocochleography (henceforth, ECochG[1]); measuring the compound VIIIth nerve action potential;
2. the Brainstem-Evoked Response (henceforth, BSER) (1-to-10 milliseconds [msec]);
3. the Frequency Following Response (henceforth, FFR).

It will also discuss in somewhat less technical detail the *mediated* procedures:

---

[1] ECo*ch*G will be used since *Ecog* means *electrocorticography* to neurosurgeons.

114

1. middle ear muscle reflexes;
2. Electrodermal Response Audiometry (henceforth, EDR);
3. middle- and late-evoked potentials (10 to 500 msec); and
4. two other emerging procedures: cardiotachometry and respiration audiometry.

DIRECT VERSUS MEDIATED INDICES

The procedures listed above either assess some portion of the auditory nervous system *directly* or use some *mediator* to give the observer insight into a child's auditory function. The so-called *direct* procedures measure the responses that suprathreshold auditory stimuli elicit from the appropriate structures; the *mediated* responses can be activated by either auditory or nonauditory systems or conditions. For example, in ECochG, the characteristic synchronous discharge of many VIIIth nerve fibers can be elicited *only* by auditory means. In contrast, the change in a child's heart rate used to signal audition by inference, while it can be elicited by the auditory stimulating signal, can also be elicited by changes in alertness, a deep breath, or a generalized body motion. As another example, in certain evoked potential paradigms, sleep interferes with the recording of the response. The diagnostician should be aware that, if he relies solely on physiological indices of audition, he can make two broad types of errors:

1. He can call a child "deaf" when, in fact, there is considerable residual auditory function.
2. He can call a child "normal" when there is essentially no capacity for auditory function.

The physiological techniques that use *mediated* functions are generally susceptible to *both* types of errors; the *direct* procedures (especially ECochG) are generally vulnerable only if a response is *absent.*[2]

TECHNICAL BACKGROUND

Preamplifiers

Preamplifiers (see glossary) are necessary because most of the electrophysiological responses to be measured are of small amplitude. For example, depending on the site of recording, the compound VIIIth nerve action potential can be less

---

[2]Poor electrode contact, trigger failure, or related equipment shortcomings are generally at fault here; however, pseudo FFRs may sometimes appear via induction or by tissue compression from high-intensity signals (see Davis, 1976).

than a microvolt (μv; 1 microvolt = 1 millionth of 1 volt). In addition, this small potential is embedded in considerable obstructive electrical *noise* including muscle activity, electrocardiographic (EKG) activity, and the atmospheric electrical activity of radio stations, fluorescent lights, and 60-Hz fluctuating line power. Because of these obstructions, the preamplification stage for 0.1–1.0 microvolt potentials should be a *differential*, or push-pull, preamplifier, with high input impedance and good *common mode rejection*.

Common Mode Rejection and the Differential Amplifier. A three-conductor electrode array is the usual hallmark of a common mode rejection system. The target electrode (see glossary) is placed as near the source of the desired potential as possible; its companion should be placed somewhat further away in similarly configured tissue. Thus, target and companion electrodes, with reference to the third electrode (ground), will be subjected to similar *ambient* electrical activity simultaneously; the target electrode should also carry the desired response. The target and companion electrodes bring their common information to the preamplification unit, and the preamplification unit amplifies only the algebraic *difference* between the two electrodes; therefore, we have a system in which undesired ambient electrical signals (those not emanating from the target source) are cancelled by the preamplifier, ideally leaving the target response unaffected. See Fig. 4-1 in which the target voltage is a 1-microvolt signal embedded in 100 millivolts (mv; 1 millivolt = 1/1000 volts) of undesired noise.

Common mode rejection is usually frequency-sensitive; as the frequency rises, the effectiveness of the common mode rejection generally falls. Therefore, specifications of preamplifiers should be reviewed carefully to determine the frequency at which common mode rejection is cited. Acceptable common mode rejection at 60 Hz is in the 80 to 100dB range. ECochG and BSER need a low-level input sensitivity (1 to 10 microvolts) and preferably a low noise figure of 5 to 10 microvolts RMS (see glossary) with reference to the input.

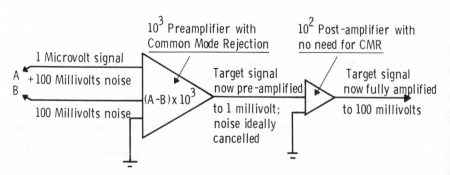

Fig. 4-1. Schematic of Common Mode Rejections

Amplifiers

Once the physiologic signal has been preamplified to a suitable level, a post-amplification stage of 10^1 or 10^2 is recommended for most purposes. This usually brings smaller signals to levels large enough to be recorded onto data recorders or brought to signal-processing computers. The amplifiers should have the same frequency response as the preamplifiers and are often packaged with companion preamplifiers. Single-ended amplification (see glossary) is now appropriate using only the output from the differential preamplifier.

Electrodes

Whenever a common mode rejection system is used, the target and companion electrodes must "see" similar voltages through similar resistances. Let us take an example. Assume two electrodes were in a field in which there were 100 millivolts of fluorescent-light noise; one electrode is attached to the skin with a 10,000-ohm resistance; the other electrode is attached to an area with either substantially more or less than 10,000 ohms. Then the induced currents in the electrodes, which should ideally be equalized, would be unbalanced and common mode rejection would be inefficient. Thus, it is important that special care be taken to monitor electrode resistance. Needless to say, the ground electrode, to which the two other electrodes will be referenced, must be firmly in place and have equally good electrical contact with the skin.

Auditory Stimuli

It is in the use of auditory stimuli that we find the biggest differences between procedures to be discussed. Some responses (ECochG and BSER) can *only* be elicited by clicks or brief transients. Others (FFR, for example) are best elicited by low-frequency stimuli; still other responses (EDR, middle-ear muscle reflexes, late evoked potentials, heart rate change, and respiratory changes) can be elicited by audiometric tones *or* speech. Some writers suggest that speech or speech-like stimuli are the most powerful elicitors of human auditory nervous system response. One author (Eisenberg, 1975) is devoting the bulk of her work in cardiotachometry to the study of peripheral and central specializations which underlie the development of verbal communication. This sophisticated goal cannot, at present, be achieved with any of the so-called direct measures cited in this chapter. Cardiotachometry, middle- and late-component electroencephalography (EEG), contingent negative variation (CNV, see glossary), and hemispheric EEG differences in responsivity may be more promising in giving investigators insight into the development of speech processing. However, the *absence* of such high-level responses (assuming they can be reliably and validly detected and recorded) may signify any combination of cerebral deficit, brainstem deficit,

117

cochlear or VIIIth nerve deficit, or even middle-ear pathology; such techniques may ultimately have to be combined with some form of more peripheral assessment to be of precise diagnostic value. The CNV, however, is much more likely to yield measures of "hearing" in the sense of a higher cortical function than are ECochG or BSER.

The Principles of Digital Averaging

If a small biological voltage is to be measured in the presence of interference (noise), the additive function of a digital computer can be used to help improve the signal-to-noise ratio (see glossary). The signal eliciting the response, the response itself, and the onset of the computer sweep must *all* be in fixed-time registration. When all three events are related in time, the small microvoltage from the sources will be added in the computer linearly; any activity *not* time-locked to the onset of the stimulus will be added as the square root of the number of sweeps. Thus, if one takes only a single look at ongoing electrical activity, the signal-to-noise ratio will be 1. One hundred sweeps will improve the signal-to-noise ratio by 10. Ten thousand sweeps will improve the signal-to-noise ratio by 100.

Figure 4–2 idealizes a set of bins or addresses to be found in most such computers. A scanner is sent through each address at the onset of the stimulus trigger and is instructed to dwell at each address for a specified amount of time. While it is dwelling at that address, the scanner digitizes any voltages occurring at that "time bin" and translates those voltages into a vertical height proportional to the voltage coming from the source. If we know how long the scanner dwells at each address, we can convert the dwell time into *elapsed time*, or latency (see glossary) from the onset of the stimulus simply by counting the number of addresses. For example, in Fig. 4–2 you see an idealized waveform as typically seen on a computer readout. If the point at the peak of the waveform is the nineteenth address, and the dwell time of the scanner at each address were 80 microseconds

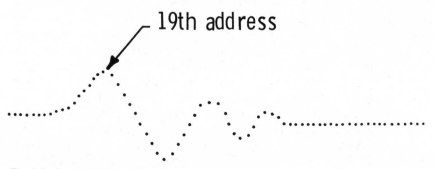

Fig. 4–2. Sample Display of Computer "Addresses"

(μsec), we can then conclude that the elapsed time, or latency, of the peak of this response from the onset of the trigger is 1.52 milliseconds (Address Number $\times$ Dwell Time = Latency).

The amplitude of the voltage can be handled in a similar fashion. Let us assume the digital converter in the computer uses a 9-bit digitizer,[3] which breaks up incoming voltages into 512 parts (2^9). Put another way, a full-scale display of 8 volts is broken up into 512 steps and the computer can resolve only about 16 millivolts (8 volts divided into 511 parts, one part being lost to the necessity of making each step discrete). If one uses a total of 10^6 amplification, then the resolution will be $16 \times 10^{-3} \times 10^{-6}$, which equals about .016 microvolts per step, a figure adequate to outline a 0.1 microvolt ECochGic response.

The correct choice of digital averager should permit the observer to have at least ten addresses available to outline the basic waveform of interest in the time domain. Thus, in ECochG, where the major waveform occurs within 1.5 milliseconds of stimulation and is completed after 3 milliseconds have passed, we recommend 200 or more addresses in the full sweep of the averager, and a dwell time per address of no longer than 100 μsec.

Magnetic Recorders

Most of the physiological events to be described in this chapter can be recorded on frequency-modulated (FM) recorders (see glossary), traditionally recommended for biological signals. To use the recorded data validly, one must first understand the frequency limitations of these data recorders with respect to the dominant frequency of the target's biological response. The critical principles are much like those of frequency response limitation in audio tape recorders and hearing aids. Most FM magnetic data recorders have response limits from dc to 1000 Hz at tape speeds up to about 3¾ inches per second. Responses higher than 1000 Hz usually require faster tape speeds, and these are possible with current electronics; it is also theoretically and practically possible to record ECochGic data (but not slow-wave EEG) on standard audio tape recorders. If the recording is done for reanalysis and replay into some form of computer system, the most critical aspect after recording the raw data involves the recording and reproduction of the trigger in proper time alignment to the data channel. If the playback unit has uneven playback speed, then responses which occurred in *real* time at, say, 1.5 milliseconds from the trigger may fluctuate in their time position on playback. This would weaken the signal averaging capability of the computer considerably; therefore, the two main considerations after frequency response in the use of recorders should be time-locking the trigger to the data channel and reproducing the two channels with stable

---

[3]For those unfamiliar with binary digit notation ("bit" is a short form of "binary digit"), a brief program is attached in the Appendix at the end of this chapter.

temporal relationship. In the parlance of the hi-fi addict, there should be good frequency response and minimal "wow" and "flutter."

In the Appendix, each of the major procedures will be listed with respect to the requisite preamplifiers, postamplifiers, common auditory stimuli, etc. A tabulation will be offered of the unique benefits and the limitations of each physiological index of auditory function. In the rest of this chapter, we will discuss the techniques of collecting each of these indices and their applications in sample patients.

A CAVEAT

In the ensuing discussion of direct vs. mediated indices of auditory function, the superficial reader may come away with the notion that certain techniques (especially ECochG and BSER) are infallible indices of "hearing." Although the repeatable presence of these responses is strong evidence against total peripheral deafness, I would be remiss if I encouraged you to make critical decisions based on any *one* test alone. As can be seen from the illustrative cases at the end of this chapter, I strongly endorse the cross-check principles outlined by Jerger and Hayes (1976) and applied in empathy and by common concern in our group's related works (Berlin et al., 1974; Berlin and Gondra, 1976, pp. 457–469; Cullen et al., 1976). However, others do not always share our opinions (see later section entitled, "Dissenting Opinions on ECochG as an Audiometric Tool").

DIRECT INDICES OF AUDITORY FUNCTION

Electrocochleography (ECochG); Recording the Human VIIIth Nerve Action Potentials

Procedure. The subject is placed in a reclining position and the target electrode is placed as close to the cochlear nerve fiber source as possible. The electrode position depends upon the biases, professional training, and expertise of the tester as well as the subject's permission. Simmons (1975) has rightfully concluded that the most dependable, accurate, and sensitive site is the promontory of the cochlea. This preferred placement requires an otologist, who is surgically and medically responsible for the trans-tympanic placement of the electrode and its recovery.

In children, anesthesia is necessary and a trans-tympanic electrode is ideal. In cooperative adults, general anesthesia is not necessary and either no anesthetic, local anesthetic, or iontophoresis—forcing of anesthetic material into tympanic membrane and canal wall tissues by mild, direct electrical current (Echols, Norris

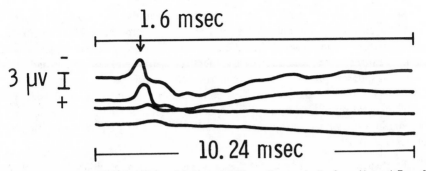

Fig. 4-3. Compound Action Potential Recorded Trans-Tympanically from Normal Ear of an Otherwise Impossible-to-Test Child

and Tabb, 1975)—can be used.[4] Where trans-tympanic placement is inappropriate, or where patients do not give permission (see Case 6), adequate recordings can usually be obtained from external auditory canal positions using silver or silver-chloride electrodes wrapped in saline-impregnated cotton (Cullen et al., 1972), or expandable clips (Coats and Dickey, 1970). Ground and indifferent electrodes can be placed on the forehead and mastoid, respectively. Moore (1976) has shown that even an earlobe-clip-to-nose configuration leads to a discernible response; the major principle involves separating electrodes sufficiently. Even Moore agrees, however, that somewhat less sensitive results are obtained when ground and companion electrodes are placed remotely from the cochlea, and the interested reader is referred to Simmons (1975) and Simmons and Glattke (1975) for a review.

The stimuli must be repetitive (usually 10 per second) and of a nature that elicits large numbers of synchronous auditory nerve discharges. Depending upon the available configuration, either a field transducer or earphone transducer is used. The action potential, shown in Fig. 4-3, can only be elicited if the rise time (see glossary) of the stimulus is faster than 1 millisecond (Goldstein and Kiang, 1958). Therefore, it is virtually mandatory that clicks or tone bursts be used for ECochG.

This requirement introduces a classical problem in auditory stimulus control: the time-frequency uncertainty principle (see glossary). Basically, the principle says that when any stimulus is abruptly gated on, it must, of necessity, contain many frequency components and cannot be a "pure tone." Licklider (1951, pp. 992, 993) gives a most scholarly analysis of this principle (see also Berlin and Lowe, 1972; Berlin and Gondra, 1976; Davis, 1976, Chapter 9).

---

[4]I and one of my colleagues have experienced and prefer the single, sharp pain of the promontory electrode to the three separate injections traditionally used to anesthetize the external canal. Iontophoresis seems to work for me, but not for him.

Specifying the intensity of such acoustic transients is not simple. Ordinary sound level meters are unsatisfactory because their mechanically controlled galvanometers do not rise or fall at rates fast enough to respond to transient stimuli. Furthermore, as I specified earlier, transients tend to have broad frequency responses, proportional to their rise time and shaped by the transducers into which they are generated. This complication introduces related spectral problems with respect to frequency responses of ordinary meters. I recommend one of the following techniques for measuring the intensity of transients used in ECochG or BSER.

1. Measure maximum positive "peak pressure" with a sound-level meter that has a "sample and hold" characteristic, such as the B&K, Model 2209.

2. Monitor the output of the recording microphone on the oscilloscope screen and match the peak-to-peak voltage of the transient coming off the microphone to the peak-to-peak voltage of a continuous sine wave at or near the resonant frequency of the transducer. When you have acquired a matching, continuous sine wave, measure *its* sound pressure level (SPL); the transient of similar amplitude can be said to have "peak equivalent SPL" identical in value to the SPL of the matched, continuous sine wave. Note that, because of duration and spectral differences, *the 90dB transient will not be as loud as a 90dB SPL tone.* A 90dB peak equivalent sound pressure click in our laboratory is about 65 to 70dB hearing level (HL), whereas the 4 kHz sine wave to which it is matched would be about 85dB above audiometric threshold.

3. Least desirable is running a group of normal subjects under relatively consistent listening conditions and searching for the mean group threshold. The accuracy depends upon group size and sampling procedures, and the technique seductively invites subsequent results to be interpreted in audiometric terms.

The Response

The compound action potential vs. the single unit action potential. Fig. 4–3 shows a *compound* action potential recorded trans-tympanically from the normal ear of an otherwise impossible-to-test child. This *compound* potential represents the sum of many *single* unit discharges, all of which occurred almost synchronously following the arrival of an acoustic stimulus at the ear. The careful reader should have noted that this compound action potential is only recordable in response to a click or tone burst with a rapid rise time; continuous tones, or tones with slow rise times, will not elicit a response *even though the tones are audible to the listener.* This is not to say that individual VIIIth nerve action potentials do not operate during the transmission of continuous sine waves, but only that the *synchronous* discharge of many fibers at once (the compound action potential) is not visible.

The underlying principles. While the apparent magnitude of the response is somewhat labile depending upon tissue resistance, distance from the source, etc. (Rosenblith and Rosenzweig, 1951), most workers have found the latency to be an extremely reliable and stable index of the response. Fig. 4–4 shows some data from the work of Mouney et al. (1976) that trace the mathematical regression lines for human ear latencies (see glossary) to tones of 2, 4, 6, and 8 kHz, as well as a click resonating a TDH–49 earphone placed approximately 1 foot from the external auditory canal. It is axiomatic in the nervous system that as the amplitude of the stimulation continues to rise above threshold, neural responses occur at shorter and shorter latencies. However, there is a minimum time

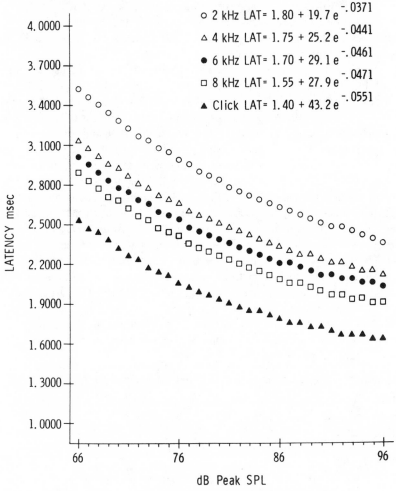

$$\circ \ 2 \text{ kHz LAT} = 1.80 + 19.7 \, e^{-.0371}$$
$$\triangle \ 4 \text{ kHz LAT} = 1.75 + 25.2 \, e^{-.0441}$$
$$\bullet \ 6 \text{ kHz LAT} = 1.70 + 29.1 \, e^{-.0461}$$
$$\square \ 8 \text{ kHz LAT} = 1.55 + 27.9 \, e^{-.0471}$$
$$\blacktriangle \ \text{Click LAT} = 1.40 + 43.2 \, e^{-.0551}$$

Fig. 4-4. Latency-Intensity Function for Tones and Click (from Mouney et al.)

period within which discharges cannot occur, hence the flattening of the curve at high intensity. This 1.5-millisecond value is thought to encompass the period during which mechanical and electrochemical events take place between the hair cell and the unmyelinated portion of the spiral ganglion fiber (see Bobbin, 1976 for programmed text).

It has been suggested that most of the auditory nerve fibers innervate *inner* hair cells, and only about 10% are activated by outer hair cells (Spoendlin, 1973). This paradoxical circumstance leads to the prediction that the gross magnitude of the compound action potential would not grow linearly with intensity, but that its latency would remain roughly constant if outer hair cells are missing. Yoshie (1968) has shown that up to about 50 to 60dB sensation level there is a relatively slow growth of response magnitude, whereas above that level the response grows more sharply; Wang and Dallos (1972) and Berlin et al. (1974) have shown normal latency in the presence of outer hair cell loss which would be analogous to a moderate sensorineural loss.

It is important to review basilar membrane mechanics as we discuss interpretation of ECochG. The traveling wave of the basilar membrane always moves from base to apex, and the velocity of that wave is uneven. The wave moves much more rapidly at the basal end, discharging many more hair cells and nerve fibers synchronously, than at the apical end, where the speed and stimulating arc of the traveling wave both reduce. Couple that fundamental principle with the earlier statement that signals with rise times of 1 millisecond or less are the only ones suitable for ECochG and you see one of the major shortcomings of the ECochGram. Since the travel time of the basilar membrane is between 3 and 7 milliseconds, depending upon species, a compound action potential elicited 1.5 milliseconds after high-intensity stimulation *must evolve from mechanical events occurring primarily at the basal turn.* At low intensities, ECochG cannot easily assess regions of the cochlea below 1000 to 2000 Hz without concomitant spectral splash or contamination from basal turn elements. Keep in mind also that even for low-frequency tones, portions of the basal turn may participate in the coding process. Thus, a person with a normal basal turn may give a normal ECochGram to a click and still have some audiometric difficulty in low frequencies, although a *total* low-frequency loss in the presence of *normal* high-frequency hearing is physiologically impossible.

Interpretation. There are three parameters that can be used for clinical interpretation:

1. The latency of the response
2. Its amplitude
3. Its waveform.

To a great extent, both amplitude and waveform may be affected by auditory and nonauditory constraints such as tissue and electrode impedance, current paths, and such. Latency, on the other hand, is least labile to these inter-ferences, and we have found it to be the most useful measure of the action potential.

The presence of a synchronous whole nerve action potential must rule out total peripheral deafness, at least the sort that is commonly associated with hair-cell and nerve-fiber loss. It is fair to say that the subject must have reasonably normal input in certain narrow ranges of the auditory spectrum (see Elberling, 1973; Berlin et al., 1974; Simmons and Glattke, 1975; Mouney et al., 1976; Ruben, Elberling, and Salomon, 1976) if the response is large at high intensities, reduces in magnitude, lengthens in latency (in typical fashion), and finally is barely detectable after 1000 or so very low-intensity stimuli.

Because the test-retest reliability of the latency for an VIIIth nerve action po-tential is remarkably high, it is possible to develop a template and norms for ears with conductive and sensorineural as well as mixed hearing losses. Using click stimuli, we (Berlin and Gondra, 1976) found that patients with conductive hear-ing losses basically showed an abnormally lengthened latency, patients with mixed losses tended to show normal latency at high intensities but a characteris-tically lengthened latency at low intensities, and patients with mild-to-moderate sensorineural losses showed essentially normal latency but reduced amplitude and a loss of the response at levels well above normal. Our findings only con-firmed earlier work by Yoshie and Ohashi (1969), Aran (1971), Eggermont et al. (1974), and others.

One of the unique benefits of ECochG is that it enables us to study each ear independently (masking is obviously never necessary); thus ECochG can help select the better of two ears for a hearing aid or, if surgery is contemplated or necessary, it can aid the surgical decision-making process. We have also found it useful to get permission to perform ear surgery before the ECochGic procedure begins. Our surgeon often finds middle-ear fluid or debris in the patient's ear. Not only can the ECochGic measurements be done, but with surgical permission in hand, the child's ear can be treated and pre- and post-treatment ECochGic information can be acquired.

ECochG can also be done via bone conduction (Berlin et al., 1977), again without need for masking, and can aid in making certain surgical decisions on children too young for traditional audiometric tests. This gives us still another opportunity for early detection and intervention even in patients with mild con-ductive hearing losses.

A Brief Digression into Effects of Mild Conductive Hearing Loss on Auditory Development. It has been intimated by Goetzinger (1965), Holm and Kunze (1969), Northern and Downs (1975), and others that even minimal conductive hearing losses may have adverse effects on speech and language development. Two of my colleagues have recently completed animal studies showing degenera-tion in certain brainstem auditory nuclei after both surgically induced conductive hearing loss and controlled sound isolation (Webster and Webster, 1976). They have also found similar dystrophies in brainstem nuclei of humans with long-standing hearing losses. Recently, *physiological* changes following conductive hearing loss have also been shown at the level of the cat's brainstem (Clopton and Silverman, 1976; Silverman and Clopton, 1976). The adverse effect of being raised in darkness on the development of central visual structures is well known. We should not be surprised, therefore, to find the suggestion that peripheral, even somewhat benign-appearing, sensitivity deficits may have effects on the rest of the auditory nervous system. This provocative suggestion only heightens the importance of the *early* detection and management of hearing and ear disabilities.

Dissenting Opinions on ECochG as an Audiometric Tool. Up until now, I have offered physiologic, acoustic, and deductive evidence for questioning the validity of an ECochGram as a *substitute* for an audiogram. Briefly, my arguments are these:

1. A continuous suprathreshold tone, which does not have a rise time shorter than 1 millisecond, will not elicit a compound action potential. Thus, one can "hear" stimuli that can't elicit an ECochGram (see 3, below).
2. The acoustic constraints of a short tone-burst are such that an uncontaminated sine wave cannot be easily generated unless at least two periods of the signal pass during the rise time. This basically restricts the use of "clean" signals to frequencies of about 2000 Hz and upward.
3. Audiometric tones have slow rise times and are continuous; they do elicit single-unit activity, but the single-unit activity is not synchronous enough for us to average a compound action potential. Therefore, relating an audiometric tone to an ECochGic stimulus is at best tenuous.

Despite these theoretical objections, a number of workers have demonstrated remarkably good agreement between voluntary thresholds and ECochGic thresholds to tone bursts ranging from 500 to 8000 Hz (Coats, 1976; Eggermont, Spoor, and Odenthal, 1976; Mouney et al., 1976; Naunton and Zerlin, 1976a,b). While individually convincing audiograms are presented by each of these reporters, scattergrams of the data of at least one extensive study (Eggermont et al., 1976) show total disagreement as great as 45dB at 8000 Hz, 35dB at 4000 Hz, 30dB at 2000 Hz, 30dB at 1000 Hz and a surprisingly small 20dB at 500 Hz. Eggermont et al. (1976) conclude that, compared with the voluntary audiometric threshold, the ECochG threshold is somewhat poorer at low intensities and somewhat better at high intensities.

Using tone bursts alone has some inherent problems in assessing frequency specificity; however, methods are being applied that use either high-pass filtered noise or masking of a click by a continuous tone, followed by subtraction of the residual action potential (Eggermont et al., 1974). These must be considered as important additional contributions to the ECochG armamentarium.

Perspective. Although I have had limited experience using tone-burst ECochG for clinical purposes, I have never seen a case in which normal-click ECochG was not confirmed by tone-burst ECochG. The routine addition of the tone-burst ECochG for five frequencies, however, would lengthen our test procedure and increase the anesthetic risk by almost five times. On the other hand, I have never chosen to do tone-burst ECochG in the absence of a response to a high-intensity click, and Case 6, to be discussed later, will show how that may well be a short-coming in my methodology.

In looking back on my own experience with ECochG, I began using extra-tympanic ECochG and clicks because they were most expedient. Now, with more extensive experience, I believe that, for diagnosing young children, trans-tympanic ECochG is ideal; I have no doubt that in the years to come, with still more experience, I will reconsider the value of tone-burst ECochG for approxi-mating audiometric thresholds. However, at this time, I find it intellectually un-satisfying to view the auditory nervous system as a relatively simple cable that, when stimulated synchronously enough to generate a compound action potential made up of single-unit synchronous discharges, transmits "all the information necessary to hear." When that compound action potential is not visible, does that show "no hearing has taken place"?[5]

One other issue that must be raised concerns the safety of ECochG. Crowley, Davis, and Beagley (1975) have reported on a worldwide survey of 3,696 sub-jects on whom ECochG has been used. Only half of the procedures were done transtympanically, and of these, fewer than 0.1% showed undesirable effects (two cases reported of otitis media and one case reported of tympanic mem-brane perforation). There was about 1% incidence of general anesthetic compli-cations (nausea, vertigo, or vomiting: 17 cases; laryngospasm or bronchospasm after Ketamine: 4 cases; extrapryamidal motor syndrome: 1 case; excessive mucus production: 2 cases). There were no deaths.

Virtually all experienced users of ECochG report the gratitude of parents and referring agents when a definitive and unequivocal answer can be given about the physiological state of the patient's ear. Subsequent rehabilitation is usually rapid and unhampered by differences of opinion (see Case 1). Consider-ing the negligible risk, ECochG is especially useful with neonates or with young

---

[5] For example, what is the state of spontaneous discharge of the VIIIth nerve just before a given stimulus comes to the ear? It is statistically possible that large numbers of units will be refractory at one time, but responsive at another, because of pre-existing spontaneous activity. (See, for example, Kiang, Moxon, Kahn, 1976, or Coats, 1976, and Elberling and Salomon's 1976 experiment with computer simulation of audiograms and VIIIth nerve action potential (pp. 439–455), and reread arguments 1 and 3 in this section.)

children whose complex neurological or behavioral problems make definitive auditory assessment difficult, if not impossible.

Brainstem-Evoked Response (BSER)

Workers in electrophysiology have long sought an EEG-related evoked potential synonymous with the "moment of hearing" (Davis, 1976). Unfortunately, most of the earlier forms of evoked-response audiometry had low reliability because the results changed during sleep, under sedation, or under general anesthetic. This labile state of the subject primarily affected the evoked potentials seen from 50 to 300 milliseconds. Jewett, Romano, and Williston (1970) and Sohmer and Feinmesser (1970) were among the first to record earlier 1.0- to 10-millisecond brainstem responses unaffected by sleep or sedation.

Procedure. The subject can be either awake or asleep, since this response is essentially unaffected by sleep stage and most drugs. The target and companion electrodes are usually placed at the vertex and earlobe, respectively, with a ground at the forehead. Stimuli are repeated between 2½ to 10 times per sec (although rarely they are repeated faster) and should be clicks or rapid-rise tone bursts. In this respect, all procedures are identical to trans-tympanic ECochG except the placement of the target electrode. In fact, the techniques are so similar that many European workers, including Sohmer, Feinmesser, and Szabo (1974) and Thornton (1975a), call the procedure "surface ECochG." The major drawback with such a labeling is that the cochlear portion of the response is rarely visible below 60 or 70dB HL and, while the presence of a normal fifth wave (see next section) can be taken to infer adequate cochlear function, the absence of the normal fifth wave gives us no cochlear information (see Case 4).

The Response. Fig. 4–5 shows a sample of these responses recorded from my own scalp and compared to my own ear-canal ECochGram. The presumed source of each of these responses, reading from left to right, is as follows:

1. The first peak is the compound VIIIth nerve action potential presumably arising from synchronous discharge of single units in the VIIIth nerve.
2. The second peak is presumed to come from the cochlear nucleus;
3. The third from the contralateral olivary bodies;
4. The fourth from the ventral nucleus of the lateral lemniscus and pre-olivary region; and
5. The fifth (and most consistently used for studies of auditory sensitivity) is presumed to come from the inferior colliculus.
6. The subsequent waves probably come from the medial geniculate and primary auditory cortex.

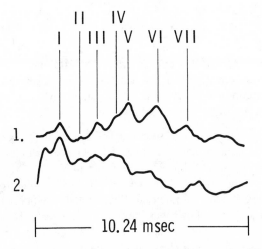

1. Potentials recorded from vertex 2048 clicks
2. N_1 recorded from external canal

Note: Latencies of 1.5 msec for N_1's in both tracings

Fig. 4-5. Brainstem-Evoked Response (top trace and ear canal ECochG; bottom trace from same subject)

Underlying Principles. The synchronous depolarization of the VIIIth nerve itself is thought to lead to the subsequent synchronous discharge of many units in the major auditory nuclei. The vertex electrode records all the synchronous potentials from the "far field," and the source of the "far-field potentials" was originally assigned to the major nuclei by virtue of their latency (Jewett and Williston, 1971). Subsequent studies (e.g., Lev and Sohmer, 1972; Buchwald and Huang, 1975; Thornton and Hawkes, 1976; Martin and Moore, 1977) support this interpretation, but caution must be exercised in concluding that the sources are accurate and the stimulation is *serial.* Case 4 shows what may be either: (1) very late waves 4 and 5, with no wave 6, or (2) missing waves 4 and 5, and nearly normal wave 6.

In any event, it is appealingly simple but premature to view BSER as a straightforward series of waves, each of which depends upon its predecessor. Only the first wave seems to be mandatory; even it is often not seen at low sensation levels, though the fifth wave is visible (see Ino, 1976). For example, Meunier and May (1976) concluded, after measuring ear-canal ECochG simultaneously with BSER, that

... in contrast to vertex (derived) N_5, vertex-(derived)-N_1 is small and more variable in waveform despite its high correlation with the ear canal recording.

Fig. 4-6 is taken from their report and shows the fifth wave (here pointing downwards) still present at 46dB peak equivalent SPL (about 10dB HL for their stimulus). The N_1 recorded from the ear canal is no longer visible in the BSER at 66dB peak equivalent SPL; thus, the series analogy cannot be visualized even in the normal subject at low sensation levels.

Interpretation. Workers agree that the so-called fifth wave in the series is the most useful one for audiometric purposes (e.g., Sohmer and Feinmesser, 1970; Hood, 1975; Davis, 1976; Galambos, 1976; Meunier and May, 1976). The fifth wave follows an orderly regression with reduction in intensity similar to, but not identical to, the whole nerve action potential. Meunier and May (1976) have calculated this regression; Fig. 4-7 shows its relationship to intensity. Most workers to date (e.g., Galambos, 1976; Sohmer and Cohen, 1976) agree that in the presence of conductive losses, there is a clear-cut and dramatic shift towards longer latencies. Such shifts are not seen in peripheral sensorineural losses, and available data suggest various latency, magnitude, and waveform changes with sundry pathologies in the central auditory system (see Hecox and Galamobos, 1974; Starr and Achor, 1975; Galambos, 1976; Sohmer and Cohen, 1976; Starr, 1976; Thornton and Hawkes, 1976).

Schulman-Galambos and Galambos (1975) showed that as gestational age increased, there was a developmental decrease in fifth-wave latency in a group of premature infants. They agree with others when they conclude that, because the response is not subject to fatigue or sleep-stage, it is useful in evaluating auditory function in high-risk, newborn infants. However, their conclusion concerning latency shift with age must be tempered; although there may indeed be a fifth-wave developmental trend with gestational age, these infants are prone to middle-ear mesenchyme, which also tends to resorb with gestational age (see later section entitled Middle Ear Muscle Reflexes). This disappearance of mesenchyme could cause a developmentally receding conductive hearing loss that could account for, or *add* to, the latency shifts seen at the fifth wave. My evidence for this supposition comes from examination of the normal ECochGic responses of two newborns; the responses were of normal latency in two of the four ears tested. Two ears were filled with mesenchyme and generated an ECochGic latency about 1 millisecond later than normal. That amount of shift can account for most of the main effects in their report. While I doubt that this is a serious objection, it must be considered in the prediction of normal fifth-wave latency of neonatal BSER (see Hecox and Galambos, 1974). Jerger[6] is presently preparing a summary of his extensive pediatric clinical experience using BSER and should have some information to add to this area.

[6]Personal communication with Dr. J. Jerger, 1976.

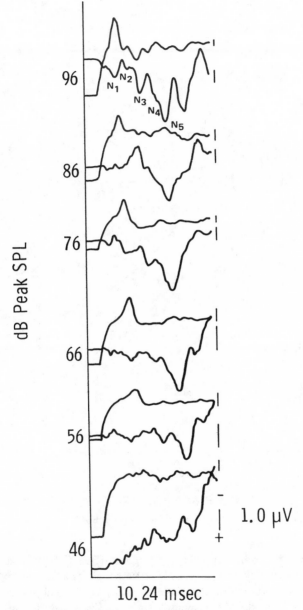

Fig. 4-6. Simultaneous BSER ECochG from Normal Subject

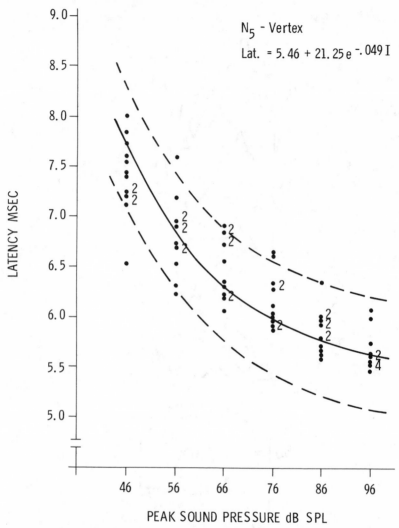

PEAK SOUND PRESSURE dB SPL

Fig. 4-7. Latency-Intensity Function for Fifth Wave of BSER

The BSER is primarily an onset response (Hecox, Squires, and Galambos, 1976) whose latency changes in only some people as a function of positive- vs. negative-going polarity of the acoustic pulse. Ornitz and Walter (1975) have shown that in adults the responses are only slightly shifted in time when a positive- vs. a negative-going pulse is used. In contrast, they show autistic children whose responses are 180 degrees out of phase to the positive- vs. negative-going pulse in some places. Our experience with autistic children (see Case 4) suggests that there may be some brainstem anomalies in these children. Thus,

BSER may be useful not just audiometrically, but also to aid in the diagnosis of various other problems which simulate or complicate deafness.

Thus, the BSER technique is extremely promising in the pediatric assessment of acoustic function for a number of reasons:

1. Abnormalities may aid in neurologic as well as audiologic assessment.

2. Anesthesia, while not necessary, apparently does not affect the response (Ketamine may be an exception).

3. Because surface electrodes are used, none of the expense, anesthetic, or other risks inherent in trans-tympanic ECochG are involved.

4. When a normal fifth wave is seen, information is presumably transmitted to the level of thalamus (medial geniculate bodies).

5. The response is stable and repeatable over time (e.g., Schulman-Galambos and Galambos, 1975).

However, there are drawbacks to the *exclusive* use of BSER with children.

1. At the level of the fifth wave, the observer is really never sure which ear has contributed to the response. If the stimulation is at high intensity, trans-cranial transmission has taken place and some spurious interpretations may be drawn, for example, for ear choice with a hearing aid.

2. Bone conduction, while possible, yields similar problems unless masking is used; and then certain decisions must be made about masking parameters that require unavailable audiometric thresholds.

3. Electrode-shielding, common mode rejection, muscle artifact, and ambent electrical activity problems can either obscure any good recordings and/or confound the easy identification of the key responses.

4. Finally, since both sides of the auditory system are being stimulated at levels above the cochlear nucleus, it is conceivable that, in certain cases, out-of-phase responses from either side can interact and confound the interpretation of the recordings. Thus, having a single source followed by multiple generators along the auditory pathway may preclude simple interpretation.

These objections, however, should not be taken as particularly serious; BSER promises to be the most widely used response in the audiologists' armamentarium, since it requires minimum dependence on other specialists and under ideal circumstances can give much of the same data produced by trans-tympanic ECochG. When used for children, in concert with ECochG, tympanometry, and middle-ear muscle reflexes, the *combination is probably the most powerful battery available to the hearing diagnostician to date* (see case discussions at end of chapter; also, as examples, Picton et al., 1974; Sohmer, Pratt, and Feinmesser, 1974; Hyde, Stephens, and Thornton, 1976; Thornton, 1976; Skinner and Glattke, 1977).

Hood (1975) recently commented that the BSER had, perhaps, been over-looked because of overconcern for early myogenic responses. In fact, some of the BSER responses had already been reported in the physiologic literature (see, for example, Teas and Kiang, 1964) but were inadvertently obscured by clinical workers using EEG amplifiers whose frequency responses, sensitivities, and gains were not suitable to record the BSER potentials. It is probably premature to say that all the major potentials that can be seen by surface recordings have been identified. As more daring researchers develop new sites of recording or broader frequency response and as greater sensitivity and more rapid digitizing rates become available, I suspect additional potentials will be uncovered and noted. It may be only coincidental that there is a major auditory nucleus corresponding to each one of the BSER waves. On the other hand, the responses are separated by about 1 to 1½ milliseconds, which is a reasonably well-accepted refractory period for neural elements in the human nervous system. Whether new responses will be discovered in this time epoch or interactive responses will be uncovered remains to be seen. However, the future for BSER is extremely bright, not only for pediatric evaluation but for neurologic assessment of lesions that have only limited effect on the peripheral pure-tone audiogram (Starr and Achor, 1975; Starr, 1976).

Frequency Following Response (FFR)

In ECochG and BSER, clicks and tone bursts are necessary and, therefore, the assessment has only limited audiometric value for frequencies below 1000 to 2000 Hz. Since units of the auditory nervous system discharge in synchrony with given phase angles of sine waves (Rose et al., 1967), it is conceivable, with proper averaging technique, that one might be able to record these synchronous firings to low-frequency tones. Marsh and Worden (1968) first reported the FFR; they later showed that there are both ipsilateral pathways to the colliculus from the superior olivary complex and a contralateral path from the cochlear nucleus directly to the colliculus, *without* passing through the olivary bodies.[7] Thus, because of its low-frequency responsivity, FFR may yield data in the very frequency range where ECochG and BSER have limitations.

Procedure. Subjects are seated in comfortable chairs and a target electrode is usually fixed at the vertex. Indifferent electrodes have sometimes been fixed to each earlobe and a ground electrode to the leg. Researchers were interested in comparing monaural to binaural stimulation and in acquiring data about voltage differences between the vertex and the two ears (Moushegian, Rupert, and Stillman, 1973; Gerken et al., 1975; Daly, Roeser, and Moushegian, 1976). In clinical applications, Stillman, Moushegian, and Rupert (1976) used only a vertex

---

[7] Here is further evidence to question the *serial* number of the BSER.

target electrode, a right earlobe electrode as a companion, and a ground electrode placed on the opposite earlobe. Here, as in BSER and ECochG, a high-gain and high-frequency response preamplifier is necessary. However, in contrast to ECochGic and BSER recordings, a lower-frequency limit was set on the preamplifier to allow for passage of the low-frequency synchronous discharges.

The response reportedly is most obvious to tones of 500 Hz and below and can be elicited to a tone whose rise time is as slow as 4 to 5 milliseconds.

A considerable number of sweeps is generally needed to see a response; studies have used from 999 up to 3000 events, 6 to 16 milliseconds in duration, presented at rates ranging from 1 per second to 15 per second.

The Response. Fig. 4-8 shows a sample of the response obtained from a colleague's vertex. The response is ascribed to frequency-locked synchronous discharge of many fibers in the auditory nervous system to low stimulating frequencies. Let us take an example. Imagine a stimulus of 250 Hz presented to the auditory system, first at the level of the cochlea. It is well known that, in addition to the characteristic place array of fibers, neural elements will discharge at even multiples of stimulating frequencies. In addition, there are many fibers that will discharge at the reciprocal of their most sensitive frequency (Kiang, 1965); thus, a 250-Hz stimulus can elicit a group of synchronous firings from units at the cochlear level every 4 milliseconds (4 milliseconds being the period of a 250-Hz signal). If the stimulation were at 500 Hz, the units would tend to discharge every 2 milliseconds; if it were at 1000 Hz, every 1 millisecond, and so forth. This sort of frequency-following begins to taper off drastically above 1000 to 2000 Hz but is most easily seen at low frequencies. Thereafter, it is presumed

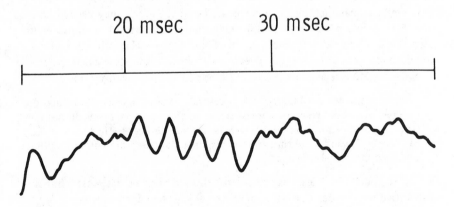

2048 sweeps of a 4-cycle, 500-Hz tone burst

Fig. 4-8. Sample FFR to 500 Hz Toneburst

other auditory nuclei may perform similarly, discharging in phase with the cochlear stimulation.

The source of the response is essentially unclear, but evidence points to its close relationship to the fifth wave in the BSER complex.

Note in the figure that the response seems to ride on a pedestal, which helps make the identification of the response more precise. The actual frequency-following "bumps" in the response usually occur somewhere above 40dB sensation level; however, the pedestal on which these responses ride usually occurs within 20dB of the patient's threshold.

Interpretation. The FFR has perhaps been subject to premature criticism for a number of reasons. First, it has been suggested the response can arise from basal-turn elements of the cochlea and, therefore, offers *no* added or complementary information to ECochG or brainstem potentials (Davis, 1976). Criticisms have also suggested that the responses could be "artifactual": a "microphonic," an induction artifact, or volume-unit conduction artifact (see glossary). I have not had any direct clinical experience recording the response, and therefore have only academic familiarity with the data. However, I am satisfied with the controls and individual experiments the following authors have performed using sound-conducting tubes on subjects with unilateral hearing losses (Daly, Roeser, and Moushegian, 1976), using monaural and binaural stimulation (Gerken et al., 1975), and with masking (Moushegian, 1976).

For example, Stillman, Moushegian, and Rupert (1976) concerned about artifacts, used short tone bursts of 4 milliseconds in studies of hard-of-hearing subjects. Their logic was as follows: they knew they would need high intensities for the hearing-impaired subjects, and they also knew that at high intensities they would risk induction and related artifacts; therefore, they elected to use a brief stimulus, which was completed before the expected response would begin. This, of course, introduced the problem of spectral splash, but under the circumstances they answered the objections of acoustic purists adequately.

Stillman, Moushegian, and Rupert (1976) added a provocative note:

> ... responses were obtained from several persons having "learning disorders". .... These responses are aberrant in that the waveforms do not contain frequency-following peaks even at intense levels of stimulation (70dB SL). Latencies and amplitudes of the response, however, are within the limits observed in normal subjects.

Not all subjects with "learning disorders" showed aberrant responses, but it is provocative to consider that some of these subjects had dyssynchrony of neural firing in their brainstems. If early conductive losses do change the organization of some brainstem structures (see earlier discussion on work of Clopton and Silverman, 1976; Silverman and Clopton, 1976; Webster and Webster, 1976), the phenomenon may be revealed by FFR studies. Thus, in addition to the physiological assessment of auditory sensation, especially in the low frequencies, FFR may also add information about the integrity of the brainstem for synchronous firing to low-frequency stimuli. Whether or not the same phenomena could be assessed by studies of the BSER directly remains to be seen.

Summary of Direct Measures

We've reviewed three direct measures well suited for assessing children's auditory function, each of which complements the other quite well. The ECochGram gives ear-specific information to clicks and rapid-rise tone bursts. The BSER, which uses similar clicks and tone bursts, gives information about each of the major nuclei in the child's auditory nervous system, provided the cochlea is intact. The FFR may be related to the BSER in ways we do not understand at present, but seems to complement ECochG and BSER because it is responsive to low-frequency tones; both BSER and FFR may also yield information about synchrony of discharge along the medullary neural axis—important to understanding children's "disorders of learning" that may have auditory perceptual bases.

MEDIATED RESPONSES

Middle-Ear Muscle Reflexes

The tensing of the stapedius muscle in the human constitutes the major recordable activity related to the middle-ear muscle reflexes, while the tensor tympani muscle is probably not involved (Djupesland, 1975). A child's reflexes are measured without invading its middle ear space by using instruments that infer action of the stapedius muscle by changes in impedance of the total middle-ear system (see Northern and Downs, 1974, Chapter 6; Feldman, 1975; Jerger, 1975) for updated reviews of the instrumentation).

Procedure. The reflex is elicited by placing a probe tone in the child's ear, checking first to see if both middle ears are normal (inferred by a normal tympanogram), and then stimulating either ear with tones, noise, or speech. Only certain tones are used if the probe and stimulus are presented to the same ear. An increase in the stiffness of either ear as a result of the stimulus affects the amount of probe tone reflected; this change in probe tone can be observed on either a galvanometric needle or a stripchart recorder. Stimulating one of two normal ears usually generates a reflex in both ears between 75 and 85dB HL. The presence of the reflex generally rules out *total* peripheral deafness; however, because of the familiar recruitment phenomenon, the presence of the reflex signal at normal hearing levels does not rule out a considerable hearing loss.

The Response and Its Interpretation. If one uses indirect instruments, three conditions are required in order to "see" the middle-ear muscle reflex:

1. The middle ear ossicles and tympanic membrane must be structurally normal; thus, *tympanometry will be normal.*
2. *The reflex arc must be intact.*
3. *The eliciting signal must be "loud" enough.*

The next section will discuss each of these prerequisites.

The normal middle ear by tympanometry. In order to establish that the middle ear is normal, tympanometry is a critical adjunct. Tympanometry is the measurement of transmission efficiency of a probe tone under varying air pressure. Current scholarly reviews on technique and instrumentation are available (Feldman, 1975; Jerger, 1975), as are programmed-instruction devices for the novice (Berlin, 1976). Depending on the type of measuring device used, whether a stiffness meter like the Madsen or American Electromedics (Berlin and Cullen, 1975), or an otoadmittance meter like the Grason-Stadler, tympanograms generated from normal ears will resemble each other. The most efficient probe-tone transmission point in the normal middle ear will occur when the ear is being studied under normal atmospheric pressure. Transmission efficiency should drop when the ear is being studied under either negative or positive pressure conditions. Pathological middle ears generally will show very little transmission if they are too stiff, or will show too much acceptance and dissipation of energy if they are too flaccid. Some ears will work exceptionally well when subjected to negative pressure, since the impressed external negative pressure essentially brings the ears into pressure equalization.

While there is some disagreement on the organization under which these tympanograms should be classified (see, for example, Feldman, 1975; Jerger, 1975; Seidemann, Byers, and Sisterhen, 1976), all workers agree that a normal tympanogram is a prerequisite to a reflex, and reflexes should then be visible (all other things being equal) with adequate stimulation. Sometimes, however, children have normal tympanograms but no recordable reflex. This paradox—not uncommon in Rubella babies—is often traceable to any one, or all, of these problems:

1. Otosclerosis or malleolar fixation
2. Other anomalies of the middle ear which can obscure the reflex (e.g., adhesions, congenital anomalies, or postsurgical ear changes that are not reflected in the tympanometry)
3. Congenital or acquired dysfunction of a portion of the reflex arc, including facial nerve palsy, brainstem dysgenesis, etc.
4. Deafness

Thus, the absence of the reflex in the presence of a normal tympanogram is not *always* a sign of deafness in the peripheral sense. Cases 3 and 4 discuss the danger of depending upon any single test, like middle-ear muscle reflexes, for this decision. There is, however, one important principle to restate: some people do not have any reflex even though they have normal hearing; the astute diagnostician will always try to elicit a reflex by nonacoustic means (for example, stroking the external ear canal or portions of the face; see Djupesland, 1975, Chap. 5).

The reflex arc must be intact. When an adequate stimulus is delivered to one ear, the normal child has equal and bilateral stapedius muscle reflexes. Borg (1973) has recently outlined the middle-ear muscle reflex pathways for both ipsilateral and contralateral activation. The cochlear nucleus in this arc projects to the ipsilateral and contralateral medial superior olives, but only to the *contralateral* medial nucleus of the trapezoid body for purposes of reflex activation of the VIIth nerve. This, then, is the structural basis for comparing ipsilateral to contralateral reflexes. If a child has normal contralateral reflexes, we expect and should see normal ipsilateral reflexes, providing the signals to each ear are "loud" enough. However, when the child has absent contralateral reflexes, but present ipsilateral reflexes, we can often implicate fourth ventrical structures related to the pathway from the cochlear nucleus to the contralateral trapezoid body. Case 4 at the end of the chapter may have such a problem.

The eliciting signal must be "loud" enough. It has become a matter of convenience to say that the signals used for acoustically eliciting the stapedius muscle reflex must be "loud enough" (for example, see Northern and Downs, 1974, p. 183). There is considerable evidence that the acoustic reflex is not a simple index of loudness, but may be related to density of neural discharge (e.g., Anderson and Barr, 1966; Ross, 1964; Margolis and Popelka, 1975; Scharf, 1976; Denenberg and Altshuler, 1976).

It has also been suggested that the degree of sensorineural hearing loss can be predicted by comparing the child's acoustic reflex threshold elicited by tones to his reflex thresholds elicited by wide-band noise (see Niemeyer and Sesterhenn, 1974; Jerger et al., 1974). The Jerger et al. application, called SPAR (Sensitivity Prediction from the Acoustic Reflex), depends on the principle that the intensity of a pure-tone necessary to elicit a middle-ear muscle reflex is at least 20dB greater than the intensity of *broad-band noise* needed to elicit the same reflex. If the reflexes elicited to tone and noise were to appear at almost the same levels, the child in question would be likely to have a sensorineural loss. Thus, according to Jerger et al., the first recommended step is to compare reflex thresholds for tone vs. noise stimuli.

The basis of SPAR's predictive ability in children is as follows: the loudness of a broad band of noise is made up of the sum of the loudnesses of each of the critical bands in that noise; the tone itself presumably is made up of only one critical band (by critical band here I mean a frequency range within which two simultaneous signals will interfere with each other's monaural audibility). Let us now imagine two separate signals—one a broad-band noise, the other a pure-tone, both capable of eliciting identical reflexes from a hypothetical child. If the intensity of the equally effective signals were measured, the noise would be about 20dB less intense overall than the tone; the "loudnesses" of the individual components in the broad-band noise are adding up (not interfering with one another) to equal the loudness of the narrow-band tone. Therefore, less *total* energy is registered on the sound-level meter. In contrast, in a patient with a sloping sensorineural loss, the high bands do not contribute to "loudness," and the critical bands are thought to widen (Jerger, 1975). Thus, *more* noise is necessary to elicit the reflex; however, if recruitment is taking place, the tone will elicit a reflex at the same levels as in a normal child (see Jerger et al., 1974). The convergence of these two principles then reduces the difference between the reflex threshold to noise and the reflex threshold to tones.

I recommend as a second screening step presenting high-intensity stimuli (100 to 110dB) quickly at 8000, 4000, 2000, 1000, and 500 Hz, respectively. This procedure is especially useful if only a brief period of testing is likely in a difficult-to-test child. The absence of the response at the high frequencies with its emergence at low frequencies is a powerful index of sloping sensorineural loss (see later, the same principle at work in the section on Electrodermal Response Audiometry entitled Unconditioned Response Audiometry).

The major limitation in the interpretation and use of middle-ear muscle reflexes occurs in the presence of an abnormal tympanogram. Patients with sensorineural losses are not immune to middle-ear disease and sometimes middle-ear disease can coexist with pre-existing sensorineural hearing loss or mixed hearing losses on either or both sides. On other occasions, patients may have damaged ears as a result of trauma, and neither tympanometry nor reflexes can be adequately measured (see Case 5 of a comatose child with traumatic injury to the external and middle ears; the surgeon wanted to know whether the damaged ear was still functioning before performing surgery). Jerger and Hayes (1976) cite an appropriate case in which a pathological tympanogram in one ear, accompanying a perforation in the other, obscured the nature of the sensorineural hearing loss in a 2-year-9-month-old boy.

Special Problems with Infants. Mesenchyme, an embryonic tissue which helps to give rise to connective tissue, is often an obstruction in neonatal ears. The material can cause hearing loss, obstruct tympanometry, and, of course, obstruct recording of middle-ear muscle reflexes. Hence, impedance audiometry in neonates may present some inherent difficulties, but it has been pursued with a modicum of success (see Robertson, Peterson, and Lamb, 1968; Keith, 1973; Jerger et al., 1974; also see earlier section re BSER).

Whether a child is anesthetized, sedated, or struggling, it is often difficult to place the stimulating earphone properly over his ear-canal opening. Artificially collapsed canals or misplaced earphones are not uncommon. Whenever we fail to find a reflex in a child, we try again after rechecking the earphone and placement and, if necessary, we hold the phone slightly away from the child's ear.

In addition, since the reflex can be elicited and/or obscured by vocalization, crying children are difficult to assess. Sedation does not interfere with reflexes, but some barbiturates might; my experience with Ketamine-anesthetized children indicates the reflex is unaffected either by that drug or by halothane or penthrane. However, if a child indulges in prolonged crying, the peak efficiency of its ear may appear at *positive* pressures in contrast to the more common negative pressure peak. It is for this reason we try to complete both tympanometry and reflexes before anesthesia. A positive-peaked tympanogram would have the same obstructive effect on the reflex as a negative pressure peak and is usually resolved by a yawn or swallow. In such cases, trans-tympanic penetration for ECochG often produces an audible "pop" in the operating room.

In summary, middle-ear muscle reflexes are extremely powerful physiological indices of audition, but must be interpreted with caution, since they are mediated responses. The presence of the response is mediated via the VIIth and VIIIth nerves and portions of the brainstem whose damage does not necessarily generate reports of audiometric difficulties. The responses, of course, can be obscured by middle-ear pathology which, in itself, need not necessarily impair hearing severely.

Electrodermal Response Audiometry (EDR)

Introductory Comment re "Conditioned" vs. "Unconditioned" EDR. Bordley, Hardy, and Richter (1958) were among the first to suggest that the so-called galvanic skin response (GSR; for our purposes the same as EDR) could be used as a mediated index of "hearing." In my experience using the technique with humans as well as animals (Berlin, 1963; Berlin, Gill, and Leffler, 1968; Gill and Berlin, 1968), I found it useful to keep two major points clearly in mind. The change in skin conductance which is the characteristic precursor of *the EDR can be elicited by virtually any supra-threshold auditory or non-auditory stimulus with or without conditioning.* By "conditioning" I mean the very strict pairing of tone with shock events, and the use of a criterion for conditioning before an actual search for audiometric threshold begins. In 1959, I was first introduced to the power and efficiency of conditioned EDR by two rigorous, precise, and demanding colleagues, Drs. Joseph Chaiklin and Ira Ventry. It is appropriate, therefore, that I quote from Ventry (1975, p. 220) regarding the use of EDR, or GSR, as we all called it then:

The adequate definition of a response [to an audiometric stimulus] is at the heart of successful GSR audiometry. In all likelihood, failure to use appropriate criteria for response definition has led to more errors in GSR audiometry than any other single procedural factor.

Unless strict and rigorous criteria are adopted for rejecting spurious "responses," and unless rigorous criteria for both conditioning and threshold determination are set in advance, it is easy to mistakenly conclude that an acoustic stimulus was "heard" because 1.5 to 3.5 seconds after the stimulus was given, an EDR appeared on the stripchart recorder (Michels and Randt, 1947). Case 6, for example, may have been called "normal" in part because of this error in procedure.

Procedure

Conditioned response audiometry. Target and companion electrodes are attached to the child's meticulously cleaned fingertips on the nonpreferred hand, with a ground on either the arm or leg. Equipment arrays usually impress a small voltage between the electrodes, and any change in skin resistance is monitored as a change in current flow in the circuitry of the galvanometer. Shock electrodes are usually strapped to the other hand or some other available extremity, and the intensity of the shock is set to a level of discomfort, admittedly difficult to establish in the hard-to-test, typically nonverbal child. A 40% reinforcement schedule (two-fifths of the audible tone events are paired with a shock 0.5 seconds after the tone onset) is recommended. Unconditioned EDR levels might be used as a guide for estimating whether a given tone were audible, and hence suitable as a "conditioned stimulus," but even Ventry (1975) has suggested that this elaborate procedure is not really suitable for the young, difficult-to-test child.

Unconditioned response audiometry. Few authors would suggest the use of *unconditioned* GSR audiometry as an index of auditory sensitivity. However, some of my research in animals (Berlin, Gill, and Leffler, 1968; Gill and Berlin, 1968) had led me to believe that the amplitude of the unconditioned GSR might be proportional to the density of neural fibers available in response to a given sine wave (Finck and Berlin, 1965).

An unconditioned stimulus, by definition, is a stimulus that is capable of eliciting a response (like EDR) without being paired with any other stimulus. By contrast, a conditioned stimulus is defined as a stimulus that, by itself, is incapable of eliciting an EDR but which, after skillful pairing with the unconditioned stiumulus, ultimately becomes capable of eliciting the EDR. The problem with this description of the EDR in relation to testing with tones is clear to the careful reader; *intense* tones which are also *loud* can elicit EDR's *without* any previous pairing with shock. Using this principle, unconditioned EDR might help screen for some correlate of loudness without the use of noxious shock. Here shock electrodes are not necessary, nor are earphones, unless some form of ear specificity is desired.

Signals along a presumed equal-loudness contour (100dB SPL) are administered from a descending sequence starting at 8000 Hz and going down to 250 Hz at 30-second intervals. In normal subjects, this equal-loudness contour would elicit roughly equal-sized EDRs were it not for response habituation. By response habituation I mean the reduction of the size, and occasionally temporary disappearance, of the EDR due to repeated unreinforced administrations of the tone. Thus, in the normal subject, the first tone elicits the largest response; the others elicit successively smaller EDRs. The effectiveness of this screening technique comes through if one considers a subject who has essentially normal low-frequency hearing, but absent high-frequency hearing; in this case, there will be *no* unconditioned response to the first tones, starting at 800 Hz. Only where the tones fall into the 1000-Hz range and below will an unconditioned EDR appear. The screening procedure is biased so that at the end of a run the normal subject should give the smallest response. Thus, one might uncover patients with sharp slopes to their audiograms because the first three stimuli in the series would be inaudible and the *last* three stimuli would elicit the largest responses.

I completed this study in the hopes of showing that in normal subjects one might get a rough estimate of loudness by measuring the magnitude of unconditioned EDR to tones along an equal-loudness contour (Berlin et al., 1968). In the mid-60s, this technique was useful with difficult-to-test children, but for me, it has been superseded by the widespread availability of middle-ear muscle reflex technology, EcochG, BSER, etc. However, the technique was reviewed here for those readers who still have EDR equipment available to them and would like to apply it to the study of children with external ear canal atresias, for example, who cannot be tested with ECochG or impedance audiometry.

Response Interpretation and Limitations. Conditioned EDR is especially difficult in children because:

1. Some people do not have an EDR because of absence of sweat glands in the skin;
2. The reflex arc for the drop in skin resistance is not completely understood and may be obliterated by brainstem or spinal injuries;
3. Virtually any event affecting the subject (a light flash, a breeze, a sneeze, a cough, a movement, or a deep breath, to name a few) can elicit an EDR;
4. Conditioning is complicated and lengthy, requiring both the subject's cooperation and the examiner's insight into the subject's pretest hearing.

There is no question that the unconditioned EDR is suitable only as a screening procedure for high-tone hearing loss, as a useful adjunct to middle-ear muscle reflexes, and for other physiologic tests; it is not a threshold level assessing device.

Therefore, with the exception of the use of the unconditioned EDR as a screening tool for high-frequency loss, we concur with Ventry (1975) when he says:

> The outlook is bleak for the use of EDA with difficult-to-test children, at least in its traditional form, modeled after classical conditioning procedures. The noxious shock, the long test sessions, the conditioning procedures, and so on, all mitigate, in my opinion, against the widespread use of EDA with children (p. 245).

In adults or cooperative children who can tolerate the earphones, the unconditioned stimulus (the shock), and the protracted time necessary to avoid habituation and acquire criterion responses, EDR is still an excellent technique for assessing audiometric thresholds. Unconditioned EDR screening may have some limited application in children with bilateral atresias or other anomalies which prevent the use of ECochG or impedance audiometry.

EDRs have been collected on thousands of children from the late 1950s to the present, and I stressed EDRs here more because of my experience with the technique than because of any important future applications. An astute but anonymous critic of this work concluded that:

> There is no reason to generate great optimism for EDR or middle, late, and CNV responses for the assessment of difficult-to-test children. Of the two, however, the electroencephalic responses offer more.

I must concur. The next section shows why.

Middle- and Late-Evoked Potentials

Problems in Terminology. Until 1971, most workers called the responses occurring from 10 to 50 milliseconds after stimulation the "early responses." The development of the BSER response discussed earlier necessitated a change of terminology, and responses from 10 to 50 milliseconds are now called "middle responses" (see, for example, McRandle, Smith, and Goldstein, 1974; Goldstein and McRandle, 1976).

The responses to be described also have various characteristic waveforms: some have dominant high frequencies, others dominant low frequencies. The literature has traditionally called the high-frequency responses "fast responses" and the low-frequency responses "slow responses." It is an unfortunate coincidence from a semantic point of view that *early* responses are also called "fast responses" and *late* responses are also called "slow responses." It is relatively easy for the superficial reader to confuse the intent of the labels *early* and *fast* vs. *late* and *slow*. Fast and slow refer to frequency content of the waveform; early and late refer to latency after stimulation.

Middle Responses (10 to 50 Millisecond Latencies).

Procedure. The EEG activity is usually recorded from an electrode placed on the vertex (the target), a reference electrode (the companion) on the mastoid, and a ground on the forehead. Stimuli are clicks or tone bursts similar to those used in ECochG and BSER. However, in this case the EEG activity that is analyzed is high-pass filtered above 150 to 200 Hz and below 20 Hz. Usually 500 or so clicks are used and rates of 5 to 9 per second have been used with no apparent effect of stimulus repetition rate within this range.

The response itself is minimally affected by natural sleep. Fig. 4-9 shows a recording of this response from my own vertex elicited at about 60dB HL with clicks repeated at a rate of 5 per second. In this recording, positive is upward; the response occurred at about 25 milliseconds from stimulation. This particular response is difficult to separate from a so-called myogenic, or sonomotor, response (Bickford, Jacobson, and Cody, 1964). Thornton, (1975b), has even attempted to use the sonomotor response, or as he called it, the post-auricular muscle response, as an audiometric tool. Here we see the attractiveness of a physiologic index of "hearing" so great that researchers are willing to use a mediated response as labile as muscle tension to predict hearing losses.

Mendel, Adkinson, and Harker (1977) studied these components in infants. The study was designed to include 18 subjects, but they had to test 50 infants to acquire these 18. Of the 50 subjects, 9 were excluded for failure to sleep the required 40 minutes, 3 were excluded because of equipment failure or experimenter error, and 15 were excluded for failure to meet predetermined health

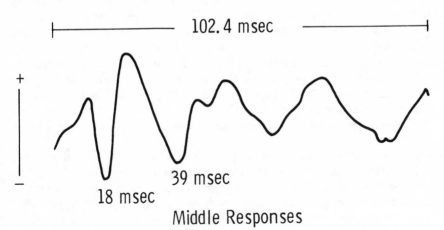

Fig. 4-9. Sample Middle Response

criteria. The balance were discarded for a number of other reasons to achieve a design that studied 6 children at each of the following ages: 1 month, 4 months, and 8 months, plus or minus 2 weeks.

Using a system whose total gain was 4×10^5, and filters band-passed from 25 to 175 Hz, 400 samples of EEG activity were taken. They presented 1000-Hz tone bursts in the open field at levels of 15, 30, 45, and 60dB re normal adult tone burst threshold, and reported that judges agreed that virtually all of the infants showed a response at 60dB HL. The latencies of the major peaks occurred at approximately 16, 26, and 39 milliseconds, respectively, after stimulus onset. Therefore, the authors quite correctly conclude that the middle components of the auditory-evoked potential offer promise as a diagnostic tool. However, this tool must be used with caution until reliability and validity data can be acquired near threshold.

In trans-tympanic ECochG the failure to get adequate recordings is virtually nil. Diagnosticians have control over the subject by virtue of general anesthesia and, if equipment is adequately maintained, the presence or absence of a response is a firm and reliable observation. The state of the subject's skin, brain tissue, muscle activity, etc. are not serious obstacles. In contrast, Mendel, Pals, and Harker (1976) show that in 10 of 108 cases they were unable to have the subjects acquire successful sleep. In reviewing 73 patients, they found 21 patients in whom threshold levels could not be determined. Technically, poor recordings were blamed in 3 cases, abnormal EEG blamed in 3 more cases, and no response was identified in 12 cases. In 2 patients, 1 of whom was autistic and the other severely retarded, the middle components seemed to exaggerate the amount of hearing impairment when compared to subsequent behavioral testing. In order to overcome the effects of abnormal EEG on the middle components, Mendel, Pals, and Harker (1976) have begun to record BSER responses along with the middle component information. They feel this combination offers a powerful approach for testing patients who are difficult to assess in a voluntary audiometric mode. Here again, the utility of BSER and ECochG as validating procedures is critical. Starr (1976), for example, has recently shown that, in patients with complete brain death, the whole nerve action potential (ECochG) is still functioning while the rest of the EEG is iso-potential. The importance of having some information on the VIIIth nerve action potential, therefore, is inescapable if one wishes to determine the incidence of a peripheral hearing loss.

Middle vs. Late Components. This response and the subsequent evoked responses to be discussed probably have a number of major drawbacks with their respective application in children. The response itself can be either obscured or distorted by random muscle activity, poor common mode rejection, poor electrode contact, and related conditions that abound when one tries to test young or severely handicapped children. The middle components may permit some audiometric assessment (Davis, 1976; Mendel, Pals, and Harker, 1976; Mendel,

Adkinson, and Harker, 1977), but the test-retest reliability is still unclear (Skinner, 1977). Mendel et al. (1975) compared the middle to the late components in adult auditory evoked potentials during sleep. The research was done independently in two laboratories and both groups agreed as follows: the middle responses were basically unaffected by sleep, and a single set of voltage and magnitude criteria could be used for all stages of waking and sleeping. However, the late responses were affected by sleep and required different criteria for judging their appearance at various sleep stages. During deep sleep, clearly positive responses were often not attained at levels 30dB above the patient's voluntary thresholds and, therefore, they concluded that threshold was indeterminate. During light sleep and while awake, middle responses usually gave thresholds somewhat more sensitive than the late responses by 10 to 15dB, and also gave fewer trials whose results could not be interpreted.

The authors suggested the middle responses might be used for audiometric purposes even though 1 of their 28 normal subjects failed to yield any identifiable middle response. It is fair to say that any physiological evaluation of the subject in a test situation in which almost 4% of normal subjects might fail to generate a response is potentially dangerous when applied to young infants and otherwise difficult-to-test children. However, it would be premature and unfair to dismiss middle- and late-evoked potential responses as basically unimportant because they are mediated responses and not directly applicable to problems of audiometry. As we will see later, the so-called late responses can give very powerful insights into the ability of a listener to discriminate important features of the signal; in addition, McRandle, Smith, and Goldstein (1974) report that preliminary testing on high-risk children with the middle responses yielded deviant patterns in at least one of three children. Thus, like FFR, the response pattern itself may be used to tell us something about the integrity of the central auditory nervous system.

Late, Slow Cortical Responses (50 to 300 Millisecond Latencies)

Procedure. The same electrode configuration as for middle responses is used. These responses require amplification of about 10^4 or 10^5, but a bandpass in the preamplifiers not much higher than 15 Hz. The signals can be either tones or speech, and are best given at rates not exceeding 1 to 2 per sec. In contrast to ECochG and BSER, late responses *are* subject to drugs and sleep and cannot be reliably averaged. Let me clarify that statement with an example. As you recall in the earlier section on digital averaging, we mentioned that any event that occurs in a time-locked relationship to the onset of the computer sweep will be added linearly. If a sleep stage or drug stage shifts the onsets of discharges of neural groups, then it is conceivable that discernible peaks will be obliterated with prolonged averaging as the latency of characteristic peaks shifts. Since the responses are highly unreliable when the subject is asleep—and therefore of dubious value audiometrically—the literature is replete with attempts to relate the slow potentials (sometimes called "V" potentials or vertex potentials) with loudness, auditory-discrimination ability, cross-modality stimulation, maturation, and utility for audiometry (e.g., Goldstein and Kendall, 1963; Price and Goldstein, 1966; Davis et al., 1967; Davis, Bowers, and Hirsh, 1968; Onishi and Davis, 1968; Davis and Onishi, 1969; Gjerdingen and Tomsic, 1970; Hay and Davis, 1971; Hirsh, 1971; Davis, 1973, 1974; Osterhammel et al., 1973; Davis, et. al., 1975). However, using the slow responses, Russ and Simmons (1974) concluded, after subjecting the obtained responses to three independent readers, that electric response audiometry (ERA) using these potentials was not a reliable tool and should be considered as only part of diagnostic audiometry; they recommended avoiding clinical judgments made solely on the basis of ERA.

The Contingent Negative Variation (CNV)

Procedure. If a subject receives a warning signal and understands that a subsequent target is to follow, the expectation of the target generates a slow, direct current (dc) shift of the baseline of the EEG about 300 or so milliseconds after the warning signal is received.

In order to record the CNV, the preamplifiers must be able to pass the dc potentials and, of course, if this activity is to be recorded on tape, an FM unit is imperative. The CNV can be recorded from any place on the skull and, therefore, can be acquired as part of any other surface recording. The technique requires adequate bandpass in the preamplifiers and sufficient amplification.

While the CNV presently has had little application in audiometry, it has some intriguing possibilities. A stimulus of light could be given, let us say, as a warning for an upcoming tone or speech stimulus. The light itself could elicit a response that makes a stable baseline for evoked potential measurement, presuming we do not have a blind child. Subsequent to the warning light flash, either tone burst or speech can be presented, and the infant may associate a light with the auditory signal and present a CNV. On the other hand, if the auditory signal is not perceived, no CNV will be seen. Potential further refinements, for example, could include the presentation of a light or tone as a warning signal for various classes of speech events. If adequate paradigms can be developed, it may be possible to use a CNV to get insight into children's ability to discriminate speech sounds, male or female voices, environmental noises, etc.

Cardiotachometry and Respiration Audiometry

Eisenberg (1975) and Bradford (1975) have covered these two emerging techniques in much more detail and depth than this chapter permits. However, I should not like to imply criticism by virtue of allocating only limited space to these techniques. Like CNV, both have intriguing possibilities of shedding light on higher-level processing of speech and related stimuli.

Cardiotachometry. In this procedure either the absolute rate, the change in rate, or the interval between heart beats is studied as an index of audition. Schulman (1973), using an index of *change* in heart rate rather than a count of beats per minute, concluded that the level of stimulation required to elicit a response was too variable to allow use of cardiotachometry with neonates, but it may be useful by 6 weeks of age. Eisenberg (1975) used heart-rate interval analysis to determine whether or not response to auditory stimulation had taken place. She found a characteristic deceleration of heart rate with *speech* but not with non-speech stimuli.

She candidly states:

There is little reason to suppose that heart rate measures can be refined for clinical use within the immediate future . . . [she goes on to say few of the current physiologic tests are amenable to the disclosure of central problems and adds that evoked potential audiometry is . . .] . . . extremely expensive and fraught with special difficulties relative to movement artifacts, changing maturational patterns, and effects of arousal level. By comparison, then, cardiotachometry has some specific advantages. It has been found to yield valid data on newborns, infants and even such difficult-to-test subjects as autistic teenagers. It is relatively inexpensive as compared with such alternatives as evoked cortical response audiometry. It is almost totally free of movement artifact and, consequently, well suited to telemetric procedures. It is past the stage of purely preliminary exploration (p. 343). [I should like to add that because of the apparent sensitivity of the response to speech and speech-like stimuli, it should gain some important applications in the audiologists' armamentarium.]

Respiration Audiometry. Bradford (1975, Chap. 8), has recently presented some superficially convincing arguments about the utility of respiration audiometry. Using methods developed by Rousey, Snyder, and Rousey (1964), he outlined three basic signs of a respiratory response to tonal stimulation:

1. A reduction in the amplitude of the excursion of the response;
2. What he called the jamming or M-shaped pattern;
3. The flattening of the response cycle.

Fig. 4-10 is redrawn from his presentation. He states that a reduction of amplitude occurs most frequently with presentation of pure-tone stimuli. I could not find any descriptions of "control events," pictures, or counts of the number of times in which the so-called responses to tones occurred during silent intervals.

The cases Bradford presents are primarily psychiatric in nature and he himself recognizes that unless a child is quiet and relatively placid, the technique is of limited value for audiometric purposes. In his case reports, other physiological corroborative tests such as ECochG, tympanometry, and middle-ear muscle reflexes were not available (see Case 6). He appeared to make major decisions

A   "M"
Response

B   Flattening
Response

C   Reduction in
Amplitude

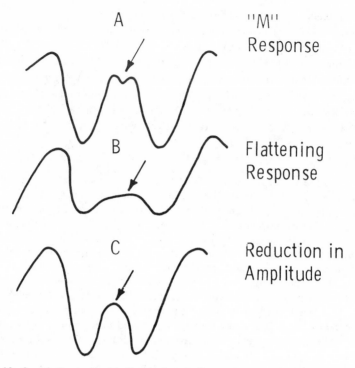

Fig. 4-10. Sample Traces Used in Respiration Audiometry

based primarily on respiration audiometry, and subsequently "confirmed" some of them himself by voluntary audiometry (Bradford, 1976[8]). The voluntary results acquired from a subject could have been biased by staff members' investment in the so-called true results obtained by respiration audiometry.

The absence of published control events, independent reader studies of the records, and such makes it difficult to evaluate the technique. But because of its benign, noninvasive, and inexpensive character, it would be premature to dismiss respiration audiometry at this stage. There is not enough information on its failure rate to be definitive about any conclusion.

SUMMARY

ECochG, BSER, tympanometry, and middle-ear muscle reflexes constitute the most definitive battery in my armamentarium for assessing the physiological function of a child's auditory system. The cases to follow show some of our group's experience applying the techniques.

[8] Personal communication with Dr. L.J Bradford, 1976.

ILLUSTRATIVE CASES—THE CROSS-CHECK PRINCIPLE IN ACTION

We have been able to make accurate predictions about auditory behavior in difficult-to-test children by combining our ECochGic procedures with tympanometry, middle-ear muscle reflexes, and BSER. In a follow-up study of almost 50 children seen for extra-tympanic ECochG, we have found *none* whose subsequently recordable hearing measurements are inconsistent with the ECochGram-tympanometry-reflex-BSER combination. The cross-check of recordable hearing measurements with tympanometry and reflexes gave us some low-frequency-specific information which complemented the high-frequency-biased information of the ECochGram (Cullen et al., 1976). Up to this point we have not found it necessary to use FFR, EDR, middle or late ERA, cardio-tachometry, or respiration audiometry on any of the 295 subjects currently in our "hard-to-test" pediatric patient pool.

Case 1

Normal ECochG, tympanometry, reflexes, and BSER in a child who gave inconsistent results to behavioral tests

Three-year-old Lavonne had been alternately diagnosed as "deaf," "hard-of-hearing," and "retarded." She was reportedly difficult to test and inconsistent in her responses. Trans-tympanic ECochG to clicks showed normal responses down to 9 and 19dB HLs in both ears. Middle-ear measurements indicated normal tympanometry, and contralateral stapedial reflexes were present at normal levels. BSER also showed normal latencies and responses of the fifth wave. Voluntary screening audiometry was subsequently obtained by an outside source; the child showed consistent responses at 25dB HL from 500 to 4000 Hz, bilaterally.

Lavonne was an ideal patient for ECochGic recording; because of the inconsistency and disagreement coming from various evaluative agencies, her parents were confused and she was not being treated. The physiological findings permitted rapid and rational rehabilitative measures.

Case 2

A "deaf-appearing" child with normal reflexes, normal ECochG, but abnormal visual and auditory late responses (Using late-evoked potentials alone might have labeled this child "hard-of-hearing.")

Robin, a 4-year-old girl, stopped talking after a high fever at 1 year of age, was not developing speech and language, and failed to respond to any overt environmental stimuli. She had been consistently evaluated as being behaviorally deaf in three separate clinics. She was brought to us for ECochG, which, at the time, we were performing only extratympanically. We found repeatable ECochGic responses all the way down to about 10dB HL in both ears. Tympanometry and reflexes were all within normal limits. We were not aware of the BSER procedure at the time and referred her elsewhere for middle- and late-evoked potentials. These findings showed abnormal, late responses to both visual and auditory stimuli. As part of our follow-up procedure, we were fortunate to have another independent audiologic clinic evaluate this child for what may be called unbiased audiologic assessment. In August 1976, Robin passed pure-tone air-conduction screening at 20dB HL, but still had no speech. Neuropsychological evaluation showed dull-normal intellectual function with mild left hemiparesis.

Case 3

An "autistic" child where absent reflexes were misleading

Rhonda, age 4½, had been diagnosed as retarded and autistic when she was 18 months old. Two years after the diagnosis, she was studied by another agency with sound-field observation (no responses), tympanometry, and reflexes; trans-cranial reflexes were absent when the right ear was stimulated. She would not cooperate further, and testing from the other ear was not completed. This led the diagnosticians to rightfully question how much auditory function the child might have, especially since both ears showed normal tympanometry.

When we performed middle-measurements we found Type A tympanograms bilaterally and *absent stapedial reflexes bilaterally to both contralateral and ipsilateral stimulation.* This usually is a harbinger of severe sensorineural deafness. However, trans-tympanic ECochG revealed consistent, repeatable responses on the left side down to 26dB HL but no response in the right ear. BSERs were obtained and showed abnormally long latencies of the fifth wave. Our report read as follows:

"Rhonda appears to have a severe-to-profound sensorineural hearing loss in her right ear. Peripherally, the left ear appears to have adequate reserve for communicative purposes. However, the absence of stapedial reflexes upon left-ear stimulation reflects possible central involvement."

It is clearly unusual to have a normal ECochGram and absent ipsilateral reflexes at 1000 and 2000 Hz. The possible explanations include a reflex-testing artifact, mild conductive loss, a brainstem lesion, and/or a severe high-frequency loss in the left ear; this latter observation is not consistent with ECochGic results. Reflexes were checked three times on Rhonda (they were present to nonacoustic stimuli), and the machine was used to elicit my own normal reflexes. Basically, then, we conclude, *by exclusion,* that in addition to her other problems, Rhonda probably has:

1. An inoperative right ear;
2. A left ear that, while it may not be entirely normal, has enough sensitivity to permit speech and language development;
3. Brainstream involvement in addition to (or possibly as a cause of) her autistic behavior.

Case 4

Tympanometry and trans-cranial reflexes alone suggest deafness; ECochG and BSER suggest a central anomaly

Cecilia, age 2, was referred to us for failure to develop verbal language. Her mother reported that pregnancy was full-term and uncomplicated with no natal or neonatal problems. Aside from lack of speech, developmental milestones appeared normal. The child seemed to have normal vision, was easily disciplined, and was cared for by the maternal grandparents in the mother's absence. At age 2 she showed a Vineland Social Maturity Scale social age equivalent near the 1½-year level. Type A tympanometry was seen with *no* trans-cranial reflex to acoustic stimuli; reflexes were present to nonacoustic stimuli. Ipsilateral reflexes were not available to us at the time. Because of these findings, she had received a hearing aid from another agency and balked at its use.

Extra-tympanic ECochG by air conduction revealed responses in both ears down to 20dB HL for the clicks used. Bone-conduction ECochG showed normal bone-conduction responses in both ears, and BSERs were then taken on this child by moving the extra-tympanic electrode from the ear canal under the scalp at the vertex. Figure 4-11 shows Cecilia's ECochGic and BSER responses. There was an aberrant BSER dyssynchrony at approximately 5 milliseconds, which was repeated consistently throughout the test procedure and which suggests some form of interruption to the central auditory pathways. Note the absence of a synchronous wave immediately after N_2, but two consistent waves about 2.5 milliseconds after the hiatus. Would the hearing aid, if she had been forced to use it, have given her peripheral loss as well? (See Case 6.)

---

10. 24 msec

Ecoch G

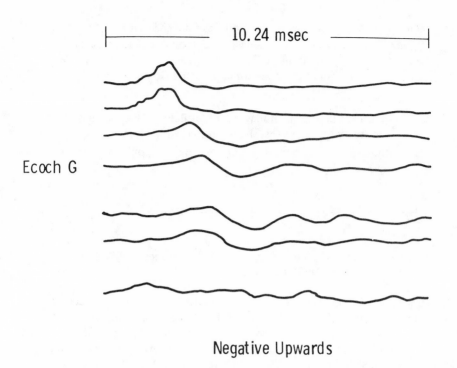

Negative Upwards

BSER

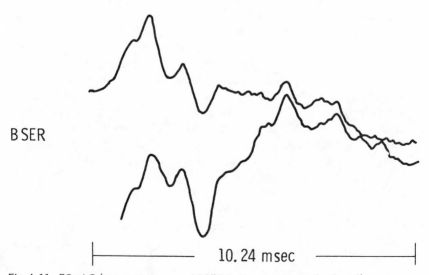

10. 24 msec

Fig. 4-11. ECochG (top seven traces and BSER bottom two traces for Case 4)

Case 5

An operating room emergency with no chance for other tests

Quintril, a 2-year-old boy, had a repeated history of self-inflicted injuries to his left ear. On the occasion of this test, the resident on duty called me late one evening saying he had an emergency procedure on a little boy. It seemed Quintril had reinjured the ear, which was now leaking perilymph. The resident surgeon was preparing to close the leak and, because the injury had destroyed some of the ossicular chain, he wished to know whether reconstruction of the ossicular chain should be attempted for hearing-conservation purposes. The critical issue was, did this boy have any residual auditory function in that ear? ECochG was done through the traumatically induced opening in the boy's canal; excellent responses were recorded from the ear despite the perilymphatic leak. The surgeon repaired both the leak and the middle-ear injury. When I first saw the boy, he was already in the operating room and under anesthesia; this is one of the few cases in which ECochG was the only procedure done. Some months post-operatively, other tests showed the validity of the ECochGic observations.

Case 6

My most unusual case, in which the limitations of ECochG, tympanometry, reflexes, and other procedures are highlighted

Harriet was 22 years old when I first saw her. I am including her in the review of pertinent cases to show what would have happened if I had seen her as an infant and had relied upon tympanometry, reflexes, and ECochG for my predictions regarding her management. For reasons which will become clear later, tympanometry, reflexes, and ECochG would have indicated that she was severely deaf. As the case unfolds you will see how and why this was only a restricted and basically fragmentary conclusion.

Harriet had been brought to audiologists and otolaryngologists around age 4 when she was diagnosed as being severely hard-of-hearing and/or deaf. However, in subsequent test procedures, she manifested some unusual behavior that prompted astute diagnosticians to alter their initial impressions. Among the most unusual was her ability to respond to speech, behind her back in the open field, at hearing levels as low as 30dB. Note, please, that the speech was presented without earphones. Under earphones she generally failed to respond until about 50 or 60dB HL, but even that was grossly inconsistent with her voluntary pure-tone averages around 90 to 100dB HL. In addition, she showed a *deaf* voice, but *very precise and meticulous high-frequency articulation* and *excellent timing in her connected speech.* Finally, by age 12, because of repeated speech detection thresholds at around 30 to 40dB in spite of her insistence that she heard virtually no pure-tones in the speech frequency range, Harriet was diagnosed as having a "hysterical hearing loss." She was treated for ten years by psychologists and psychiatrists and in that time the only physiologic test that was done was GSR audiometry, which showed her to have "normal hearing"; no discussion was made of the criteria by which the so-called normal responses were obtained.

When I saw Harriet for her first evaluation I did a speech-detection threshold under earphones and in open fields. Under earphones, she acquired a speech-detection threshold close to 40dB HL, and in the open field, with a sound level meter held close to her ear to measure the level at which my voice reached her ear, she responded by detecting my speech accurately at about the sound pressure equivalent of 35dB HL. However, *despite normal tympanometry, and reflexes present to nonacoustic stimuli, she showed no reflexes to any of the tones presented. Extra-tympanic ECochG revealed hair-cell responses but no synchronous compound action potential.*

I was stunned at these results because I, too, had first suspected she had much better hearing than she volunteered. However, the physiological tests corroborated clearly that, in the ranges under test, she had little residual auditory function. I asked Harriet, "What did you hear during the electrocochleographic tests?" (See Simmons and Dixon, 1964, on the importance of asking the patient "What do you hear?") She told me she *heard the clicks* during the ECochGram, but they were very far away and *very high-pitched.* I asked her if she would submit to trans-tympanic ECochG, but she would not, so I decided to test her hearing above 8000 Hz. Using an ultrasonic system improvised from laboratory equipment, I found her hearing to be approximately 55dB SPL at 10000 Hz and slightly better at 14000 Hz.

Her high-frequency hearing was the apparent source of her excellent sibilant articulation, her ability to detect speech in the open field at such low levels (she was responding to the articulatory hiss and burst), and her ability to follow the time-code of speech. With this type of hearing loss, she would not have been able to use the telephone, and certainly would have been hurt by a hearing aid because of its obstructive nature with respect to her limited high-frequency residual hearing. Among the so-called signs of hysterical hearing loss were her refusal to use the telephone and her insistence that hearing aids did her no good, despite her ability to detect speech in the open field at such low levels.

This unusual case has been cited in a preliminary report (Cullen et al., 1976), and she and I and her referring audiologist, Bob Findlay, will be preparing a more complete report in the near future.

In Harriet's case, I am certain that her fine speech and timing are traceable directly to her excellent high-frequency hearing, all of which would have been missed for failure to include high-frequency tone bursts or high-frequency click spectrum in our stimuli. *Does a profoundly deaf oral child with excellent speech have the occult advantage of ultra-audiometric high-frequency hearing?* Certainly if good "deaf" speakers have that advantage, we should know about it; James Jerger, Sharon Smith, Kathy Wexler, and I have already found three such patients during a two-day visit to an oral deaf school in Houston.

The question still remains: Had I seen Harriet when she was a year old, how would I have interpreted the results of her test? Sad to say, I would have recommended to her parents that she get a hearing aid and be treated as a severely to profoundly deaf child. Here, I would have made an invalid assumption that the click in ECochG was broad enough to cut into the ultra-audiometric range. Tympanometry and reflexes would have supported the ECochGic results, but they, too, were limited in frequency. It was fortunate, then, for Harriet that she was misdiagnosed as having a hysterical hearing loss. The end result of such a fortuitous misdiagnosis was to deny her a hearing aid, which would have, in fact, obstructed her already minimal high-frequency acuity and *probably destroyed it by acoustic trauma.* She was forced to function in a primarily oral environment that precisely suited her most bizarre and unusual hearing loss.

RESEARCH NEEDS

We have reviewed the principles of electrophysiological assessment in pediatric audiology. The combination of impedance audiometry, ECochG, BSER, case history, and clinical observation have proven to be a most powerful mixture. However, even with that battery available to us, the last case presented shows how easily we can make a serious error.

Thus, there is probably no substitute for being able to ask a child directly, "What do you hear?" Until we get an electrophysiological tool that can ask that question and generate an unequivocal answer, there is more work to be done in electrophysiological indices of audition.

GLOSSARY

companion electrode (see also target electrode.) *"Target" and "companion" electrodes* are the notations I use for so-called "hot" and "indifferent" electrodes in a common mode rejection system. The target (hot) electrode should be placed as close to the source as possible; the companion (indifferent) electrode is best placed nearby in tissue with similar resistive properties. Their purpose is to bring a [(signal + noise) – noise] condition to the common mode rejection portion of the preamplifier so that the algebraic difference (signal alone) can be passed through.

contingent negative variations (CNV)   A slow dc shift in the EEG seen 300 milliseconds or so after a warning signal is presented. The CNV usually implies some conscious awareness on the part of the subject that a signal is approaching or that some appropriate event is about to take place.

FM recorders   FM means *frequency modulated.* The FM recorder changes the frequency of a carrier, let us say 1 million Hz, proportional to the frequency of the recorded signal; thus, if one were recording a 200-Hz tone, it would be recorded mixed with the 1 million Hz carrier which would then generate *a sum and difference signal* of 1 million *plus 200* and 1 million *minus 200* Hz. The carrier would then be filtered or cancelled out, leaving only the remaining 200 Hz as a residual.

induction artifacts   These occur when the electrical activity of the stimulating transducer cuts across the electrodes and electromagnetically induces a current in the target electrodes and can be mistaken for a response.

latency   is elapsed time between arrival of the stimulus and response.

preamplifier   In this case a sensitive, generally small, device that strengthens weak biological signals to levels suitable for processing by either other amplifiers or recorders.

pure-tone and time-frequency uncertainty   Whenever a signal is gated on abruptly it is likely to have sidebands containing many other frequencies. Any stimulus that is activated abruptly is subject to this fundamental law; thus, small noise-makers, which have clappers or strikers attached to them, used in many audiology clinics are likely to give spectral splash in addition to the dominant frequency content which the audiologist hoped for as the intended stimulus. The shorter the rise time, the broader the frequency splash is likely to be until one reaches the limits of resonation of a given transducer. Once these limits of resonation are reached, no matter how much briefer the stimulus, the resonator still produces the same spectrum. Thus, in our ECochG system, a 100-microsecond transient will generate a resonant peak in a TDH-39 earphone at around 4000 Hz, but so will a 50-microsecond transient.

rise time   The time from the start of the stimulus to the point at which it reaches 75% of its maximum height (see also *pure-tone and time-frequency uncertainty*).

RMS Stands for "root-mean-square," which essentially means taking the peak-to-peak voltage of any signal and dividing it by the square root of two.

single-ended amplification This is used, in contrast to the common mode rejection amplifiers or differential amplifiers, to signify simple addition without any cancellation or subtraction.

signal-to-noise ratio Whenever a signal must be identified, it is rarely isolated and clearly defined. Signals or targets often occur embedded in or surrounded by *noise*. The intensity relation between the signal and the noise is called the signal-to-noise ratio. Noise in this specific sense, then, does not mean acoustic noise but rather unwanted electrical disturbances, muscle tension, or mechanical interference, all of which are *undesired.*

target electrode See *companion electrode.*

time-frequency uncertainty principle See *pure-tone and time-frequency uncertainty.*

volume-unit conduction artifact Compression and rarefaction of molecules or synchronized motion of electrodes, even in Jello, can generate electrical currents which can be confused for neural events; these are sometimes called volume-unit conduction artifacts. (See also *induction artifacts.*)

ACKNOWLEDGMENTS

This work was supported by National Institutes of Health, USPHS Grant No. NS-11647 (Program Project), The Deafness Research Foundation, and The Kresge Foundation. I am indebted to the anesthesia staff of Charity Hospital of Louisiana in New Orleans and to my colleagues, Dennis Casey, Jeff Chicola, Jack Cullen, Mike Elam, Jerry Fourrier, Maria Gondra, Jim Jerger, Herbert Marks, Jim May, Tom Meunier, Dan Mouney, Ed Ross, Sharon Smith, Kathy Wexler, and Diane Wilensky, who participated in some of the data collection. I thank Yvonne Beck, Gae Decker, Pamela Weaver, Charles Wiesendanger, the Louisiana State University Developmental Disabilities Unit, the Louisiana State University Medical Center's Department of Audiology and Speech Pathology, and the students, staff, and principal of the Houston School for the Deaf for their unique contributions.

REFERENCES

Anderson, H., and B. Barr, "Conductive Recruitment," *Acta Oto-laryngologica,* 62 (1966), 171–184.

Aran, J-M., "The Electro-cochleogram: Recent Results in Children and in Some

Pathological Cases," *Archive fur Klinische und Experimentelle Ohren- Nasen- und und Kehlkopfheilkunde,* 198 (1971), 128–141.

Berlin, C.I., "Hearing in Mice via GSR Audiometry," *Journal of Speech and Hearing Research,* 6 (1963), 359–368.

Berlin, C.I., "Impedance of the Ear, Part I: Tympanometry," a self-instructional materials program developed for distribution by the Health Sciences Consortium, Chapel Hill, N.C., 1976.

Berlin, C.I., and J.K. Cullen, Jr., "The Physical Basis of Impedance Measurement," in *Handbook of Clinical Impedance Audiometry,* edited by J. Jerger. Dobbs Ferry: American Electromedics Corporation, 1975, pp. 1–20.

Berlin, C.I., J.K. Cullen, Jr., M.S. Ellis, R.J. Lousteau, W.M. Yarbrough, and G.D. Lyons, Jr., "Clinical Application of Recording Human VIIIth Nerve Action Potentials from the Tympanic Membrane," *Transactions of the American Academy of Ophthalmology & Otolaryngology,* 78 (1974),401– 410.

Berlin, C.I., J.K. Cullen, Jr., M.I. Gondra, and D.G. Fourrier, "Clinical Experience with Electrocochleography: Special Applications in Bone Conduction," Birmingham: Aesculapius Publishing Co., 1977.

Berlin, C.I., A. Gill, and M. Leffler, "Hearing in Mice by GSR Audiometry: I. Magnitude of Unconditioned GSR as an Index of Frequency Sensitivity," *Journal of Speech and Hearing Research,* 11 (1968), 159–168.

Berlin, C.I., and M.I. Gondra, "Extratympanic Clinical Electrocochleography with Clicks," in *Electrocochleography,* edited by R.J. Ruben, C. Elberling, and G. Salomon. Baltimore: University Park Press, 1976, pp. 457–469.

Berlin C.I., and S.S. Lowe, "Temporal and Dichotic Factors in Central Auditory Testing," in *Handbook of Clinical Audiology,* edited by J. Katz. Baltimore: Williams & Wilkins Co., 1972, pp. 280–312.

Bickford, R., J. Jacobson, and D. Cody, "Nature of Averaged Evoked Potentials to Sound and Other Stimuli in Man," *Annual of the New York Academy of Science,* 112 (1964), 204–223.

Bobbin, R.P., "Auditory Physiology, Topics 1–8," a self-instructional materials program developed for distribution by the Health Sciences Consortium, Chapel Hill, N.C., 1976.

Bordley, J.E., W.G. Hardy, and C.P. Richter, "Audiometry with the Use of the Galvanic Skin Resistance Response," *Bulletin of Johns Hopkins Hospital,* 82 (1958), 569.

Borg, E., "On the Neuronal Organization of the Acoustic Middle Ear Reflex. A Physiological and Anatomical Study," *Brain Research,* 49 (1973), 101–123.

Bradford, L.J., "Respiration Audiometry," in *Physiological Measures of the Audio-Vestibular System,* edited by L.J. Bradford. New York/ San Francisco/ London: Academic Press, Inc., 1975, pp. 249–317.

Buchwald, J.S., and C-M. Huang, "Far-Field Acoustic Response: Origins in the Cat," *Science,* 189 (1975), 382–384.

Clopton, B.M., and M.S. Silverman, "Latency Changes for Unit Responses at Rat

Inferior Colliculus after Early Auditory Deprivation," *Journal of the Acoustical Society of America,* 60 (1976), S82.

Coats, A.C., "Evaluation of 'Click Pips' as Impulsive yet Frequency Specific Stimuli for Possible Use in Electrocochleography: A Preliminary Report," in *Electrocochleography,* edited by R.J. Ruben, C. Elberling, and G. Salomon. Baltimore: University Park Press, 1976, pp. 387–406.

Coats, A.C., and J.R. Dickey, "Non-surgical Recording of Human Auditory Nerve Action Potentials and Cochlear Microphonics," *Annals of Otology, Rhinology and Laryngology,* 29 (1970), 844.

Crowley, D.E., H. Davis, and H.A. Beagley, "Survey of the Clinical Use of Electrocochleography," *Annals of Otology, Rhinology and Laryngology,* 84 (1975), 297–307.

Cullen, J.K., Jr., C.I. Berlin, M.I. Gondra, and M.L. Adams, "Electrocochleography in Children: A Retrospective Study," *Archives of Otolaryngology,* 102 (1976), 482–486.

Cullen, J.K., Jr., M.S. Ellis, C.I. Berlin, and R.J. Lousteau, "Human Acoustic Nerve Action Potential Recordings from the Tympanic Membrane without Anesthesia," *Acta Oto-laryngologica,* 74 (1972), 15–22.

Daly, D.M., R.J. Roeser, and G. Moushegian, "The Frequency-following Response in Subjects with Profound Unilateral Hearing Loss," *Electroencephalography and Clinical Neurophysiology,* 40 (1976), 132–142.

Davis, H., "Classes of Auditory Evoked Responses," *Audiology,* 12 (1973), 464–469.

Davis, H., "Relations of Peripheral Action Potentials and Cortical Evoked Potentials to the Magnitude of Sensation," in *Sensation and Measurement,* edited by H.R. Moskowitz. Dordrecht-Holland: D. Reidel Publishing Company, 1974, pp. 37–47.

Davis, H., "Principles of Electric Response Audiometry," *Annals of Otology, Rhinology and Laryngology,* Supp. 28, 85 (1976).

Davis, H., C. Bowers, and S.K. Hirsh, "Relations of the Human Vertex Potential to Acoustic Input: Loudness and Masking," *Journal of the Acoustical Society of America,* 43 (1968), 431–438.

Davis, H., S.K. Hirsh, J. Shelnutt, and C. Bowers, "Further Validation of Evoked Response Audiometry (ERA)," *Journal of Speech and Hearing Research,* 10 (1967), 717–732.

Davis, H., and S. Onishi, "Maturation of Auditory Evoked Potentials," *International Audiology,* 8 (1969), 24–33.

Davis, H., P.A. Osterhammel, C.C. Wier, and D.B. Gjerdingen, "Slow Vertex Potentials: Interactions among Auditory, Tactile, Electric, and Visual Stimuli," *Electroencephalography and Clinical Neurophysiology,* 33 (1975), 537–545.

Denenberg, L.J., and M.W. Altshuler, "The Clinical Relationship between Acoustic Reflexes and Loudness Perception," *Journal of the American Audiology Society,* Baltimore: Williams & Wilkins Co., 2 (1976), 79–82.

Djupesland, G., "Advanced Reflex Considerations," in *Handbook of Clinical Impedance Audiometry*, edited by J. Jerger. Dobbs Ferry: American Electromedics Corporation, 1975, pp. 85–126.

Echols, D.F., C.H. Norris, and H.G. Tabb, "Anesthesia of the Ear by Iontophoresis of Lidocaine," *Archives of Otolaryngology*, 102 (1975), 418–421.

Eggermont, J.J., D.W. Odenthal, P.H. Schmidt, and A. Spoor, "Electrocochleography: Basic Principles and Clinical Application," *Acta Oto-laryngologica*, 316 (1974), 1–84.

Eggermont, J.J., A. Spoor, and D.W. Odenthal, "Frequency Specificity of Tone Burst Electrocochleography," in *Electrocochleography*, edited by R.J. Ruben, C. Elberling, and G. Salomon. Baltimore/London/Tokyo: University Park Press, 1976, pp. 215–246.

Eisenberg, R.B., "Cardiotachometry," in *Physiological Measures of the Audio-Vestibular System*, edited by L.J. Bradford. New York: Academic Press, 1975, pp. 319–348.

Elberling, C., "Transitions in Cochlear Action Potentials Recorded from the Ear Canal in Man," *Scandinavian Audiology*, 2 (1973), 151–159.

Elberling, C., and G. Salomon, "Action Potentials from Pathological Ears Compared to Potentials Generated by a Computer Model," in *Electrocochleography*, edited by R.J. Ruben, C. Elberling, and G. Salomon. Baltimore/London/Tokyo: University Park Press, 1976, pp. 439–456.

Feldman, A.S., "Acoustic Impedance-admittance Measurements," in *Physiological Measures of the Audio-Vestibular System*, edited by L.J. Bradford. New York: Academic Press, 1975, pp. 87–146.

Finck, A., and C.I. Berlin, "Comparison between Single Unit Responses in the Auditory Nerve and GSR Determined Thresholds in Mice," *Journal of Auditory Research*, 5 (1965), 1–9.

Galambos, R., Panel Discussion—"Electric Response Audiometry (ERA): Present Status and Problems," *Journal of the Acoustical Society of America*, 60 (1976), S15.

Gerken, G.M., G. Moushegian, R.D. Stillman, and A.L. Rupert, "Human Frequency-following Responses to Monaural and Biaural Stimuli," *Electroencephalography and Clinical Neurophysiology*, 38 (1975), 379–386.

Gill, A., and C.I. Berlin, "Hearing in Mice by GSR Audiometry: II. Magnitude of Unconditioned GSR as a Function of Intensity and Frequency Interactions," *Journal of Speech and Hearing Research*, 11 (1968), 169–178.

Gjerdingen, D.B., and R. Tomsic, "Recovery Functions of Human Cortical Potentials Evoked by Tones, Shocks, Vibration, and Flashes," *Psychonomic Science*, 19 (1970), 228–229.

Goetzinger, C.P., "Effects of Small Perceptual Losses on Language and on Speech Discrimination," *Volta Review*, 64 (1965), 408.

Goldstein, M.H., and N.Y.-S. Kiang, "Synchrony of Neural Activity in Electric Responses Evoked by Transient Acoustic Stimuli," *Journal of the Acoustical Society of America*, 30 (1958), 102.

Goldstein, R., and D.C. Kendall, with the technical assistance of B.E. Arick, "Electroencephalic Audiometry in Young Children," *Journal of Speech and Hearing Disorders*, 28 (1963), 331–354.

Goldstein, R., and C.C. McRandle, "Middle Components of the Averaged Electroencephalic Results to Clicks in Neonates," in *Hearing and Davis: Honoring Hallowell Davis*, edited by S.K. Hirsh, D.H. Eldredge, I.J. Hirsh, and S.R. Silverman. St. Louis: Washington University Press, 1976, pp. 445–456.

Hay, I.S., and H. Davis, "Slow Cortical Evoked Potentials: Interactions of Auditory, Vibro-tactile and Shock Stimuli," *Audiology*, 10 (1971), 9–17.

Hecox, K., and R. Galambos, "Brain Stem Auditory Evoked Responses in Human Infants and Adults," *Archives of Otolaryngology*, 99 (1974), 30–33.

Hecox, K., N. Squires, and R. Galambos, "Brainstem Auditory Evoked Responses in Man. I. Effect of Stimulus Rise-Fall Time and Duration," *Journal of the Acoustical Society of America*, 60 (1976), 1187–1192.

Hirsh, S.K., "Vertex Potentials Associated with an Auditory Discrimination," *Psychonomic Science*, 22 (1971), 173–175.

Holm, V.A., and L.H. Kunze, "Effect of Chronic Otitis Media on Language and Speech Development," *Pediatrics*, 43 (1969), 833–839.

Hood, D.C., "Evoked Cortical Response Audiometry," in *Physiological Measures of the Audio-Vestibular System*, edited by L.J. Bradford. New York/San Francisco/London: Academic Press, Inc., 1975, pp. 349–370.

Hyde, M.L., S.D.G. Stephens, and A.R.D. Thornton, "Stimulus Repetition Rate and the Early Brainstem Responses," *British Journal of Audiology*, 10 (1976), 41–50.

Ino, T., "Comparison of the Response Threshold between ERA and EcoG," in *Electrocochleography*, edited by R.J. Ruben, C. Elberling, and G. Salomon. Baltimore/London/Tokyo: University Park Press, 1976, pp. 247–256.

Jerger, J., ed., *Handbook of Clinical Impedance Audiometry*. Dobbs Ferry: American Electromedics Corporation, 1975.

Jerger, J., P. Burney, L. Mauldin, and B. Crump, "Predicting Hearing Loss from the Acoustic Reflex," *Journal of Speech and Hearing Disorders*, 39 (1974).

Jerger, J., and Hayes, D., "The Cross-Check Principle in Pediatric Audiometry," *Archives of Otolaryngology*, 102 (1976), 614–620.

Jerger, S., J. Jerger, L. Mauldin, and P. Segal, "Studies in Impedance Audiometry: II. Children Less than Six Years Old," *Archives of Otolaryngology*, 99 (1974), 1–9.

Jewett, D.L., M.N. Romano, and J.S. Williston, "Human Auditory Evoked Potentials: Possible Brain Stem Components Detected on the Scalp," *Science*, 167 (1970), 1517–1518.

Jewett, D.L., and J.S. Williston, "Auditory-Evoked Far Fields Averaged from the Scalp of Humans," *Brain*, 94 (1971), 681–696.

Keith, R., "Impedance Audiometry with Neonates," *Archives of Otolaryngology*, 97 (1973), 465–467.

Kiang, N.Y.-S., "Discharge Patterns of Single Fibers in the Cat's Auditory Nerve," Research Monograph No. 35, Cambridge, Mass: M.I.T. Press, 1965.

Kiang, N.Y.-S., E.C. Moxon, and A.R. Kahn, "The Relationship of Gross Potential Recorded from the Cochlea to Single Unit Activity in the Auditory Nerve," in *Electrocochleography*, edited by R.J. Ruben, C. Elberling, and G. Salomon. Baltimore/London/Tokyo: University Park Press, 1976, pp. 95-115.

Lev, A., and H. Sohmer, "Sources of Averaged Neural Responses Recorded in Animal and Human Subjects during Cochlear Audiometry (Electrocochleography)," *Archive fur Klinische und Experimentelle Ohren- Nasen- und Kehlkopfheilkunde*, 201 (1972), 79-90.

Licklider, J.C.R., "Basic Correlates of the Auditory Stimulus," in *Handbook of Experimental Psychology*, edited by S.S. Stevens. New York and London: John Wiley & Sons, 1951, pp. 985-1039.

Margolis, R., and G. Popelka, "Loudness and the Acoustic Reflex," *The Journal of the Acoustical Society of America*, 58 (1975), 1330-1332.

Marsh, J.T., and F.G. Worden, "Sound Evoked Frequency-following Responses in the Central Auditory Pathway," *Laryngoscope*, 78 (1968), 1149-1163.

Martin, M.E., and E.J. Moore, "Scalp Distribution of Early (0-10 msec.) Auditory Evoked Responses," *Archives of Otolaryngology*, 1977.

McRandle, C.C., M.A. Smith, and R. Goldstein, "Early Averaged Electroencephalic Responses to Clicks in Neonates," *Annals of Otology, Rhinology & Laryngology*, 83 (1974), 695-702.

Mendel, M.I., E.C. Hosick, T.R. Windman, H. Davis, S.K. Hirsh, and D.F. Dinges, "Audiometric Comparison of the Middle and Late Components of the Adult Auditory Evoked Potentials Awake and Asleep," *Electroencephalography and Clinical Neurophysiology*, 38 (1975), 27-33.

Mendel, M.I., C.D. Adkinson, and L.A. Harker, "Middle Components of the Auditory Evoked Potentials in Infants," *Annals of Otology, Rhinology & Laryngology*, 86 (1977), 293-299.

Mendel, M.I., L.A. Pals, and L.A. Harker, "Two Years Clinical Experience with the Middle Components of the Auditory Evoked Potentials," presented at the Annual Convention, American Speech and Hearing Association, November 20-23, 1976, Houston, Texas.

Meunier, T.J., Jr., and J.G. May, "Simultaneous Averaging of Acoustic Nerve and Brainstem Auditory Potentials in Humans," *ASHA*, 18 (1976), 658.

Michels, M.W., and C.T. Randt, "Galvanic Skin Response in the Differential Diagnosis of Deafness," *Archives of Otolaryngology*, 75 (1947), 302-311.

Moore, E.J., "Recording the Electrocochleographic (ECochG) Response in Humans: A Reply to A. C. Coats [J. Acoust. Soc. Am. 56 (1974), 708-711]," *Journal of the Acoustical Society of America*, 59 (1976), 1504-1505.

Mouney, D.F., J.K. Cullen, Jr., M.I. Gondra, and C.I. Berlin, "Tone Burst Electrocochleography in Humans," *Transactions of the American Academy of Ophthalmology & Otolaryngology*, 82 (1976), 348-355.

Moushegian, G., Panel Discussion–"Electric Response Audiometry (ERA): Present Status and Problems," *Journal of the Acoustical Society of America,* 60 (1976), S15.

Moushegian, G., A.L. Rupert, and R.D. Stillman, "Scalp-recorded Early Responses in Man to Frequencies in the Speech Range," *Electroencephalography and Clinical Neurophysiology,* 35 (1973), 665–667.

Naunton, R.F., and S. Zerlin, "Human Whole-Nerve Response to Clicks of Various Frequency," *Audiology* 15 (1976a), 1–9.

Naunton, R.F., and S. Zerlin, "Basis and Some Diagnostic Implications of Electrocochleography," *Laryngoscope,* 86 (1976b), 475–482.

Niemeyer, W., and G. Sesterhenn, "Calculating the Hearing Threshold from the Stapedius Reflex Threshold for Different Sound Stimuli," *Audiology,* 13 (1974), 421–427.

Northern, J.L., and M.P. Downs, *Hearing in Children.* Baltimore, Md: Williams & Wilkins Co., 1974.

Onishi, S., and H. Davis, "Effects of Duration and Rise Time of Tone Bursts on Evoked V Potentials," *Journal of the Acoustical Society of America,* 44 (1968), 582–591.

Ornitz, E.M., and D.O. Walter, "The Effect of Sound Pressure Waveform on Human Brain Stem Auditory Evoked Responses," *Brain Research,* 92 (1975), 490–498.

Osterhammel, P.A., H. Davis, C.C. Wier, and S.K. Hirsh, "Adult Auditory Evoked Vertex Potentials in Sleep," *Audiology,* 12 (1973), 116–128.

Picton, T.W., S.A. Hillyard, H.I. Krausz, and R. Galambos, "Human Auditory Evoked Potentials. I. Evaluation of Components," *Electroencephalography and Clinical Neurophysiology,* 36 (1974), 179–190.

Price, L.L., and R. Goldstein, "Averaged Evoked Responses for Measuring Auditory Sensitivity in Children," *Journal of Speech and Hearing Disorders,* 31 (1966), 248–256.

Robertson, E.O., J.L. Peterson, and L.E. Lamb, "Relative Impedance Measurements in Young Children," *Archives of Otolaryngology,* 88 (1968), 162–168.

Rose, J.E., J.F. Brugge, D.J. Anderson, and J.E. Hind, "Phase-Locked Response to Low-Frequency Tones in Single Auditory Nerve Fibers of the Squirrel Monkey." *Journal of Neurophysiology,* 30 (1967), 769–793.

Rosenblith, W.A., and M.R. Rosenzweig, "Electrical Responses to Acoustic Clicks: Influence of Electrode Location in Cats," *Journal of the Acoustical Society of America,* 23 (1951), 583–588.

Ross, S., "On the Relation between the Acoustic Reflex and Loudness," *Journal of the Acoustical Society of America,* 43 (1964), 768–779.

Rousey, C., C. Snyder, and C. Rousey, "Changes in Respiration as a Function of Auditory Stimuli," *Journal of Auditory Research,* 4 (1964), 107–114.

Ruben, R.J., C. Elberling, and G. Salomon, editors, *Electrocochleography.* Baltimore/London/Tokyo: University Park Press, 1976.

Russ, F.M., and F.B. Simmons, "Five Years of Experience with Electric Response Audiometry," *Journal of Speech and Hearing Research,* 17 (1974), 184–193.

Scharf, B., "Acoustic Reflex, Loudness Summation, and the Critical Band," *Journal of the Acoustical Society of America,* 60 (1976), 753–755.

Schulman, C.A., "Heart Rate Audiometry. Part I. An Evaluation of Heart Rate Response to Auditory Stimuli in Newborn Hearing Screening," *Neuropädiatrie,* 4 (1973), 362–374.

Schulman-Galambos, C., and R. Galambos, "Brain Stem Auditory-evoked Responses in Premature Infants," *Journal of Speech and Hearing Research,* 18 (1975), 456–465.

Seidemann, M.F., V.W. Byers, and D.H. Sisterhen, "A System for Reporting Tympanometric Results," *Journal of Speech and Hearing Disorders,* 41 (1976), 520–522.

Silverman, M.S., and B.M. Clopton, "Critical Period for the Development and Maintenance of Binaural Interaction," *Journal of the Acoustical Society of America,* 60 (1976), S82.

Simmons, F.B., "Human Auditory Nerve Responses: A Comparison of Three Commonly Used Recording Sites," *Laryngoscope,* 85 (1975), 1564–1581.

Simmons, F.B., and R.F. Dixon, "On the Importance of the Question: What Do You Hear?," *Archives of Otolaryngology,* 80 (1964), 167–169.

Simmons, F.B., and T.J. Glattke, "Electrocochleography," in *Physiological Measures of the Audio-Vestibular System,* edited by L.J. Bradford. New York/San Francisco/London: Academic Press, 1975, pp. 147–176.

Skinner, P., "Electroencephalic Response Audiometry," in *Handbook of Clinical Audiology,* 2nd ed., edited by J. Katz. Baltimore: Williams & Wilkins Co., in press.

Skinner, P. and T.J. Glattke, "Electrophysiologic Response Audiometry: State of the Art," *Journal of Speech and Hearing Disorders,* 42 (1977), 179–198.

Sohmer, H., and D. Cohen, "Responses of the Auditory Pathway in Several Types of Hearing Loss," in *Electrocochleography,* edited by R.J. Ruben, C. Elberling, and G. Salomon. Baltimore/London/Tokyo: University Park Press, 1976, pp. 431–437.

Sohmer, H., and M. Feinmesser, "Cochlear and Cortical Auditory Responses Conveniently Recorded in the Same Subject," *Israeli Journal of Medical Science,* 6 (1970), 219–223.

Sohmer, H., M. Feinmesser, and G. Szabo, "Sources of Electrocochleographic Responses as Studied in Patients with Brain Damage," *Electroencephalography and Clinical Neurophysiology,* 37 (1974), 663–669.

Sohmer, H., H. Pratt, and M. Feinmesser, "Electrocochleography or Evoked Cortical Responses: Which is Preferable in Diagnosis of Hearing Loss?," *Revue de Laryngologie,* 95 (1974), 7–8.

Spoendlin, H.H., "Innervation Densities of the Cochlea," *Acta Oto-laryngologica,* 73 (1973), 235–248.

Starr, A.S., "Auditory Brain-stem Responses in Brain Death," *Brain,* 99 (1976), 543–554.

Starr, A., and J. Achor, "Auditory Brainstem Response in Neurological Disease," *Archives of Neurology,* 32 (1975), 761–768.

Stillman, R.D., G. Moushegian, and A.L. Rupert, "Early Tone-evoked Responses in Normal and Hearing-impaired Subjects," *Audiology,* 15 (1976), 10–22.

Teas, D.C., and N.Y-S. Kiang, "Evoked Responses from the Auditory Cortex," *Experimental Neurology,* 10 (1964), 91–119.

Thornton, A.R.D., "The Measurement of Surface-recorded Electrocochleographic Responses," *Scandinavian Audiology,* 4 (1975a), 51–58.

Thornton, A.R.D., "The Use of Post Auricular Muscle Responses," *Journal of Laryngology and Otology,* 89 (1975b), 997–1010.

Thornton, A.R.D., "Statistical Properties of Electrocochleographic Responses and Their Use in Clinical Diagnosis," in *Electrocochleography,* edited by R.J. Ruben, C. Elberling, and G. Salomon. Baltimore/London/Tokyo: University Park Press, 1976, pp. 257–276.

Thornton, A.R.D., and C.H. Hawkes, "Neurological Applications of Surface-recorded Electrocochleography," *Journal of Neurology, Neurosurgery, and Psychiatry,* 39 (1976), 586–592.

Ventry, I.M., "Conditioned Galvanic Skin Response Audiometry," in *Physiological Measures of the Audio-Vestibular System,* edited by L.J. Bradford. New York/San Francisco/London: Academic Press, 1975.

Wang, C.-Y., and P. Dallos, "Latency of Whole-nerve Action Potentials: Influence of Hair-cell Normalcy," *Journal of the Acoustical Society of America,* 52 (1972), 1678–1686.

Webster, D.B., and M. Webster, "Brainstem Auditory Nucleus After Sound Deprivation," *Journal of the Acoustical Society of America,* 59 (1976), S91.

Yoshie, N., "Auditory Nerve Action Potential Responses to Clicks in Man," *Laryngoscope,* 78 (1968), 198–215.

Yoshie, N., and T. Ohashi, "Clinical Use of Cochlear Nerve Action Potential Responses in Man for Differential Diagnosis of Hearing Losses," *Acta Oto-laryngologica,* 252 (1969), 37–69.

TABLE 4-A-1. Brief Analysis of Responses Acquired by Averaging Neuroelectric Activity

	Direct			Mediated	
	EcochG	BSER/FFR	Middle	Late	CNV
Latency of major waves in msecs	1.5–3.5	5–7.5/5+ multiples of period (FFR).	10–50	75–275	300
Common mode rejection Pre-amp. Bandpass Frequency (Hz)	100 to 3000	100–3000/ 0.2–3000 (FFR).	20–150	1–15	direct current
Gain	10^3	10^3	10^3	10^5	10^5
Add'l amplifier gain	10^2	10^2	10^2	Not needed	Not needed
Best audio stimulus	Clicks or tone bursts rising in 1 msec or less.	Same for BSER; 500 Hz and below for FFR.	Clicks or tonebursts.	Clicks, but any slow-rise all right.	Precede target with warning.
Sedation or anesthesia necessary in children?	Yes	Preferred, but may not always be necessary.	Preferred	Undesirable	Undesirable
Affected by: Sleep	No	No	Unclear	Yes	Yes
Drugs	No	No	Unclear	Yes	Yes
Br. Inj.	No	Unclear	Unclear	Yes	Probably
Age	No	Slightly	Yes	Yes	Probably

Observer agreement on response	Virtually perfect.	Very good for wave 5. Pedestal useful for FFR.	Uncertain	Highly unreliable.	Unclear
Major Weakness	Narrow freq. range near thresholds. Bias for ?	Narrow freq. range near thresholds.	Uncertainty of response. Narrow freq. range near thresholds.	Unreliability	Requires cooperation
Comments:	Surest, but biggest risks: however, no deaths or serious injuries reported to date. Should be a last resort procedure. (Crowley et al. 1975)	Optimum tradeoff; usually should be tried before ECochG. FFR may complement BSER & ECochG.	Best of mediated ERA for audiometry. Still has problems with respect to sleep, drugs, and interpretation.	Unreliable and relatively insensitive.	May give insight into perception, but a *direct* response should be achieved first.

Appendix

TRANSFORMATIONS FROM DECIMAL TO BINARY NUMBERS

Introduction

Binary number systems are based on the values of logarithms to the base 2. Our everyday numbers are based on a system of positions of a number *relative to a decimal point*. Thus the number 400 is quite different from the number 0.04 because of their different placement in relation to the decimal point. These everyday numbers are called *decimal numbers* because of their relationship to 10 (base 10). *Decimal* has as its root the word *Dec* which means *ten*.

1. This modified program concerns itself with the *binary* number system, which has as its root *bi*, meaning two. In this system there are only two numbers—the number 1 and the number 0. If you were told that 0 stood for the verbal concept *no*, it would be logical to assume that 1, therefore, stood for the verbal concept _____(a). Certain types of computers can handle information only when it is changed into a *yes* or *no* form. These computers cannot handle numbers such as 1,245 or 67 directly because the numbers are in decimal form rather than the *yes* or *no* form of the _____(b) number system.

Answers

(a) yes

(b) binary

2. To understand the binary system, we must briefly review logarithms. Logarithms are exponents. In the expression $10^2 = 100$ (verbally expressed as 10 squared equals 100, or 10 to the second power equals 100) the number _____(a) is the exponent or logarithm. It tells you to use the number 10 as a factor in multiplication two times like this: $10 \times 10 = 100$.

If the expression were 10^5, that would mean to use the number 10 as a factor in multiplication _____(b) times like this: _____(c) = _____(d).

170

Answers

(a) 2
(b) five
(c) 10X10X10X10X10
(d) 100,000

3. The base of the logarithm can be any number you choose. In the cases mentioned above, the base of the logarithm was the number 10, and the

logarithm told you how many times to use the _____
(a) as a factor in multiplication. In the present program we will concern ourselves with the logarithms to the base 2. If we write the expression 2^3,

that means _____ (b). The expression that means

"take two as a factor 6 times" is _____ (c).

Answers

(a) base, or the number 10
(b) Use 2 as a factor three times. This, of course, equals 8. If you wrote 2 X 3 or 6, you have probably confused simple numerical multiplication with using a number as a factor with which to multiply itself.
(c) 2^6

4. The decimal (everyday) value of the expression 2^4 is _____

_____ (a).

Answer

(a) 16. If you wrote 6, you mistakenly added 4 and 2 when you should have used 2 as a factor 4 times. If you wrote 8, you multiplied 4 times 2 and have confused simple multiplication with the message the logarithm notation transmits to you. It would be wise to reread the section on the meaning of the logarithm.

5. You will also recall that any number raised to the first power equals itself. So that $2^1 = 2$, $5^1 = 5$, $12^1 =$ _____ (a), $18^1 =$

_____$^{(b)}$, and so forth. However, remember that any number raised to the zero power equals 1, as in: $2^0 = 1$; $10^0 = 1$; $15^0 =$ _____$^{(c)}$; $22^0 =$ _____$^{(d)}$; and so forth.

Answers

(a) 12
(b) 18
(c) 1
(d) 1

If that needs clarification, see *note* below.

6. Now let us take the decimal number 2 and start with its logarithmic value at 2^0, then 2^1, then 2^2, then 2^3 and so forth. Underneath some of these expressions we have written decimal equivalents for you. Complete the table, and then copy it onto a separate sheet of paper. You will need it to complete the rest of the program. Work from right to left!

Log:	2^5	2^4	2^3	2^2	2^1	2^0
Decimal Value:	32	_____	_____	_____	2	1
		(c)	(b)	(a)		

Log:	2^{11}	2^{10}	2^9	2^8	2^7	2^6
Decimal Value:	_____	1024	_____	_____	_____	_____
	(h)		(g)	(f)	(e)	(d)

Answers

(a) 4   (e) 128
(b) 8   (f) 256
(c) 16   (g) 512
(d) 64   (h) 2048

7. Now, with respect to our averages, a "9-bit digitizer" converts incoming voltages into 2^9 parts or _____ (a) Parts. A "10-bit digitizer" would resolve incoming voltages into _____ (b) parts.

Answers

(a) 512
(b) 1024

The resolution of any digitizer is (2^n-1) with the one lost bit being redundant with respect to degrees of freedom.

Note. Explanation of why any number to the zero power equals 1: To multiply logarithms, we leave the base intact and add the exponents. For example:

$$10^4 \times 10^7 = 10^{4+7}, \text{ or } 10^{11}.$$

To divide we leave the base intact but subtract exponents. For example:

$$\frac{10^7}{10^4} = 10^{7-4}, \text{ or } 10^3.$$

Now then, any number divided by itself always equals 1:

$$\frac{1,268}{1,268} = 1, \text{ or } \frac{4,272,456}{4,272,456} = 1.$$

Therefore, it follows that an expression such as $10^4 \div 10^4 = 1$ and also equals 10^{4-4} or 10^0; therefore, $10^0 = 1$. Because a number to the zero power means the number is to be divided by itself, and because any number divided by itself equals 1, then any number raised to the zero power yields a value of 1.

CHAPTER FIVE

Tests of Hearing–
Birth through One Year

WILLIAM R. HODGSON

INTRODUCTION

The first purpose of an audiologist is to identify auditory disorder. If a hearing loss is found, its nature and magnitude must be determined. The audiologist must ask whether the disorder, as measured, is sufficient to explain observed behavior. The social, educational, and vocational implications of the disorder must be explored. Habilitative procedures must begin.

Eliciting this information when working with infants is not easy, but remarkable progress in our ability to do so has been made. Key elements in the progress are (1) the concept of evaluation as an ongoing process to assess disorders with greater precision over time and (2) the availability of a battery of audiologic tests, rather than a single procedure, so that children within a wide range of functional capacity can be accurately evaluated.

OBJECTIVES

In this chapter I explain clinical and experimental procedures used to assess auditory function in infants from birth to one year of age and discuss developmental norms and maturation of auditory behavior. I attempt to describe the variables that affect test responses and to assess the validity of procedures used in infant audiometry. My major objective is to explain the techniques that have clinical utility in assessing the auditory sensitivity of infants.

INFANT DEVELOPMENT AND RESPONSE

To assess infants with auditory disorder, you must know how normal infants behave, and what the developmental norms for motor, auditory, language, and speech acquisition are. You should observe normal infants to become familiar with their appearance and behavior. Read some good books on child development, such as Smart and Smart (1972) and Mussen, Conger, and Kagan (1974). You must be familiar with infants to feel at ease during testing, to know the capabilities of your patient, and to differentiate normal and abnormal behavior.

Some basic information about infant development is presented below. You must remember that development guidelines are averages and that a range of normal development reflects individual differences.

Neonates

The neonatal period, which includes the first five days of life, is important to us because programs for early detection of auditory disorders concentrate on infants this age. Almost all infants are in hospital nurseries at this time and are available for testing.

Determination of prematurity in neonates is important because this condition is correlated with such disorders found later on in life as increased behavioral and reading problems (Lubchenco et al., 1963) and hearing loss (Vernon, 1967). With considerable variability, neonates weigh about 7.5 pounds. If birth weight is less than 5.5 pounds, infants are considered premature. Another criterion for prematurity is gestation period less than 37 weeks. Yerushalmy (1968) suggested that a combination of these criteria is best for estimating prematurity.

The neonate can usually visually follow a slowly moving object which is directly in front of his face. Wolff (1966) found that 8 of 12 infants followed movement of a red ball within 2 hours of birth, and all responded within 24 hours. Control of motor activity in the neonate is limited. Visual responses may be slow, with jerky movements and poor coordination. Eye movement toward the source of sound (cochleo-oculogyric reflex) may be observed both independent of and in conjunction with head-turning responses. Motor behavior of the neonate, which is useful for auditory testing in ordinary clinical situations, is primarily limited to reflexive responses, and more of these responses are described below.

An eye blink in response to sound is called an auropalpebral reflex (APR) or cochleopalpebral reflex. This response is commonly observed in infants. The eyelid movement may be seen in waking or sleeping babies. Froding (1960) reported it to be the most reliable auditory response in neonates. With both infants and adults, a relatively intense signal is required for elicitation of the APR. Wedenberg (1956) reported that SPLs of 105-115dB were required for pure-tones to result in APRs in neonates. However, Northern and Downs (1974) indicated that APRs can be reliably elicited, in a quiet room, with broad-band signals (noisemakers) at 50-70dB SPL. They also indicated that APRs occur for speech signals at about 55-75dB SPL, and for warble tones at about 55-90dB above the normal human threshold of audibility. Commercially available portable sound generators intended for use in neonatal hearing screening have frequently used high frequency warble tones or narrow bands of noise, with a recommended effective SPL of 90dB. The 90dB level is considered adequate to elicit APRs in normal hearing neonates. Eisenberg, Coursin, and Rupp (1966) considered the APR a most useful response because it is common and quite resistant to extinction.

A startle response to auditory and other stimuli is frequently observed in neonates. Hardy, Dougherty, and Hardy (1959) observed startle responses in neonates from a noisemaker at a reported 64dB as measured via the B-weighting network of a sound-level meter. Northern and Downs (1974) reported expected startle responses in infants to speech at a level of about 80dB SPL.

Other arousal or orientation responses may be observed. The sucking reflex may occur—and is probably more likely when the infant is hungry—on presentation of auditory stimuli. Conversely, an infant already engaged in sucking may stop or diminish this activity when an auditory signal is presented, although Kaye and Levin (1963) did not demonstrate significant differences between experimental and control groups in this respect.

Changes in respiratory pattern can sometimes be seen on presentation of an auditory signal. In addition to the visually observable chest or abdominal movements, graphic recordings of respiratory patterns during auditory stimulation have been found useful and are described in Chapter 4. In that chapter, too, are descriptions of cardiac rate measurement (cardiotachometry) and impedance audiometry. The latter has been particularly helpful in corroborating information about auditory response and indicating the status of the peripheral auditory mechanism. Evoked response audiometry and electrocochleography are also discussed in Chapter 4.

In addition to auditory sensitivity, other factors that influence responses to acoustic signals are the activity state of the neonate, the ambient noise level, and certain signal parameters. Activity state not only contributes to whether or not the neonate responds, but also to the type of response he makes. State may be described in terms of level of activity: deep sleep, light sleep, awake and quiet, or awake and active. Classifications and descriptions of activity states vary. Deep sleep, however, is characterized by little body movements except for sporadic startle responses, little or no eye movement, and rhythmic respiration. In light sleep there is considerable body and eye movement, with occasional flutter of the eyelids. Respiration is less regular than in deep sleep. Awake and quiet is characterized by open eyes and some movement of the head and limbs. Infants in the awake and active stage engage in generalized body movement, breathe irregularly, and vocalize. Northern and Downs (1974) suggested that deep and light sleep may be differentiated by flicking the eyelashes or touching the infant's eyelid lightly. The deeply sleeping infant does not respond, but the lightly sleeping infant responds with eye and other small body movements.

The type of response made by the infant not only varies according to state, but also seems to follow the law of initial value (Bench, 1970). That is, the quieter the prestimulus state, the greater the increase in activity upon stimulation; the more active the prestimulus state, the greater the decrease in activity. Thus, a startle or body movement is a more likely response from quietly sleeping infants; reduction or cessation of movement is more probable from an active infant.

There is evidence suggesting that, especially for neonates, light sleep may be the best state for auditory assessment. False positive responses are likely to be reduced, and more responses may be observable than at other activity levels. Eisenberg et al. (1964) observed a higher percentage of responses to noise-makers from neonates in light sleep or less than full wakefulness than from those either deeply asleep or fully awake. Bench and Mentz (1975) reported a similar finding when neonates, 6-week-old, and 6-month-old infants were stimulated with broad-band noise at 90dB SPL. However, they found some interesting interactions between signal intensity, activity state, and age. That is, the neonates responded to the 90dB SPL signal better when sleeping than when awake, but they responded better to a 60dB signal when awake. An increase in signal complexity enhanced response. All groups responded better to broad-band than narrow-band signals. There was a relatively better response to a speech signal from infants in the 6-month-old group than from the younger subjects.

Older Infants

Growth and motor development are extensive during the first year; by the end of a year the infant may weigh about 24 pounds. Motor development is summarized in Fig. 5-1. Important milestones are the ability to hold the head erect while sitting (3-4 months), to sit alone (6-7 months), and to walk alone (soon after the first birthday).

Several new responses that are useful in auditory evaluation develop during the first year. The developing ability to locate the source of sound is probably the most useful. Orienting responses in the first weeks of life may show crude localization attempts but are more commonly and noticeably manifested by reduction in general motor activity. Localization efforts mature with motor development and experience in hearing.

In normal infants localization efforts—searching for the source of sound—can be expected to begin by 3 months. By then motor control is sufficient for the baby to hold his head erect and make controlled if wobbly head movements to the right and left. Murphy (1969) reported maturation of localization as shown in Fig. 5-2. By about 3 months, the infant may localize on a horizontal plane, but does not look below or above his eye level for the source of sounds unless an additional visual component directs him there. By 5 months a horizontal localization effort may terminate in a vertical head movement toward a sound source originating below eye level. This inefficient movement may progress to an arc by 6 months and to efficient direct localization by 7½ months. Quick and accurate localization of sound requires both motor coordination and listening experience.

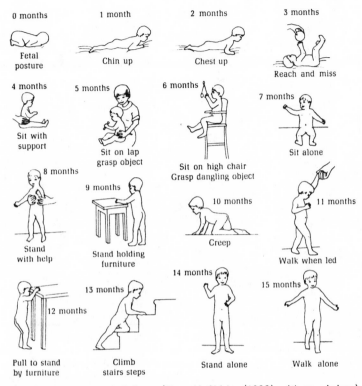

Fig. 5-1. Motor Development in Infants. (From M. Shirley (1933), with permission.)

Therefore, usefulness of this orienting response is limited in infants either with motor retardation or with hearing loss, which reduces their auditory experience.

Experimenters have long demonstrated that neonates and other infants under 1 year can be conditioned to respond to auditory signals by classical or instrumental conditioning procedures. For example, Aldrich (1928) paired presentation of an acoustic signal and a pin-scratch on the foot of a 3-month-old infant. After 15 trials the infant withdrew its foot on presentation of the acoustic signal only. Marquis (1931) successfully conditioned 7 out of 8 infants from 1 to 10 days of age to respond by sucking when they heard a signal that had been previously presented along with the infants' bottles. Fulton, Gorzychi, and Hull (1975) attempted to establish auditory stimulus-response control for pure-tone audiometry in twelve children 9–25 months of age, with a median age of 12 months (mean = 13.8 months). Edible reinforcers were used, and subjects responded by pressing a bar. The investigators successfully conditioned 7 of the 12 subjects to respond to low-level signals near expected normal threshold or at screening levels of 15dB (ANSI). The 7 who were successfully conditioned ranged in age from 12 to 25 months, with a median age of 14 months (mean =

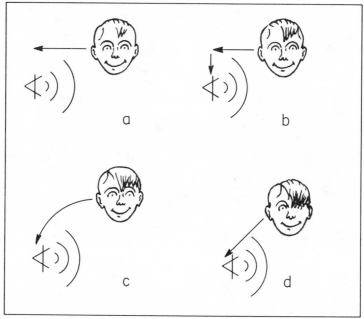

Fig. 5-2. Stages in the Development of Auditory Localization. (a) 3 months: Head movement along horizontal plane, generally toward sound source. (b) 5 months: Inefficient horizontal, then vertical orientation toward sound source. (c) 6 months: Improvement in moving head toward sound source. (d) 7½ months: Direct and efficient localization of a sound source below eye level. (After Murphy, 1969.)

16.4 months). The number of training sessions averaged 11.4, with a mean time of 11.5 minutes per session.

To summarize, numerous investigators have established responses from normal hearing infants under 12 months of age using classical or instrumental conditioning procedures under laboratory conditions. The clinical utility of these procedures with hearing-impaired infants under 1 year has not been demonstrated. However, as I'll discuss later in this chapter, use of reinforcement principles to strengthen and maintain auditory behavior already present in infants has shown clinical utility.

In addition to measures of auditory sensitivity, some information about auditory discrimination ability in infants also exists. Bronstein and Petrova (1967) demonstrated frequency discrimination in neonates. They obtained sucking responses on presentation of an auditory signal. Habituation occurred after repeated presentation, and the responses stopped. When the frequency of the signal was changed, the responses reoccurred. Butterfield and Hodgson (1969) demonstrated different sucking behavior in neonates when presentation of music was contingent on the infants sucking or not sucking.

Reduction of response through habituation must also be considered a form of auditory discrimination. Eisenberg, Marmarou, and Giovachino (1974a) found cardiac deceleration in neonates at least 70% of the time on presentation of the vowel *ah* at 68dB SPL. In a companion article (1974b), these authors reported differences in habituation rate between normal and high-risk infants. They feel this phenomenon may be useful in detecting infants in whom subtle auditory problems may later become evident.

AUDITORY ASSESSMENT

Now that we have had a brief look at infant development and the responses that babies are capable of, let's turn our attention to some actual test procedures and philosophies. We will begin by looking at the question of identification audiometry with neonates—programs that try to detect hearing loss in newborn infants.

We once thought that newborn babies couldn't hear. Spock (1968, p. 232) wrote, "A newborn baby seems to be deaf the first day or two because of fluid in his inner ear. . . . A few babies remain deaf for a number of weeks, apparently because the fluid in the ear is slow to absorb." With better attention to anatomy, Pratt (1965) wrote that hearing may be impaired in neonates because of amniotic fluid in the middle ear. Of course, there is no question that the neonate can hear. In fact, the presence of even prenatal response to sound is well established (Elliot and Elliot, 1964; Bench, 1968). The routine response to sound by thousands of neonates in screening programs is described in the following pages.

According to Jaffe (1972), the external ear canal of the neonate can be expected to contain blood and vernix caseosum, the waxy substance which coats the skin of the newborn. However, Jaffe continued, these materials dehydrate in a few hours. Keith (1976) obtained tympanograms on 60 neonates. He had the vernix removed from the canals of 20 infants between 2½ and 20 hours of age, but did not clear the canals of the older neonates. Results were similar to normal tympanograms in older children, with maximum compliance near atmospheric pressure. Fourteen infants had tympanograms with a notch-shaped curve and two points of maximum compliance near atmospheric pressure. Keith concluded that the results ". . . are virtually incompatible with an ear full of fluid or mucous and the normal tympanogram indicates that middle-ear mobility is normal almost from birth. The findings of normal compliance measurements and well aerated middle ears . . . would contradict statements in the literature that the middle ear is filled with a mucous cushion or mesenchymal tissue at birth" (p. 73). Bennett (1975) successfully obtained tympanograms from all 98 of his subjects between 5 and 218 hours of age. The tympanograms generally indicated normal middle-ear pressure although a fairly large number showed a notched tympanogram similar to that described in the study by Keith. Bennett felt that this notch was associated with the hypermobile neonatal tympanic membrane, and that it disappears with maturation. No attempts were made to remove the vernix caseosa in Bennett's study, and it did not appear to interfere with obtaining the tympanograms.

To repeat, there is no question that the neonate can hear. The questions needing answers are: What are the least intense sounds he can hear? How useful does he find his hearing? And, most important for our purposes, how can we detect those newborn infants who do not hear well? Possible answers to this last question are discussed below.

Neonatal Hearing Screening Programs

Large-scale efforts to detect hearing loss through neonatal audiometric screening got underway in the 1960s. Downs and Sterritt (1964) stimulated 117 neonates with high-frequency narrow-band noise at 90dB SPL and looked for motor responses. Four infants failed to respond and follow-up testing indicated that one of the four was most probably deaf and the other three were likely "false positives"—infants with normal hearing in whom responses were not observed during the screening procedure. No effort was made to determine if there were "false negatives"—deaf infants to whom responses were attributed and who therefore passed the screening test and were not identified.

Neonatal hearing screening programs subsequently became popular. Most were based on the format Marion Downs developed. That is, a moderately intense high-frequency signal was delivered to the infant in the hospital nursery while one or more observers looked for a motor response. Many of the programs were probably not as well controlled nor executed as the Downs program, and most were not very successful. We soon learned that the programs were not identifying deaf infants very successfully, and that the large number of false positives were causing unnecessary parental anxiety and costing a lot of time and money. Subsequently, in 1970, a joint committee of the American Speech and Hearing Association, the American Academy of Ophthalmology and Otolaryngology, and the American Academy of Pediatrics recommended that routine neonatal screening programs for hearing loss be discontinued. They urged that controlled experimental programs continue to investigate useful stimuli, response patterns, environmental factors, status of the neonate during testing, and behavior of observers. In a supplementary statement in 1973 the joint committee recommended the use of a high-risk register to identify neonates in whom the probability of hearing loss could be expected to be higher than normal. Criteria for the register were: (1) history of hereditary childhood hearing impairment in the family; (2) rubella or other nonbacterial intra-uterine fetal infection; (3) defects of ear, nose, or throat, or other craniofacial anomalies; (4) birthweight less than 1500 grams (3.3 pounds); and (5) bilirubin level greater than 20 milligrams per 100 milliliters serum. As discussed below, subsequent experimentation has seen development of new techniques for identification audiometry as well as refinement and validation of the high-risk register.

Table 5-1 summarizes the results of some neonatal identification studies. We believe the incidence of congenital deafness to be about one per 1000 live births. If this is the case, three of the four studies summarized in Table 5-1 were very efficient. Results of the fourth led its authors, Feinmesser and Tell (1976), to conclude that the conventional procedure of observing motor responses of awake infants was not sensitive enough to detect deafness in neonates. That is, the high number of false positives and false negatives indicated that the procedure was inefficient and invalid. Conversely, the two programs which used arousal from light sleep as the criterion response identified approximately the expected number of deaf infants. Furthermore, an acceptably low number of false positive results occurred (18 in Downs, 1976) as well as a low number of false negatives (1 in Mencher, 1974). My conclusion from looking at the results of these studies is this: So far we have demonstrated valid and efficient identification of deaf neonates only when they are tested in a quiet room and arousal from light sleep is the criterion response.

The studies summarized in Table 5-1 also evaluated effectiveness of a high-risk register. As would be expected, there was a high percentage of false positives. Stated differently, many infants at risk for deafness because of prenatal or neonatal hazards were not actually deaf. The number of false positives depended on the stringency of the high-risk register. The effectiveness of the high-risk registers used by the different investigators also varied. Feinmesser and Tell (1976) initially used a high-risk register which designated 20% of the test population at risk and included 18 of the 25 deaf children in the population. Through modification of the register, they reduced the number of neonates included to 6 to 7% of the population and retained 15 of the 25 deaf neonates within the register. Their restricted high-risk register included familial deafness, rubella during pregnancy, birthweight of 1500 grams (3.3 pounds) or less, congenital craniofacial malformations, Apgar score of 1-4, hyperbilirubinemia (bilirubin level of 20 milligrams per 100 milliliters or more), and neonatal sepsis. Their original high-risk register, which resulted in an unacceptably high number of false positives, also included consanguinity (blood relationship) in parents and a birthweight of 1900 grams (4.2 pounds) or less.

Downs (1976) reported about the same false positive rate (7.8%) as Feinmesser and Tell. All of the infants found deaf by her identification audiometry program were included on her high-risk register. She used the register proposed by the Joint Committee on Infant Hearing Screening, described earlier in this chapter.

Because of findings such as those just discussed, authorities meeting at a conference on early identification of hearing loss (Mencher, 1976) made some recommendations regarding neonatal screening and high-risk registers. The conference recommended that a high-risk register for deafness be universally insti-

TABLE 5-1. Summary of Neonatal Identification Studies

Author	Response	No. Screened	No. Screened Found Deaf	False Positive	False Negative	No. High Risk (%)	No. High Risk Found Deaf
Downs (1976) (Arousal)	Arousal	3,681	5	18*	DNT	(7.8%) 288	5†
Mencher (1974)	Arousal	10,000	9	?	1	?	5
Rossi and Guidotti (1976)	Numerous	5,304	5	?	2	(36.8%) 1,954	3
Feinmesser and Tell (1976)	Motor Responses From Awake Infant	17,731	6	307	19‡	(20%)§ 3,546	18

*Actually 18 or fewer. At least two children were lost to follow-up.
†Same 5 as identified by screening.
‡Authors concluded "Apriton" test not sensitive enough for neonatal screening.
§Recommended restricted high risk register (6–7% of population), would detect 15 of the deaf infants.

tuted. The register chosen was one instituted by the Joint Committee on Infant Screening. The register suggests that neonates should be considered at risk for deafness if any of these conditions obtain: (1) history of hereditary familial childhood hearing impairment; (2) rubella or other nonbacterial intra-uterine fetal infection, such as cytomegalovirus or herpes infections; (3) abnormalities of the otorhinolaryngeal system; (4) birthweight less than 1500 grams; and (5) bilirubin level greater than 20 milligrams per 100 milliliters serum. I think application of this high-risk register is a defensible and utilitarian procedure. From the studies summarized in Table 5–1 we see evidence that the majority of deaf infants can be expected to be included in this register, and it provides a beginning place to look for deafness both without direct attention to the entire population of neonates and without the necessity of examining a distressingly high number of false-positive cases.

Members of the conference also recommended that the high-risk register may be supplemented by individual behavioral screening, following a particular model: First, the ambient noise level at the time of the test should be measured and reported. I believe that the conference members also should have stipulated that the noise level not exceed 60dB SPL, as recommended by Northern and Downs (1974). The conference recommended that the infant be asleep prior to testing. One study indicated that neonates sleep 80% of the time (Mussen, Conger, and Kagan, 1974). Therefore, although requiring a pretest state of sleep will obviously complicate the test procedure, it is not an impossible criterion. I believe the evidence we have discussed justifies this requirement, and that a state of light sleep, as defined earlier, is preferable. The conference members further recommended that the test stimulus be a predominately high-frequency complex signal with a sharp rise time, a maximum SPL of 90dB, and a duration of ½ to 2 seconds with an interstimulus interval of at least 15 seconds. The arousal response they stipulated can be any generalized body movement that involves more than one limb and that is accompanied by some form of eye movement. They suggested one of two scoring criteria: that the observer not know when a signal is presented, or that two observers score the infant's response independently. Finally, they recommended that two or more responses out of eight stimuli be a passing score. I think that individual neonatal hearing screening should be done in addition to maintenance of a high-rise register *if* the procedures and criteria just presented can be met without equivocation. If not, the evidence suggests that the screening program will not be efficient or valid, and it would be better to rely on use of a high-risk register alone.

The conference we have been discussing also recommended field trials of a device that we have not yet discussed for identification of hearing loss; this device relies on an automated procedure that graphically records motor responses to auditory stimuli, which are presented at several points in time over a period of several hours. One such device is the Crib-o-gram (Simmons and Russ, 1974; Simmons, 1976). This device consists of a motion-sensitive transducer attached to a bassinet and a graphic recorder which records the measured motion, as well as timing and signal-generating equipment. Each test period consists of a 10-second prestimulus recording of bassinet activity, presentation of the test signal, and recording of activity during the subsequent 6 seconds. This cycle is repeated at desired intervals. It includes built-in control periods during which recordings are made but actual presentation of the signal does not occur. The scorer does not know which events represent control periods, and acceptance on his part of the recorded random movements as responses is an index of his tendency to accept false responses. The experimenters reported that, of 7655 neonates screened in normal nurseries, 777 have failed. Of these, 5 have proven hearing loss, for an incidence of .8 per 1000 births. Of 607 infants in intensive care units tested, 103 failed the test, and 7 were proven to have hearing loss (an incidence of 12.7 per 1000 births). As in earlier studies, best responses to the Crib-o-gram were obtained from sleeping infants.

Another automated procedure has been reported by Altman, Shenhav, and Schaudinischky (1975, 1976). The device, called an Accelerometer Recording System, is shown in Fig. 5-3. An accelerometer picks up vibrations of the crib, and samples are recorded in association with stimulus presentations. A pilot study with 400 neonates resulted in distinct responses from all but 7. Some of

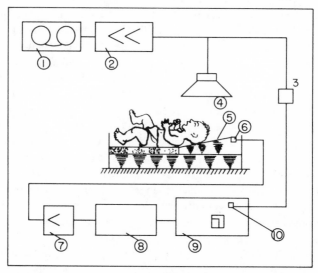

Fig. 5-3. Accelerometer Recording System. (1) Graphic recorder. (2) Timer. (3) Loud-speaker. (4) Cradle. (5) Headrest with accelerometer. (6) Preamplifier. (7), (8), and (12) Vibration-isolation device consisting of concrete slab, rubber tire, and polyurethane sheet. (9) Narrow band filter. (10) Signal source (tape recorder). (11) Audio amplifier. (From Altman, Shenhav, and Schaudinischky (1975), with permission.)

these 7 were later found to have familial history of deafness or other high-risk factors.

Automated procedures hold promise for routine use in neonatal detection of hearing loss. They are attractive in that they can be used with minimal disruption of nursery routine. Scoring of the infant's response is simplified. Validation of the procedures discussed above through field testing is still required. Refinement of test and scoring procedures is needed to reduce false positive results. When these things are accomplished, automated procedures may come into routine use in neonatal screening programs.

In conclusion, high-risk registers have been shown to be reasonably effective in identifying infants who should be considered at risk for deafness. A register has been established which strikes a fair compromise between the number of false positives and false negatives resulting from its use. I feel that its use should be routine in all nurseries. Moreover, if attention is limited to neonates at risk for deafness, some deaf babies will be missed. For this reason, I believe that hearing screening should also be conducted if a quality program can be maintained. Three final points: First authorities agree that current feasible procedures for screening neonates are sensitive only to hearing losses of about 75dB or greater (Mencher, 1974; Northern and Downs, 1974). Second, we know that at least some neonates with normal hearing at birth have progressive degenerative loss occurring early in childhood. Third, children are subject to developing and fluctuating conductive disorders. For these reasons, attention to hearing sensitivity must continue throughout childhood, with formal screening programs a good idea whenever they can be instituted and done well (for example, in well-baby clinics, nursery and preschools, regular schools).

Clinical Evaluation of Infants from Birth to One Year of Age

Clinical evaluation is required when infants at risk for hearing loss are isolated by a high-risk register, when infants fail hearing screening, or when, for any reason, auditory disorder is suspected. Screening procedures are ordinarily carried out by technicians or others trained for a nonprofessional role. Clinical evaluation is the job of the audiologist. The successful pediatric audiologist is flexible, sees evaluation as an ongoing process, and is prepared to use a battery of procedures to adapt to the capacities of a particular infant. Electrophysiological and electroacoustic procedures—particularly impedance audiometry—may be helpful, and these are discussed in Chapter 4. Other procedures with proven clinical utility for infants under 1 year of age are discussed below.

Behavioral observation audiometry with infants up to 3-4 months of age generally involves stimuli similar to those used in screening neonates, and similar responses are sought. In other words, moderately intense stimuli are presented to elicit reflexive responses. The generalizations regarding activity state referred to earlier still obtain. Two factors may make the task more difficult: First, developing cortical control may inhibit reflexive responses and make the infant in this age range less responsive than the neonate. Second, remember that the audiologist is now trying to get a more detailed measure of audition than when he is screening. Therefore more auditory stimuli must be presented over a longer time, and adaption (habituation) as well as fatigue may attenuate responses.

In spite of these difficulties, procedures have been suggested to obtain differential information about auditory function during this age range. Wedenberg (1956) established that normal neonates were awakened by pure tones of 70-75dB SPL, and APRs occurred at 105-115dB SPL. Using this information, Wedenberg (1972) concluded that his procedure could be used to differentiate infants as follows: First, of course, if the infant awakens at signal intensities of 70 to 75dB and gives APRs at 105-115dB SPL, hearing is assumed normal. Second, a cochlear problem with recruitment may be present if an APR occurs at the expected signal intensity, but the infant requires more than 75dB to awaken. Third, a conductive or retrocochlear disorder may be present if no APR occurs at 105-115dB, and if the infant awakens in response to some level above 75dB. Finally, deafness is indicated by no response. As is the case with most tests, I feel the results of this procedure alone should not be considered definitive. Along with other tests, however, it may provide useful information.

I think it is best to use electronically generated signals, even with children from 3 to 4 months of age. We are kidding ourselves when we attribute precise intensity and frequency measurements to most noisemakers. Bove and Flugrath (1973) analyzed 25 noisemakers and concluded 20 had spectra too wide for clinical use. They concluded that the other 5 had acceptable high-frequency characteristics. For better estimates and control of signal characteristics, it is probably better to use warble tones or narrow bands of noise. My colleague, Kevin Murphy, slips a cloth mask with a doll face painted on it over an audiometer earphone. He feels responses mediated in this fashion are reinforced, even for young infants, a view that has some experimental support. Studies such as the one by Fantz (1965) found that neonates spend more time looking at the picture of a face with human features than at other pictures with the same faceshaped outline but without human features.

Because infants at 3 or 4 months of age sleep much less than neonates, it may be difficult to find them quiet enough for testing. By letting them take a bottle, responses in the resultant relatively quiet state may be observed, and after eating they may fall asleep. Responses may include startle, APR, initiation or cessation of sucking, observable change in respiration pattern, or arousal. More than one observer should record responses independently. Responses should not be accepted unless they can be repeated.

From 3 or 4 months of age, as motor control develops, the orientation response mentioned earlier may develop. This response lends itself to auditory testing in sound field. The stimuli generally used are warble tones or narrow bands of noise. Some infants, especially younger ones, may respond only to speech. The disadvantage of a broad-band signal is that infants with normal sensitivity across any part of the signal's spectrum may respond; as a consequence, high-frequency losses are missed or their severity underestimated. I have had some success with filtering the speech spectrum to supply a more useful signal. I prefer to do this with live voice, using variable frequency filters in the audiometer circuit, for the additional flexibility afforded. Use of a tape-recorded signal is awkward when working with infants and young children, since constraints associated with selecting and cuing desired signals add another variable to an already complex situation.

A convenient sound-field audiometry setup is shown in Fig. 5–4. The infant is placed between two loudspeakers. The patient can either be supported in an infant seat or sit in a highchair. The head should be free to turn. It may be better for the parent not to hold the child because of distraction or inadvertent clues. However, if the infant will remain quiet only when held, he should sit on the parent's lap, facing forward, with no more support of the head and upper trunk than is necessary.

It is a good idea to have an assistant in the test room. He keeps the infant's

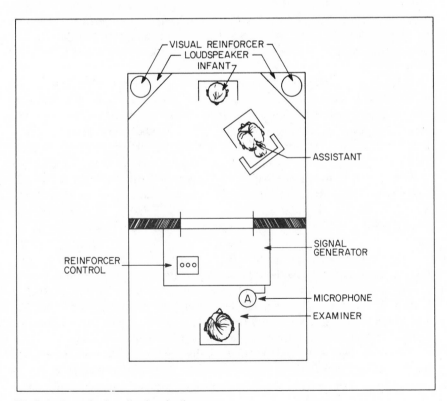

Fig. 5–4. Setup for Localization Audiometry.

attention minimally directed toward the front between signals and otherwise helps keep the test situation under control.

Attractive animated toys adjacent to the loudspeakers may provide reinforcement and reduce habituation. Moore, Wilson, and Thompson (in press) reported that use of an animated toy reinforced responses in infants between 5 and 11 months of age. However, their study showed no statistically significant differences in responses of a group of 4-month-old infants compared to a control group of infants who received no such reinforcement. The test signal is presented and, if the child looks toward the loudspeaker, the toy is activated briefly. If the child does not respond, the assistant may direct his attention toward the loudspeaker, physically moving his head if necessary. If a reliable stimulus-response pattern can be established, with accurate localization, both loudspeakers can be used. You should avoid slavish alternation between loudspeakers, to prevent anticipatory false responses. After each response, the assistant should bring the infant's attention back to midline.

Presumably because of reduced auditory experience, infants with severe or profound hearing loss may not respond consistently to sounds above their auditory threshold. If they do attempt to respond, they may not be able to localize accurately. When I see such confusion in localization attempts, I use only one loudspeaker for all signal generations. Then, if the animated toy does in fact serve as a reinforcer, the infant has only one source toward which to look for reinforcement.

The biggest limitations of sound-field localization audiometry lie in two areas: First, infants—especially those under 1 year of age—who have severe or profound loss may not respond at all in this situation. Of course, even this eventuality provides helpful information, indicating the probability of a hearing loss of considerable magnitude. Additional confirming information may be available through some of the procedures, described above, or through techniques discussed by Dr. Berlin in Chapter 4. Second, as is true with all sound-field audiometry, information obtained is almost exclusively associated with the infant's better ear. A unilateral hearing loss will probably not be identifiable. Nevertheless, an estimate of the infant's functional auditory status can be obtained.

One marked advantage of sound-field localization audiometry is that it provides a quick and easy method of substantiating functionally normal hearing sensitivity in situations where an infant's hearing, for one reason or another, is suspect. If the orientation response has developed, the infant will respond to low-intensity test signals without lengthy training sessions or much specialized equipment beyond that routinely present in an audiometric test unit.

Let us review some experimental results obtained with localization audiometry. Suzuki and Ogiba (1961) reported on a procedure they called conditioned orientation reflex (COR) audiometry. In their procedure two loudspeakers are placed some distance apart and near each is a semitransparent doll with a light behind it. A signal is presented and a second later the light behind the doll is lighted. The visual stimulus, if not the auditory, causes the child to look toward the source and the hope is to condition the child to respond to the auditory signal. If the conditioning is successful, the doll is subsequently lighted only after response to the auditory stimulus occurs—in the hope that this procedure will be reinforcing and maintain response. In this event, intensity and frequency of test signals are varied until the desired information is obtained. Suzuki and Ogiba reported that COR audiometry required an average of 5 minutes for infants under 1 year of age and was successful in 44.8% of their test sample. The success rate for older children was much higher.

Linden and Kankkunen (1969) described a procedure they called visual reinforcement audiometry (VRA). They placed loudspeakers near and on either side of the infant's head. Associated with the loudspeakers on either side were frosted glass windows on which slides of attractive pictures could be projected. They presented the test signal and visual stimuli as Suzuki and Ogiba did, described above. In addition to orientation response, Linden and Kankkunen accepted any visible response. They reported VRA could reliably evaluate infants from about 6 to 8 months of age. By plugging the ear that was not being tested and observing responses, they were able to obtain information from each ear separately when differences between ears did not exceed the attenuation characteristics of the plug plus the magnitude of the head shadow. In a group of normal infants between 3 and 11 months of age, they reported mean monaural thresholds for warble tones at octave intervals from 250 through 4000 Hz at about 30dB HL.

Haug, Baccaro, and Gilford (1967) also reported on a modification of the localization procedure that permits evaluation of each ear separately. They called their procedure the PIWI technique. PIWI stands for "puppet in the window illuminated," a description of the reinforcer they used. After testing in sound field with a procedure similar to that of Suzuki and Ogiba, they placed earphones on their subjects and continued the stimuli, hoping that the previously conditioned response would generalize to the new situation. Of eight subjects between 5 and 12 months of age, most of whom had hearing loss, the authors reported 100% success in the initial sound field segment of the test. On six of the eight subjects, they reported success in obtaining complete pure-tone air- and bone-conduction audiograms. That is, the response which generalized to earphone testing was also maintained when the test signals were delivered by the bone-conduction vibrator.

Close agreement has been reported between minimal response levels obtained from localization audiometry and air-conduction thresholds obtained under earphones. Matkin (1973) compared better ear results so obtained in a group of 26 children between 1-3 and 4-5 years of age. For 1000 Hz, 3 of the children showed no difference in the thresholds obtained by the two methods, 3 of the children showed 5dB difference, 4 showed 10dB difference, 3 showed 15dB difference, and 2, a difference greater than 15dB.

CONCLUSION

In conclusion, the following constitutes a battery of tests or procedures that should be useful in evaluating auditory sensitivity of infants under 1 year of age. The greater the number of tests applied to an individual infant, the greater the confidence that can be placed in the results.

1. Noisemakers may give useful preliminary and supplementary information. They are simple, easy to use, and sometimes may give information where more complex procedures fail. Electroacoustically obtained estimates of frequency and intensity characteristics should be available. Those who use noisemakers should remember that such measures are indeed estimates and that these soundmakers cannot be calibrated with the precision of electronic generators. They are useful in obtaining reflexive, arousal, and orientation responses in infants.

2. Localization procedures may give useful information about the better ear in infants from 3 or 4 months to 1 year and older. Speech (possibly filtered), narrow-band noise, and warble tones are good stimuli. By covering one ear or by delivering signals through earphones, a previously conditioned response may generalize to give information about each ear separately, or about bone-conduction sensitivity. Bone-conducted speech stimuli are useful for a quick estimate of cochlear levels.

3. Impedance audiometry is very helpful, giving sensitive information about the status of the conductive mechanism, and corroborative evidence about auditory sensitivity and sensorineural levels.

4. Recording of respiratory changes in response to auditory signals, evoked-response audiometry, electrocochleography, and other electrophysiologic procedures may give additional information. It is possible that these more complex procedures may not be necessary if good behavioral audiometry is done.

CASE HISTORY

The following case history demonstrates most of the techniques I have discussed. In this instance, we did some things well and some things poorly, and we were able to get an aid on the child at an early age. To our gratification he is now progressing well and using his hearing, I believe, to maximum benefit.

I first saw Gregory when he was 8 weeks old. Since 2 weeks of age, his mother had been concerned about his hearing. Normal pregnancy and birth were reported, and the otologic examination was negative. There was no familial history of hearing loss, and the child was not at high risk for hearing disorder for any other reason. The only unusual report was periodic nasal congestion. The mother's impression was that Gregory did not respond to sound at all during the first few weeks of life, but was currently responding to sound directed to the right ear. Consistent APRs were obtained when pure-tones were directed to the right ear at hearing levels of 90 to 110dB. Responses were obtained at octave intervals from 500 to 8000 Hz. No response of this sort could be obtained on the left ear. Attempts at impedance testing were unsuccessful because I could not maintain a seal on either ear.

The infant's responses together with the mother's observation suggested the possibility of a resolving conductive hearing loss. I concluded that hearing was functional—and perhaps functionally normal—on the right ear, with a probable loss on the left. I was not sufficiently convinced of the probability of permanent or handicapping hearing loss to recommend more extensive immediate testing. With the referring physician concurring, I recommended a retest in two months.

I next saw Gregory when he was 20 weeks old. The clinical picture had changed. Efforts at localization audiometry using narrow bands of noise and warble tones were unsuccessful, although the baby responded to speech in sound field at 70dB HL. APRs still resulted from pure-tone stimulation at 100 to 110dB (500 to 4000 Hz) on the right ear only. Tympanograms were Type C bilaterally and there were no acoustic reflexes. It seemed likely that my earlier impression of possible near-normal hearing on the right ear was probably in error. Current test results suggested a moderate loss on the right ear and a severe or profound loss on the left, with the possibility of a conductive component being present.

We enrolled Gregory for a period of diagnostic observation and therapy, seeing him three times each week. Our goals were to learn more about his hearing loss, to find an appropriate hearing aid, to stimulate awareness of sound, and to help his parents understand problems and solutions associated with hearing loss.

Over a period of two months we sometimes obtained Type C and occasionally Type B tympanograms. APRs could not always be elicited on stimulating the right ear, and never on the left ear. Concurrent ear, nose, and throat examinations were normal except for the observation that tympanic membrane movements were sluggish. The suspicion of bilateral secretory otitis media was established and a decongestant medication was initiated.

During this same period we began trying various moderately powerful body-type hearing aids. The child consistently responded to conversational-level speech with the aid on the right ear but never with it on the left ear. No tolerance problems were noted. When Gregory was 26 weeks old a body-type aid was recommended for the right ear, and the aid was purchased. The aid had an HAIC maximum gain of 55dB, maximum power output of 126dB, and a frequency range of 380 to 4400 Hz. With this aid, speech awareness responses at 30 to 35dB could be obtained. I did not recommend an aid with extended low-frequency response because of Gregory's demonstrated hearing across all of the speech range and my concern about possible masking of speech sounds by amplified low-frequency noise.

We began a period of hearing aid orientation for Gregory and his parents. It was fortunate that he had enough residual hearing to already be aware of the utility of sound. He must have quickly recognized the advantages of amplification, because he soon objected to removal of the hearing aid. We taught the parents how to put the aid on, adjust the controls, replace the batteries, and take care of the aid. We gradually increased the gain setting, until consistent responses were seen for low-level speech; we also increased daily use of the aid. By 34 weeks of age, Gregory was wearing the aid full-time.

When Gregory was 10 months old we instituted a home training program, teaching the parents effective methods of visual and auditory stimulation during everyday activity. We concentrated on achieving good speech-to-noise ratios. The child's vocalizations increased at an encouraging rate. At 14 months, he would wave bye-bye in response to the verbal stimulus, and look for the family pet when its name was spoken.

When Gregory was 16 months of age, the primary responsibility for his training was shifted to a local preschool center for the hearing-impaired. At the same time, working with the preschool, we began efforts to condition him to respond to pure-tones under earphones via play audiometry. By 22 months of age thresholds were tentatively established as shown in Fig. 5–5.

Because of continuing evidence of a possible conductive component, manifested in otologic examinations, by sporadically abnormal tympanograms, and air-bone gaps, ventilating tubes were inserted through the tympanic membranes when Gregory was 24 months old. Their presence was maintained for about six months. The audiogram shown in Fig. 5–6 was obtained at 28 months of age. At this time, responses to pure-tones were reliable, and I felt confident that test results approximated organic thresholds. This audiogram compares favorably with the latest obtained, at age 3 years 6 months, with no difference greater than ±10dB. Tympanograms currently are normal, with acoustic reflexes still absent.

At age 3 years 6 months, unaided SRT, obtained with spondee picture cards, is 70dB. A crude discrimination check reveals that, aided with 50dB

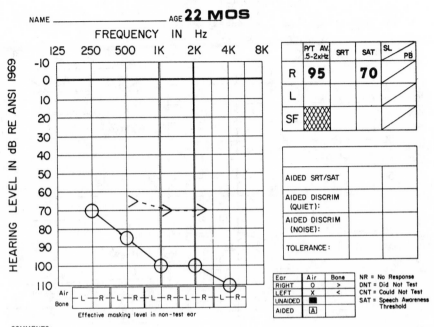

AUDIOLOGICAL RECORD

NAME _____ AGE **22 MOS**

COMMENTS:

Fig. 5-5. Tentative Thresholds Established by 22 Months of Age. (There was no response to A/C signals in the left ear or to 8000 Hz in the right ear. Bone conduction responses were unmasked.)

HL presentation, the child can discriminate 8 of 10 monosyllabic words. At the time of this evaluation he achieved a receptive vocabulary age of 2 years, 2 months on the Peabody Picture Vocabulary Test.

In preschool Gregory has made very good progress in language and speech development. He was originally enrolled in a Total Communication program but his excellent development of verbal language prompted his teacher to move to an exclusively oral-aural model. His spontaneous speech now consists of two- and three-word sentences. His voice quality is good, his rate and accent pattern quite good. He routinely produces vowels correctly but omits many consonants.

I should also mention that, during the time described above, Gregory has gone through three hearing aids of the same model. A strong and active child, he simply demolished the aids.

We were fortunate to recommend from the beginning a hearing aid that was quite appropriate. In many cases, revision of hearing-aid recommendations is necessary as the child matures and we learn more about his hearing. We sometimes first recommend a Y-cord amplification

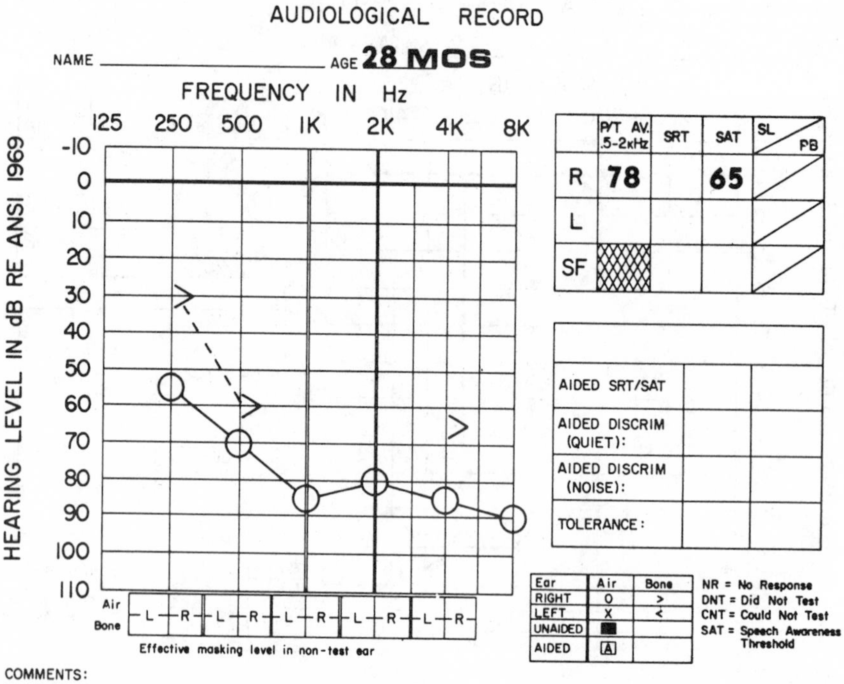

AUDIOLOGICAL   RECORD

NAME _____ AGE **28 MOS**

FREQUENCY   IN   Hz

Fig. 5-6. Pure-Tone and Speech Thresholds. (No reponse in right ear. No B/C response in left ear at 1000 and 2000 Hz. B/C response at 250 and 500 Hz may be tactile. Bone conduction threshold on thumb = 25dB at 250 Hz and 50dB at 500 Hz.)

arrangement if we cannot determine the ear best suited to amplification. Sometimes we realize the initial recommendation needs changing to achieve more or less gain. Because of this fact, flexible body aids with internal adjustments are useful. If both ears are eventually found to be appropriate for amplification, binaural aids may be recommended. I will probably eventually recommend an at-the-ear aid for Gregory, but for now, when optimum amplification is critical, a body-type aid is probably best. Gregory is learning to adjust and care for his aid himself, and this learning is probably facilitated by use of a body aid.

SUMMARY

In this chapter I have explained the procedures, clinical and experimental, that are used to evaluate auditory function in infants during their first year. When assessing hearing loss, it is important to know something about normal development and auditory responses in infants, and these areas are discussed briefly. I have reviewed the major studies of auditory assessment in infants and given my appraisal. I have tried to explain the test signals, conditions, and other variables which must be controlled for valid audiometry. The chapter is concluded with my recommendation of a battery of clinical procedures which I feel are useful in assessing auditory sensitivity of infants under 1 year of age.

RESEARCH NEEDS

Further validation is needed of tests and procedures in clinical use. More effective and efficient screening procedures are needed—ones that result in fewer false positives and false negatives and that can be universally applied with reasonable expense. Because of progressive and postnatally acquired loss we should investigate development of a system which incorporates screening procedures between birth and school age, to supplement existing neonatal and school screening.

We need better diagnostic procedures for assessment of infants who fail screening tests and tests that give more sensitive measurement of auditory threshold for each ear separately, and are applicable at an earlier age. For use with infants, we need validation and clinical adaptation of such promising procedures as evoked-response audiometry and electrocochleography. Assessment of compatible test batteries is required. The existing procedures estimate auditory sensitivity; we need ways to measure auditory discrimination ability.

We need better integration of diagnostic and habilitative services and service centers. We have not always kept up in habilitation areas with our ability to assess hearing loss. Coordination of diagnostic and habilitation programs and cooperation between specialists who operate these programs has at times been lacking, and ways to reduce this problem should be explored. Research to improve effectiveness of amplification and of training in its use is needed.

From a long-term viewpoint, exploration should be intensified in these areas: (1) better understanding of the causes of hearing loss in children, (2) prevention of hearing loss, and (3) restorative processes for the correction of conductive and sensorineural hearing losses, including cochlear implants, an area where some progress is being made.

REFERENCES

Aldrich, C., "A New Test for Hearing in the Newborn: The Conditioned Reflex," *American Journal of Diseases of Children,* 35 (1928), 36–37.

Altman, M., R. Shenhav, and L. Schaudinischky, "Semi-objective Method for Auditory Mass Screening of Neonates," *Acta Oto-laryngologica,* 79 (1975), 46–50.

Altman, M., R. Shenhav, and L. Schaudinischky, "Semi-objective Method for

Auditory Mass Screening of Neonates," in *Proceedings of the Nova Scotia Conference on Early Identification of Hearing Loss,* edited by G. Mencher. Basel: S. Karger, 1976, pp. 181-189.

Bench, J., "The Law of Initial Value: A Neglected Source of Variance in Infant Audiometry," *International Audiology,* 9 (1970), 314-22.

Bench, J., and L. Mentz, "Stimulus Complexity, State and Infants' Auditory Behavioral Responses," *British Journal of Disorders of Communication,* 10 (1975), 52-60.

Bench, R., "Sound Transmission in the Human Fetus through the Maternal Abdominal Wall," *Journal of Genetic Psychology,* 113 (1968), 85-87.

Bennett, M., "Acoustic Impedance Bridge Measurements with the Neonate," *British Journal of Audiology,* 9 (1975), 117-124.

Bove, C., and J. Flugrath, "Frequency Components of Noisemakers for Use in Pediatric Audiological Evaluations," *Volta Review,* 75 (1973), 551-556.

Bronstein, A., and E. Petrova, "The Auditory Analyzer in Young Infants," in *Behavior in Infancy and Early Childhood,* edited by Y. Brackbill and G. Thompson. New York: Free Press, 1967, pp. 163-172.

Butterfield, E., and W. Hodgson, "Tools for the Audiologic Study of Neonates." Scientific exhibit at the meeting of the American Speech and Hearing Association, Chicago, 1969.

Downs, M., "Report of the University of Colorado Screening Project," in *Proceedings of the Nova Scotia Conference on Early Identification of Hearing Loss,* edited by G. Mencher. Basel: S. Karger, 1976, pp. 77-89.

Downs, M., and G. Sterritt, "Identification Audiometry with Neonates: A Preliminary Report," *Journal of Auditory Research,* 4 (1964), 69-80.

Eisenberg, R., D. Coursin, and N. Rupp, "Habituation to an Acoustic Pattern as an Index of Differences Among Human Neonates," *Journal of Auditory Research,* 6 (1966), 239-248.

Eisenberg, R., E. Griffin, D. Coursin, and M. Hunter, "Auditory Behavior in the Human Neonate: A Preliminary Report," *Journal of Speech and Hearing Research,* 7 (1964), 245-269.

Eisenberg, R., A. Marmarou, and P. Giovachino, "Heart Rate Changes to a Synthetic Vowel," *Journal of Auditory Research,* 14 (1974a), 21-28.

Eisenberg, R., A. Marmarou, and P. Giovachino, "Heart Rate Changes to a Synthetic Vowel as an Index of Individual Differences," *Journal of Auditory Research,* 14 (1974b), 45-50.

Elliot, G., and K. Elliot, "Some Pathological, Radiological and Clinical Implications of the Precocious Development of the Human Ear," *Laryngoscope,* 74 (1964), 1160-1171.

Fantz, R., "Visual Perception from Birth as Shown by Pattern Selectivity," *Annals of the New York Academy of Science,* 118 (1965), 793-814.

Feinmesser, M., and L. Tell, "Neonatal Screening for Detection of Deafness," *Archives of Otolaryngology,* 102 (1976), 297-299.

Froding, C., "Acoustic Investigation of Newborn Infants," *Acta Oto-laryngologica*, 52 (1960), 31–40.

Fulton, R., P. Gorzycki, and W. Hull, "Hearing Assessment with Young Children," *Journal of Speech and Hearing Disorders*, 40 (1975), 397–404.

Hardy, J., A. Dougherty, and W. Hardy, "Hearing Responses and Audiologic Screening in Infants," *Journal of Pediatrics*, 55 (1959), 382–390.

Haug, O., P. Baccaro, and F. Guilford, "A Pure-tone Audiogram on the Infant: The PIWI Technique," *Archives of Otolaryngology*, 86 (1967), 435–440.

Jaffe, B., "Heredity and Congenital Factors Affecting Newborn Conductive Hearing," *Conference on Newborn Hearing Screening*. Washington: A.G. Bell Ass'n., 1972, pp. 87–101.

Kaye, H., and R. Levin, "Two Attempts to Demonstrate Tonal Suppression of Non-nutritive Sucking in Neonates," *Perceptual Motor Skills*, 17 (1963), 521–522.

Keith, R., "The Use of Impedance Measurements in Infant Hearing Programs," in *Early Identification of Hearing Loss*, edited by G. Mencher. Basel: S. Karger, 1976, pp. 68–75.

Liden, G., and A. Kankkunen, "Visual Reinforcement Audiometry in the Management of Young Deaf Children," *International Audiology*, 8 (1969), 99–106.

Lubchenco, L., F. Horner, L. Reed, I. Hix, Jr., D. Metcalf, R. Cohig, H. Elliott, and M. Bourg, "Sequelae of Premature Birth," *American Journal of Diseases of Children*, 106 (1963), 101–115.

Marquis, D., "Can Conditioned Response be Established in the Newborn Infant?" *Journal of Genetic Psychology*, 39 (1931), 479–492.

Matkin, N., "Some Essential Features of a Pediatric Audiologic Evaluation," Chap. 5, *Evaluation of Hearing Handicapped Children*. Denmark: Fifth Danavox Symposium, 1973.

Mencher, G., editor, *Proceedings of the Nova Scotia Conference on Early Identification of Hearing Loss*. Basel: S. Karger, 1976.

Mencher, G., "A Program for Neonatal Hearing Screening," *Audiology*, 13 (1974), 495–500.

Moore, J., W. Wilson, and G. Thompson, "Visual Reinforcement of Head-turn Responses in Infants under Twelve Months of Age," *Journal of Speech and Hearing Disorders* (in press).

Murphy, K., "The Psychophysiological Maturation of Auditory Function," *International Audiology*, 8 (1969), 46–51.

Mussen, P., J. Conger, and J. Kagan, *Child Development and Personality*, 4th ed. New York: Harper & Row, 1974.

Northern, J., and M. Downs, *Hearing in Children*. Baltimore: Williams and Wilkins Co., 1974.

Pratt, K., "The Neonate," in *Manual of Child Psychology*, rev. ed., edited by L. Carmichael. New York: John Wiley and Sons, 1965.

Rossi, P., and E. Guidotti, "Problems Associated with the Early Diagnosis of Deafness in Newborn Babies," in *Proceedings of the Nova Scotia Conference on Early Identification of Hearing Loss,* edited by G. Mencher. Basel: S. Karger, 1976, pp. 90–101.

Shirley, M., *The First Two Years.* Minneapolis: University of Minnesota Press, 1933.

Simmons, F., "Automated Hearing Screening Test for Newborns: The Crib-o-gram," in *Proceedings of the Nova Scotia Conference on Early Identification of Hearing Loss,* edited by G. Mencher. Basel: S. Karger 1976, pp. 171–180.

Simmons, F., and F. Russ, "Automated Newborn Hearing Screening: Crib-o-gram," *Archives of Otolaryngology,* 100 (1974), 1–7.

Smart, M., and R. Smart, *Children: Development and Relationships,* 2nd ed. New York: Macmillan Co., 1972.

Spock, B., *Baby and Child Care,* 4th ed. New York: Pocket Books, 1968.

Suzuki, T., and Y. Ogiba, "Conditioned Orientation Reflex Audiometry," *Archives of Otolaryngology,* 74 (1961), 192–198.

Vernon, M., "Prematurity and Deafness: The Magnitude and Nature of the Problem among Deaf Children," *Exceptional Children,* 33 (1967), 289–298.

Wedenberg, E., "Auditory Tests on Newborn Infants," *Acta Oto-laryngologica,* 46 (1956), 446–461.

Wedenberg, E., "Auditory Tests on Newborn Infants," in *Conference on Newborn Hearing Screening,* edited by G. Cunningham. Washington, D.C.: A.G. Bell Association for the Deaf, 1972, pp. 126–131.

Wolff, P., "The Causes, Controls, and Organization of Behavior in the Neonate," *Psychological Issues,* 5 (1966), 1–99.

Yerushalmy, J., "The Low-Birthweight Baby," *Hospital Practice,* 3 (1968), 62–69.

SUGGESTED READINGS

Eisenberg, R., *Auditory Competence in Early Life: The Roots of Communicative Behavior.* Baltimore: University Park Press, 1976.

Matkin, N., "Some Essential Features of a Pediatric Audiologic Evaluation," Chap. 5, *Evaluation of Hearing Handicapped Children.* Denmark: Fifth Danavox Symposium, 1973.

Mencher, G., editor, *Proceedings of the Nova Scotia Conference on Early Detection of Hearing Loss.* Basel: S. Karger, 1976.

Northern, J., and M. Downs, *Hearing in Children.* Baltimore: Williams and Wilkins Co., 1974.

CHAPTER SIX

Pure-Tone Tests of Hearing—
Age One Year through Five Years

ROBERT T. FULTON

INTRODUCTION

Pure-tone thresholds have long been the primary reference for defining the state of the auditory system. Even when other procedures designed for specific differential diagnostic purposes are used, their results are evaluated in relation to or in support of pure-tone thresholds. Accurate and reliable pure-tone threshold measures are equally as important—and perhaps more so—for young children than for older persons. For many young children an accurate assessment of hearing may be one of the most critical measures upon which their subsequent educational program is dependent.

CHAPTER OBJECTIVES

The development of communication skills is directly related to the capabilities of the auditory system and its cognitive relationship. Luria (1963) states that the ability to hear is a prerequisite to intellectual development, and that often ". . . a relatively inconsiderable, purely peripheral defect leads to extensive functional consequences." Even though the relationship between the auditory system and the development of communication skills has been well established and accepted by those concerned with communication disorders, there is considerable evidence that audiologists continue to use casual, inexact procedures and many times rely on a "clinical hunch" (Rosenberg, 1966) in measuring the hearing of children. ". . . In no other field of testing are the tests so poorly standardized, unobjectively administered, and poorly related to the behavior of the testee" (St. James-Roberts, 1972).

What is needed to help redirect the focus of the audiologic field is not still another test of hearing for young children, but better understanding of existing principles of behavior and measurement in auditory assessment. This chapter will examine those principles with the goal of helping the reader develop more accurate and precise skills for measuring children's auditory behavior.

The basic objective of this chapter is to inform the reader of the principles of determining pure-tone measures in young children.
More specifically, it will:

1. Discuss respondent and and operant behavior and their respective models and principles.
2. Discuss the integrity of auditory measurement.
3. Present and discuss examples of behavioral assessment of pure-tone measures with behaviorally difficult children.
4. Project the future of behavioral assessment and indicate research needs.

REVIEW OF LITERATURE

The literature indicates that only in the last few years has there been any significant effort to assess the hearing of children 3 years of age and under. Previously such assessment had been avoided because of the difficulties encountered. Most earlier studies dealt with children in the 4- to 8-year age range. Specific studies will not be reviewed here. Instead, they will be presented as they relate to topics under discussion throughout the chapter.

The literature on the auditory assessment of 1- to 5-year old children is less than comforting. Few studies with young children indicate criteria for demonstrating: (1) that the child understands the task—that is, that he demonstrates discriminative responding to an auditory stimulus; (2) that the procedural events actually have the desired operational effect on the child's behavior; (3) that the child's responses are reliable, or stable; (4) that the child was "successfully" assessed. For the most part, these functions and/or procedural operations have been established on the basis of individualized personal opinion—in other words, they represent the subjective judgment of the examiner.

Although the profession now recognizes the need for early identification and intervention and the problem of adequate assessment, few audiologists are attacking the issue with a zeal equal to their attacks on other audiologic problem areas. Perhaps this is because the problem involves coping with behavior, and behavior is often thought of as a nonquantifiable event or series of events. However, behavior can be dealt with in specific terms.

CLINICAL METHODS AND INTERPRETATIONS

Human behavior *is not static;* it is constantly varying. This is true whether you examine a biologic-physiologic response elicited by a stimulus or a volitional motor response to a stimulus. Hogan (1970, 1975) discusses the variability of the biological system, specifically the autonomic nervous system and its relation to the "law of initial values" in auditory measurement. Chapter 4 in this book also discusses biological and physiological behavior; therefore, discussion here will be directed primarily to motor behaviors.

Respondent Behavior: Classical—or Pavlovian—Conditioning

Behavior elicited by a stimulus is considered *respondent* behavior; it includes unconditioned and conditioned relfexes.

Unconditioned Reflexes. Certain stimuli will elicit specific responses in an intact organism without intervening conditioning or learning. A nipple placed against the cheek of a newborn infant will elicit head-turning and nursing behavior. Food placed on the tongue of a hungry organism will elicit salivation. These are but two examples of unconditioned reflexes. Those that have direct application to auditory assessment include the stapedial reflex to a loud stimulus, cortical or brainstem activity to a stimulus (Chap. 4), increased heart rate and respiration rate to a loud stimulus (Hogan, 1975), and the startle reflex to a loud stimulus (Chap. 5).

Relying on auditory stimuli (unconditioned stimulus) to elicit reflexes (unconditioned reflex) has two disadvantages for auditory assessment: First, many of these reflexes can be elicited only by a loud stimulus. Second, the organism tends to adapt to continued presentation of the stimulus; thus the strength of the reflex diminishes with increased presentations.

Conditioned Reflexes. It is possible to transfer the power of an unconditioned stimulus (UCS) to a neutral stimulus (NS) and elicit a response. The most familiar example of this technique is Pavlov's experiments in the 1880s in which he conditioned a dog to salivate at the sound of a bell. By pairing the sound of a bell with the presentation of food, Pavlov, after several trials, conditioned the dog to salivate in response to the bell. This procedure is commonly referred to as classical, or Pavlovian, conditioning. In the initial trials of this procedure the stimulus (in this case, the sound of the bell) is neutral and will not, of itself, elicit a response. However, if the neutral stimulus is temporally paired with an unconditioned stimulus (food), it will elicit an unconditioned response (salivation). After repeated trials, the response-eliciting power of the unconditioned stimulus will be transferred to the neutral stimulus. At this point, the neutral stimulus becomes a conditioned stimulus (CS) and the resulting response becomes a conditioned response (CR). The power of the conditioned stimulus to continue to elicit a conditioned response diminishes over time through repeated trials unless the conditioned stimulus is restrengthened by occasional re-pairing with the unconditioned stimulus.

The application of the classical conditioning paradigm to testing the hearing of newborn children was reported as early as 1928 (Aldrich). He used a dinner bell (NS → CS) and pin-scratch on the sole of the foot (UCS) to elicit a leg

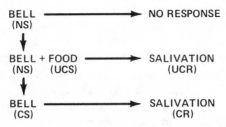

Fig. 6-1. Diagram of Classical (Pavlovian) Conditioning

withdrawal response (UCR → CR). Puffs of air on the eye (UCS) to elicit an eye-blink reflex (CR) have also been used to measure responses to auditory stimuli (CS) (Atkinson, 1959; Maietta, 1955).

The most notable application of this paradigm to the measurement of hearing has been the psychogalvanic skin response (GSR). Although Féré first noted the change in skin resistance in 1888 and Tarchenoff noted the change in skin potential in 1890, the use of the skin-resistance response in the measurement of hearing became most widely applied in the 1950s and 60s. GSR audiometry uses an electric shock as the unconditioned stimulus and measures the amplitude and/or frequency of the conditioned response, change in skin resistance, in relation to the conditioned auditory stimulus presentation. GSR has been used primarily in cases of hearing loss compensation by the Veterans Administration or with such difficult-to-test populations as the mentally retarded. Although it has been used with pediatric populations (Horton, 1952; O'Neil, Oyer, and Hillis, 1961; Statten and Wishart, 1956), it has little current support as a test for children.

OPERANT BEHAVIOR: INSTRUMENTAL—OR OPERANT—CONDITIONING

Thorndike introduced instrumental conditioning around the same time that Pavlov introduced classical conditioning. Skinner, however, is probably best known for his work with the instrumental-operant model.

To compare the two types of conditioning, in the *classical* model the response is *elicited by the conditioned stimulus;* in the *instrumental* model the response is *controlled by the consequences.* Skinner (1953) states: ". . . the term (operant) emphasizes the fact that the behavior *operates* upon the environment to generate consequences."

When a behavior generates a reinforcing consequence, there is an increased probability that similar behavior will reoccur. In this paradigm, a response is defined as a single instance of that behavior; an *operant* is defined as a class of responses that are controlled by their consequences.

Reinforcement and Punishment. Environmental events that have no specific effect on behavior are called *neutral events.* Environmental events that increase or strengthen the frequency of the behavior on which they are contingent are classed as *positive reinforcers;* events that increase the frequency of the behavior when they are withdrawn are classed as *negative reinforcers. An event can be classed as a reinforcer only when it strengthens (increases) the specific behavior under examination.* The mere application of an environmental event does not qualify that event to be classed as a reinforcer.

> Reward suggests compensation for behaving in a given way, often in sort of contractual arrangement. Reinforcement in its etymological sense designates simply the strengthening of a response. It refers to similar events in Pavlovian conditioning, where reward is inappropriate. These changes in terminology have not automatically eliminated purposive expressions (such as 'The pigeon was reinforced *for* pecking the key'), but a given instance can usually be rephrased. (Skinner, 1969, p. 109)

Punishment decreases or weakens the frequency of behavior. Careful examination of Table 6-1 is important in understanding the concepts of reinforcement and punishment. Response probability can be increased by either a positive reinforcement (that is, presenting a desired consequence, such as food, when the assigned response is completed) or negative reinforcement (that is, removing an undesired consequence, such as shock, when the assigned response is completed). Response probability can be decreased by either of two punishment procedures: presenting an undesired consequence, such as shock, for completion of a response; or removing a desired and available consequence, such as food, for completion of a response. It is often thought that presenting a desired consequence (for example, food) is the only form of reinforcement and that presenting an undesired consequence (for example, shock) is the only form of punishment. Yet, removing consequenting stimuli can also affect response probability. Removing or withholding a desired consequence for the correct responding behavior decreases the probability of continued behavior. This is called *extinction.* For example, a child who has maintained a high rate of motor behavior (button press) as a result of receiving a reinforcer (food) will decrease his motor behavior, extinguish, if the reinforcer is withheld.

TABLE 6-1. Effects on Response Probability of the Application of Consequences

Application of Consequating Event	Response Probability Effect	Procedural Name
Present	Increase	Positive Reinforcement
Present	Decrease	Punishment
Remove	Decrease	Punishment
Remove	Increase	Negative Reinforcement

Decreasing unwanted behavior by removing the opportunity for receiving a desired stimulus is called *time out*. Time out is an effective *punishment* procedure for decreasing response probability. For example, if an unwanted behavior from a child results in a delay, time out, in program continuation, or opportunity to receive reinforcement, the child will decrease the frequency of the unwanted behavior.

More specifically, *extinction* is the nonreinforcement of responses to the stimulus event under observation; whereas, *time out* precludes the occurrence of the stimulus event, thus eliminating an opportunity to receive positive reinforcement. Both decrease response probability. Extinction is often used to decrease response behavior to a specified stimulus, and time out is used to decrease random or nondiscriminative responding.

A few simple rules to remember about reinforcement are:

1. *Reinforcement controls (strengthens or increases) the response.* But every consequence following a response cannot automatically be called reinforcement.

2. *The strength of reinforcement is dependent upon the state of the organism under investigation.* More specifically, reinforcement is defined by the organism's behavior. What is reinforcing to one organism is not necessarily reinforcing to another organism. Moreover, what may be reinforcing to an organism at one time may not be reinforcing to that same organism at another time.

3. *Reinforcement is time-related.* Delays in reinforcement may affect intervening behavior.

In summary, consequation determines the effect on behavior (increase or decrease). When desired consequences are applied to behavior in the presence of an antecedent stimulus (for example, an auditory signal), the probability of that behavior's reoccurring increases.

Because of increased concern for human rights, and because it is morally and ethically appropriate, positive reinforcement procedures are usually preferred to increase response behavior, and the removal of a desired consequence is the preferred punishment to decrease unwanted behaviors.

Selecting Positive Reinforcers: Determining which consequences will result in reinforcement is critical. Remember, positive reinforcement is a consequential event that increases or strengthens the behavior under examination. In audiology we usually want to establish the strength of a specified response to a specified auditory stimulus.

More often than not, the examiner decides beforehand what agent will be used as a consequating event.

We achieve a certain success in guessing at reinforcing powers only because we have in a sense made a crude survey, we have gauged the reinforcing effect of a stimulus upon ourselves and assume the same effect on others. We are successful only when we resemble the organism under study and when we have correctly surveyed our own behavior. (Skinner, 1969, p. 109)

It is wise for examiners to reread Skinner's statement. Examiners who predetermine what agents are to be used as consequating events have often selected the agent on the basis of what they consider reinforcing, without considering the likes and dislikes of the subject. Candy is commonly used as a reinforcer. Some children do not like candy—or other edibles for that matter—unless they are subjected to a conditional state of deprivation. Small children often have small appetites and therefore are not highly reinforced by food. On the other hand, some small children have insatiable appetites for all foods. Some children are frightened by mechanical toys. The strongest reinforcing agent for some children is affection, attention, or praise; yet, others literally throw temper tantrums when spoken to or touched by anyone but their parents. In fact, some self-abusive children are reinforced by events that most persons would consider aversive. The point is, *the child being tested should select the consequating event*. If it strengthens the child's response behavior, the event is a reinforcer (S^R).

Over the years, edibles have been found to be an effective class of reinforcers. We have used candy, cereal, bits of fruits and vegetables, crackers, cookies, cheese puffs, and, for diabetics, sugarless foods. We also have used baby foods and a variety of liquids. Social praise, paired with the reinforcer, often strengthens the reinforcing event.

An effective way to determine the probable reinforcing strength of a particular item is for the examiner to display it in the palm of his hand. When the child reaches for the item, the examiner closes the fist over the item. If the child works to retrieve it, the item probably has reinforcing properties for that child. Another effective procedure is for a child to select an item from a display. These are only "preliminary screening procedures for selecting reinforcers." The proof of reinforcement lies in the demonstration of increased or strengthened response behavior.

A child old enough to understand the concept of purchasing can be asked to select a toy and told he can buy it with tokens he receives for responses to the test stimuli. Some children can be convinced to save edible reinforcers in a cup until the session is terminated—a technique that eliminates the problem of rapid satiation.

That a child indicates his choice of reinforcers on one occasion does not mean that the strength of that agent will be maintained over time or sessions. The examiner should periodically evaluate the effective strength of the consequating event.

Reinforcement Schedules. There is considerable evidence to indicate that operant behavior is more resistant to extinction under intermittent schedules of reinforcement than under continuous reinforcement schedules (CRF). Intermittent reinforcement may be either a fixed-ratio (FR) schedule, in which the subject is required to complete a predetermined number of responses for each reinforcer, or a variable-ratio (VR) schedule, in which he receives the reinforcer for a continuously varying number of responses. It is also possible to reinforce at fixed intervals (FI) or variable intervals (VI) of time; however, these schedules do not allow focus on discrete responses to stimuli, which is usually required in auditory assessment. Intermittent schedules, particularly variable-ratio schedules, are strengthened by the impact of anticipation on human behavior.

Reinforcement Delivery. Reinforcement should be delivered *immediately* upon completion of the desired response. A delay of even one or two seconds can result in the reinforcement of an unwanted intervening behavior. Suppose, for example, a child makes a correct response and then immediately picks his nose. A delayed reinforcer presented while the child is picking his nose reinforces the wrong behavior. When reinforcement cannot be delivered immediately, as happens with a food dispenser or liquids from a glass, it is advisable to use a *bridging stimulus.* A bridging stimulus may be a light or auditory signal that immediately indicates that a correct response has been made and that the primary reinforcer is forthcoming.

Attention should be directed to the placement and accessibility of reinforcement areas. Carefully planned response and reinforcement areas can enhance the efficiency and effectiveness of a procedure. Examiners should study children's motor behavior before they design a permanent delivery apparatus. This also holds true for planning response areas and the motor interactions between responses and reinforcement. Examiners should ask, for example: (1) Is the response mechanism easily accessible to the subject without strain or physical discomfort? (2) Is the accessibility to the reinforcer convenient to the subject upon completion of a response? (3) Does the subject have a comfortable resting position? A tired or confused subject is not ideal for high-performance responding.

Auditory Measurement

"Information is only as valid and reliable as the means by which it was obtained. . . . If a clinician or experimenter is unable to examine his assessment data with confidence, the tenet of his work has been violated" (Fulton, 1974, p. 11).

We all tend to approach the measurement of hearing rather casually and simplistically. More accurately, I think, we place such high priority on expedient resolution that we tend to thwart the very principles to which we wish to adhere. It is therefore appropriate to re-examine principles applicable to measurement.

Test (measurement) Instrument. Reliable measurement is a direct product of the test instrument. So first let's discuss some of the principles underlying test instrument construction. Since this chapter is focusing on the behavioral approach to auditory measurement, let's also examine this issue from the viewpoint of operant behavior.

Most of us view the operant audiometric paradigm as follows:

(Auditory Stimulus ———→ Response ————→ Reinforcer)

Such a view or reference is not inaccurate, but it leads to a simplistic and expedient view of the process. It assumes the interactions between the subject and the test instrument, the most complex component of the process, are relatively unimportant.

Applying the operant paradigm is not merely presenting an auditory stimulus, obtaining a response, and reinforcing that response. The stimulus does not "elicit" the response, which is then consequated, or reinforced. In the classical paradigm the stimulus elicits the response. In the operant paradigm the response is strengthened by the consequence—that is, the reinforcement. Then the auditory stimulus is introduced as a contingency to indicate the boundaries of the interval during which the response will result in a strengthening condition (reinforcement). Responses during the nonauditory stimulus (S^Δ) period can be consequated by extinction (nonreinforcement) or time out (nonreinforcement and punishment by delaying opportunity for next auditory signal); or by the punishment of presenting an undesirable consequence. This procedure provides differential consequation of the two stimulus conditions—auditory stimulus and nonauditory stimulus (S^Δ). When it is demonstrated that the desired response occurs during the presentation of the auditory stimulus and does not occur at other times, the auditory stimulus becomes known as a *discriminative stimulus* (S^D).

At this point two levels of control actually have been demonstrated—the level of reinforcement control (the response is under control of the reinforcer and an effective reinforcer has been established) and the level of stimulus control (the stimulus controls discriminative responding). In practice, we usually try to increase or strengthen the response at the same time that we are establishing discriminative responding, but it is important to understand the total process.

Comparatively, it is easier to bring aberrant behavior under control than it is to generate desired behavior for a given task. That is, it is easier to control response behavior of a hyperactive child than it is to generate response behavior in a nonresponsive child. Usually, with children 2 to 3 years of age and older, the problem is to channel response behavior in productive ways through contingency programs (sets of rules). With these children the application of programs to demonstrate the level of reinforcement control and the level of stimulus control can be conducted simultaneously. However, with more and more experience, we are finding that often the problem with children under 2 years of age (2 years of age is only illustrative and not definitive) is not the control of random behavior, but the lack of generative behavior. More specifically, with these children, we must first develop a productive response behavior, by increasing and strengthening that response through reinforcement, before we consider the relationship between that response and the stimulus with which we wish to assess the child. Until the desired response behavior is reliably demonstrated, there is no way to measure the child's perception of the stimulus.

Psychologists refer to this two-level total process as establishing "stimulus control." To an audiologist, the term "stimulus control" has the connotation of control of the physical parameters of the stimulus (i.e., frequency, intensity, and duration). As a behavioral audiologist, I am also interested in qualifying the response, so I am concerned with "response control." Therefore, the two issues in obtaining reliable auditory threshold measures are, first, to establish a procedure to insure that the response behavior is discriminative and, second, to insure that the discriminative stimulus contains only those acoustic properties I wish to include. I refer to such a procedure as *auditory stimulus-response control* (Fulton, 1974).

Most operantly based audiometric test instruments or procedures introduced have been modifications of the stimulus (S^D) or the consequence (S^R) events. Those procedures which introduce new or modified consequences (presumed to be reinforcers by the developer) do not direct their attention to qualifying response measurement. Instead, the proponents of this group of test instruments are in a subtle competition to demonstrate "my reinforcer is better than yours." These techniques abdicate the basic principles of reinforcement and discriminative responding.

Those test instruments which base their procedures on "novel," "less abstract," and "more meaningful" stimuli abdicate the principles of measuring the acoustic signal. They prefer to measure something of lesser or unknown quality.

The point, then, is that (1) you select the stimulus for which you wish to obtain measures and *arrange* for the control of the physical properties of that stimulus; (2) you define your response and assure (*arrange*) the integrity of that measure; and (3) you differentially consequate responses in an *arrangement* which strengthens the probability of obtaining the desired discriminative responding behavior.

Fig. 6-2 more accurately reflects the points of concern (arrangements) necessary for obtaining reliable responses to the stimulus under investigation. Again, the successful and efficient use of the operant paradigm is more than the mere occurrence of the stimulus, response, and consequential events. The control of those three events and the interactions (arrangement) between them is critical is achieving the goal of auditory stimulus-response control. The following sections discuss factors related to the arrangement interactions of the procedure.

Test Construction Criteria: Humans, children in particular, emit a variety of behaviors for a variety of reasons under a variety of conditions. The problem in

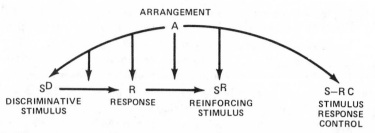

Fig. 6-2. Diagram of Stimulus-Response Control Procedure (modified version of operant conditioning model)

assuring reliable measurement is to bring the variables under systematic control by arranging contingencies. Some of the factors to be considered include:

1. Stimulus. Select and define the discriminative stimulus you want to measure. (In this chapter we are interested in pure-tones. Therefore, we will not consider the use of other stimuli—those that are presumably "less abstract" and "more meaningful" should be used only when they serve a specific purpose, never as substitutes for pure-tones.) Specifically define the physical and temporal parameters of the stimulus: frequency, intensity, stimulus duration, and stimulus presentation sequence.

   Because it is necessary to demonstrate discriminative responding between the auditory stimulus event and the nonauditory stimulus event, we must also define the nonauditory (S^Δ) event. Usually the nonauditory periods are longer in duration than the auditory stimulus periods; thus, a direct comparison of responses during these two periods is unequated. Only if specified samples of nonauditory periods (*control periods*) are observed for responses is it possible to separate discriminative responding from responding due to chance. Random, nondiscriminative responding will be evidenced by its occurrence during the control periods.

2. Response. Select the behavior you wish to define as the response and establish the criteria limits of that behavior. The response definition should clearly differentiate this behavior from other random behavior. The finer the definition of the response, the greater the likelihood of obtaining accurate information. Behavioral responses meeting carefully defined criteria are as "objective" as physiologic responses. The terms "objective" and "subjective" refer to the stringency of discriminative response criteria and should not be confused with differentiating between physiologic and behavioral responses.

3. Consequential event. The principles outlined previously dictate the relationship between this event and the effects on the response. Remember that the conditions of this event control the response; therefore, if careful adherence to these principles is not maintained, the response may be adversely affected.

4. Arrangement interactions. The interactions among the above three components are critical. Some factors to consider include:

   a. Temporal parameters. These include the temporal relationship between the stimulus presentation, the response availability period, and the delivery of the consequenting event, as well as the temporal parameters of the discriminative stimulus and the control period and their presentation schedule;

   b. Controls. Provisions must be made for mechanisms that demonstrate discriminative and/or differential responding (discussed in the section on audiometric procedures).

Data Reliability. Any test instrument should include elements for assuring that the response is reliable (stable over time) and that it measures what it purports to measure (validity, which is inferred from reliability).

The mere occurrence of a response to a stimulus does not assure that the response is reliable and not due to chance. It must be demonstrated that there is a greater differential probability of a response during stimulus presentation (S^D) than during nonstimulus presentation (control) periods. This principle is brought to to us from signal-detection theory.

Methods for demonstrating behavioral stimulus–response control include:

1. Two-interval forced-choice (2IFC). In this method the subject is taught that a specific response (R^1) indicates that the stimulus was perceived, while a different specific response (R^2) indicates that a stimulus was not perceived. The subject is then instructed that a given cue (often visual) will indicate that a stimulus trial is in effect and that he must make a decision whether he did (R^1) or did not (R^2) perceive the signal. The stimulus condition presentation must consist of one of two conditions— an audible signal (S^1) or a nonaudible signal (S^2). An analysis can then be made of the response behavior in relation to the stimulus condition.

   This differentiation seems like a simple task to most adults; however, many young children have difficulty in understanding this response task. This is an excellent procedure for long-term teaching or training of children's discrimination skills; therefore, the time spent training the task skill may be well worth the effort if a child is in a longitudinal program of discriminative training.

2. Go–No Go. The go–no go (G–NG) method is basically the same as the 2IFC procedure. However, in the G–NG, R^1 is a specific response and R^2 is the absence of R^1. Training to this procedure is difficult because many children continue to respond (R^1) to the presence of the trial cue (usually a visual cue) and disregard the primary auditory stimulus under investigation.

3. Simple detection response. In this procedure, the child is simply trained to make a well-defined response to the presence of an auditory stimulus

or a change in the auditory environment. Comparatively, this is a much simpler procedural task to train than either of the procedural tasks stated above. The $S^2 \longrightarrow R^2$ relationship mentioned above is resolved in this procedure by presenting S^2 to the subject without his awareness (no cues) and observing if R^1 occurs during that period. If R^1 does not occur during S^2, then you can assume that R^2 is under the control of S^2.

All three of these procedures can be analyzed by a chi-square analysis, tetrachoric table, as shown in Fig. 6-3. The number of stimuli and/or controls presented and the criteria for meeting stimulus–response control can be determined by the examiner. It is not necessary to complete a statistical chi-square analysis to examine discriminative control; it can be quickly analyzed by stating your criteria as the percentage of response behavior (or numbers of responses) you will accept in each cell to demonstrate stimulus-response control. The upper left quadrant indicates the number or percentage of hits, or R^1 responses, to the stimulus signal, or S^1, required to meet criteria for that particular cell. Criteria must be established for each of the other cells so that the totals equal the total number of presentations. Obviously the more stringent the criteria, the greater the reliability, and vice versa.

Establishing stimulus–response control with difficult-to-test children is not easy; however, it is essential to reliable measurements. The application of a procedure does not assure that reliable results will be obtained. It must be determined that the child understands the task by his demonstrating discriminative responding with that particular task. Statements are too often made about the auditory skills of children based on information obtained without their demonstrating discriminative responding. It has repeatedly been shown (Fulton, 1974) that retarded children can reliably discriminate a variety of signals that other investigators have believed are not within their repertoire of discriminative skills.

Reference to a specific case may clearly emphasize the point of demon-

	S^1/Signal	S^2/Control
R^1/Hit	# / % X trials	# / % Y trials
R^2/Miss	# / % X trials	# / % Y trials

Fig. 6-3. Tetrachoric Table for Determining Stimulus-Response Control

strating discriminative responding with each procedural task. Using a detection task, the subject under discussion demonstrated the ability to:

1. Provide stable repeated measure (test-retest) pure-tone auditory thresholds.

2. Detect at least 65% of the 1000 Hz signals (100 trials per each of 5 durations ranging from 14 to 112 milliseconds) presented at 10dB re pedestal tone 20dB sensation level.

3. Detect at least 50% of the interruptions of a pedestal tone (same variable as 2 above).

4. Detect frequency differentials of 6.1 Hz around 1000 Hz at least 70% of the time.

5. Detect intensity increments (re 20dB SL pedestal) of 1.2 to 1.4dB at least 46% of the time.

Because the subject had been such an excellent discriminative responder, I selected him to participate in a "two-interval forced-choice" (2IFC) task of discriminating format transitions which differed by several hundred Hz at the onset. After several sessions, the subject still demonstrated random responding. Assuming the subject might not have been able to contend with both a new procedure (2IFC) and new stimuli (format transitions), I changed the differential stimuli to white noise and pure-tones (1 KHz). After several sessions, the subject still demonstrated random responding. Using the same noise and pure-tone signals, the subject was required to *detect* the pure tone in the presence of a noise pedestal. Over 90% discrimination was demonstrated immediately. When I reversed the stimuli and required the subject to *detect* the noise in the presence of a pure-tone pedestal, the subject again immediately demonstrated better than 90% discrimination. I immediately reversed to the 2IFC procedure and required the subject to discriminate noise from pure-tone. The result again was random responding.

This example clearly indicates that the auditory system of the subject under examination could process the signals presented (detection); however, the subject did not clearly understand the 2IFC procedure (did not demonstrate discriminative responding). Had statements about the subject's auditory processing skills been made on the basis of 2IFC results, they would have been inaccurate. The subject was not under discriminative responding control during the 2IFC procedure.

Audiometric Procedures

The purpose of this chapter is to examine behavioral procedures for obtaining pure-tone hearing measures with children between the ages of 1 and 5. We have examined and discussed the inherent factors and issues (principles involved) in achieving reliable results in this goal. Relaxation of or nonadherence to these principles has an effect on the integrity of that goal or on the test instrument used to reach that goal. Now let us examine the current behavioral pure-tone assessment procedures in relation to the underlying principles stated above.

Conventional (Hand-Raising) Audiometry. Many children between 3 and 5 years of age can be auditorily assessed by instructing them to raise their hands when presented with a pure-tone signal. A variety of games have been devised to hold the attention and interest of this group of children. For example, the clinician may suggest that the child imagine that he is an astronaut or pilot and that he must signal (raise hand) each time he hears a coded message (pure-tone) through the earphones. This same type of game can be revised to have the child indicate which ear the coded message is being delivered to (ear-choice method, Curry and Kurtzrock, 1951; Lloyd, 1975). With some children a verbal response—"Yes," "I hear it," or "now"—is more reliable than hand-raising. Such children are not likely to say they heard the signal when they did not, but they are apt to raise their hand when the signal was not actually presented. In other words, verbal responses tend to reduce false-negative responses. Yet, other children are shy or withdrawn and it is very difficult for them to verbalize under any condition; for them, of course, hand-raising is the better response.

Because children of any age, particularly those younger than 5, are easily distracted from specific task performance, it is critical that the clinician be constantly alert for the loss of stimulus control and for variability in response behavior. The principles of test measurement and operant behavior, outlined above, are equally as applicable in this procedure as they are in other procedures. That is, conventional procedures tend not to be as specific in application as other procedures. Therefore, it is equally or even more important that attention be directed toward confirming that the response is discriminative or differentiated from other behavior during nonstimulus periods. The use of control periods—that is, nonstimulus-period sampling—is one way to demonstrate response reliability. More often than not, no provisions are made in conventional hand-raising or verbal-response procedures for demonstrating discriminative responding.

Remember, the strength of a response is controlled by the consequating environment. Therefore, a hand-raising response, like any other response, may weaken or extinguish without appropriate consequation. Social praise is often enough to sustain response strength; however, one should not depend upon this limited consequation.

In summary, the conventional hand-raising or verbal-response procedure is often the most expedient assessment procedure with cooperative children under good social control. However, this procedure is also subject to the behavior principles presented and the state of the children being tested.

Play Audiometry. Play audiometry is probably the most common procedure used in the pure-tone assessment of young children. In this procedure the child is instructed to engage in some activity—perhaps dropping blocks in a box, putting rings on a peg, putting pegs in holes, stacking blocks, or hitting a drum—each time he hears a signal. These activities are assumed to be interesting to the child and to reinforce his responding.

Barr (1955), credited with introducing play audiometry, indicated that "the youngest children tire comparatively quickly, and new games must be invented," and therefore recommended that a variety of activities and toys be available. Barr stated:

> Pure-tone audiometry comprises two equally important phases . . . . The first phase consists of *conditioning or learning,* the second of *threshold determination* (p. 25). . . . The moving of the marble becomes a "reward" for perception of the tone, while the "penalty" of being prevented from performing a pleasant action makes it clear to the child that he has not followed the "rules of the game" if he does not wait for the tone stimulus. Accordingly, the learning is based on traditional trial-and-error principles. (p. 40)

Personally, this is one of the most perplexing procedures used in the auditory assessment of children. I do not quarrel with the concept that play, if a variety of play activities are available, can serve as a reinforcing event for a specified response, but if moving the marble is considered the consequenting event (reinforcement), what is the response? And if moving the marble is the response, what is the consequenting event? This procedural arrangement can lead to confusion which results in noncontingent random playing.

When these questions are posed to some audiologists, I am told that the play is the response and verbal praise is the consequating event. Such a comment makes provisions for all three major elements of the operant paradigm; however, it also states that verbal praise is a reinforcing consequence for a "fun behavior" response. This is difficult for me to accept. That's like saying you will increase the probability that a child eats candy by saying "good boy" because eating the candy is a highly unstable behavior.

Play audiometry is probably often used because children who are initially shy and withdrawn can more easily be engaged in a play activity. Most clinicians, however, assume this display of extraverted behavior to be a resolution of the problem. It is not uncommon for clinicians to obtain the play behavior, then find themselves unable to control random playing. Thus the clinician must resort to a subjective judgment that "this play" is related to the signal presented but "that play" is not related. This procedure fosters a paradoxical state—a child is instructed to engage in a behavior he finds enjoyable, but then, because he enjoys it and begins playing when the clinician does not want him to, he is punished.

It is possible to translate play audiometry techniques into a functional procedure, but to do so requires adherence to the principles of the operant paradigm. Mechanical manipulation alone does not fulfill the necessary criteria. The biggest problem will be to find a consequating event that can control or strengthen play behavior, assuming the play behavior is the response.

Despite this biased view of the procedure, it is used with success by a large number of audiologists. The success rate for the procedure is acknowledged; however, the clinician should be aware of the problems that can and often do occur with the procedure.

Barr (1955) tested 135 children between the ages of 2 and 6 years with the "play" procedure, and found that the percentage of success was directly related to age. Successful tests were obtained with 16.6% of the 2- and 2½-year-olds, 55.5% of the 2½- to 3-year-olds, 70.7% of the 3-year-olds, 88% of the 4-year-olds, and 92% of the 5-year-olds. Overall successful tests were obtained with 73% of the children. Test-retest results of "successful" measures indicated no significant difference in reliability by age—82% of the test-retest measures were within ±5dB and 95% were within ±10dB. However, these results represent a small percentage of "successful" tests for children under 3 years of age. It appears the procedure is limited when assessing children under 3.

Procedures Using Picture Consequation. Dix and Hallpike (1947) introduced the "peep show" procedure which consequates responses to pure-tone signals by presenting an illuminated picture. In this procedure the child was instructed to look through a peephole in the test apparatus and press a button each time he heard a pure-tone signal presented via the speaker. Correct responses were consequated by seeing an illuminated picture.

Statten and Wishart (1956) advanced the concept of picture consequation with the construction of an elaborate doll house. The doorbell button of the doll house was the response button and a screen at the end of the hallway allowed slides to be presented for correct responses. This apparatus allowed for stimulus presentation by either earphones or a speaker. It also provided for the simultaneous pairing of a visual cue (porch light) with the auditory signal. These experimenters allowed subjects to investigate the doll house and when the subject pressed the doorbell button a slide was presented on the screen. As the response behavior developed, the auditory signal was introduced and the consequence was made contingent upon the response in the presence of the signal. The experimenters conducted 122 tests on 101 children from under 2 to 5 years of age. "Successful" audiograms were obtained with 8% of the children under 2 years of age, 43% of the 2-year-olds, and 80–93% of the children 3 years old and older.

Lloyd (1965), Miller (1963), and Shimizu and Nakamura (1957) also used slides as consequating events. Miller (1963) recommended slide sets that tell a story as opposed to unrelated pictures. Weaver (1965) used Walt Disney filmstrips. All of these procedures used earphones for presenting auditory stimuli and required a button-press response.

Liden and Kankkumen (1969a, b) did not use earphones, but placed speakers near (15 centimeters, or about 6 inches) the head. The nontest ear was plugged and slides were used as the consequence. Although their apparatus is similar in appearance to that used in conditioned orientation reflex (COR) audiometry, which will be discussed later, the experimenters indicated that it differed in response definition. They listed four types of responses: "reflexive behavior"; "investigatory responses"; "orientation responses"; and "spontaneous responses." In comparing their procedure—called visual reinforcement audiometry (VRA)—with COR audiometry, approximately the same results were obtained with children from 1 to 4 years old. After age 4, VRA was the recommended procedure.

The term "visual reinforcement audiometry" (Liden and Kankkumen, 1969a, b; Matkin and Thomas, 1974) is a misnomer based on the previously stated principles of reinforcement. Reinforcement is demonstrated by the strengthening of or increase in the response, not by labeling an event.

Procedures Using Mechanical-Toy Consequation. Conditioned orientation reflex (COR) audiometry (Suzuki and Ogiba, 1960; Suzuki, Ogiba, and Takei, 1972) is probably the most common procedure using mechanical-toy consequation. In this procedure the signal is presented through speakers mounted at approximately 45° angles on both sides of the subject. Mechanical dolls located immediately below the speakers are activated following a localization response. These investigators (Suzuki, Ogiba, and Takei, 1972) indicated they were able to obtain "satisfactory audiograms" with 38.5% of the children below one year of age and with 83 and 87% of the children ages 1 and 2 years, respectively. Success dropped to 64% for children 3 and 4 years old. Normative sound-field threshold data for the frequencies of 500Hz, 1000Hz, 2000Hz, and 4000Hz with children less than 1 year of age indicated that thresholds ranged from 25.9 to 27.8dB across frequencies. For children 2½ to 3 years of age, thresholds ranged from 11.4 to 12.5dB across the test frequencies.

Although there are several references to auditory sensory development, I find it a little difficult to accept that sensory threshold is related to age. The ear is physically and anatomically intact at birth. I feel it is more accurate to state that this change in sensory measurement is a product of the instrument or procedure used to measure sensory threshold and not a physiological phenomenon. (As used here, the measurement of the auditory sensory threshold differs from the measurement of auditory processing of complex signals. The detection of a simple auditory signal, such as a pure-tone, is processed at the peripheral level; in contrast, the processing of a complex signal, such as speech, occurs at a more central location and, in all probability, requires cognition, developmental skills, and other abilities.)

Suzuki, Ogiba, and Takei (1972) indicate that in 59% of the children "conditioning was achieved by one trial of combined tone-light stimulation" and in 80% it was achieved by two trials. This hardly constitutes a criterion for demonstrating a state of being conditioned. The state of being conditioned seems particularly questionable when the authors' own data indicate that extinction occurred within 3.0 (mean) trials at 50dB and 1.9 (mean) trials at 10dB.

This commonly used procedure has several undesirable features: (1) Sound-field stimulus-presentation techniques do not permit bilateral measurement and measure only the better ear. (2) Sound field stimuli are known to be unstable and are subject to gross intensity changes. (3) Localization responses are poorly defined and highly subjective. (4) No provisions are made for demonstrating that the responses are discriminative or that the consequence is reinforcing. Shortly after Suzuki and Ogiba introduced this procedure, Fulton and Graham (1966) used the procedure with 5- to 10-year-old retarded children, but abandoned it for the reasons stated above. Also the children quickly extinguished on the localization response, even with the exchanging of different dolls.

Matkin and Thomas (1974) used a procedure similar to COR audiometry, called visual reinforcement audiometry (VRA), with children 6 to 35 months of age. They indicated that children 24 months of age or older "conditioned" in one to four trials. They recommended the term "minimal response level" (MRL) instead of threshold and stated that this level improved with age through 23 months, then reached a plateau, but never reached adult norms. The experimenters' recommendation of the term minimal response level and their data that indicate it improves with age, point to the fact that results were probably more closely related to task performance than to the measurement of auditory acuity. Such an arrangement can lead to situations where the more skillful the subject is in task performance, the more acute his hearing sensitivity is judged to be. This condition lends support to the issue raised previously: Although auditory acuity is not a product of physiologic development, task performance for a given procedure may be related to development and age.

Thompson and Thompson (1972), in assessing 45 children from 7 to 36 months of age, found that play audiometry led to more responses than COR audiometry. They used a variety of stimuli (pure-tone, speech, filtered speech, noise, and filtered noise) and indicated that the children responded best to the speech signal and the 3000 Hz signal produced fewer responses than any other stimuli.

The PIWI (puppet in window illuminated) technique is modeled after the COR but uses earphones and requires a 90-degree localization response to the window (Haug, Baccaro, and Guilford, 1967).

The Pediacoameter (Guilford and Haug, 1952; O'Neill, Oyer, and Hillis, 1961) requires the child to press a button when a signal is presented through earphones. The consequence is a jack-in-the-box apparatus with seven dolls, one for each frequency. Guilford and Haug paired the auditory stimulus with a light during initial conditioning trials. O'Neill, Oyer, and Hillis indicated that with children 28 to 105 months of age, GSR was never successful when the operant (Pediacoameter and rear-screen slide projector) procedures were unsuccessful.

Other mechanical consequences have included a toy train (Ewing, 1930), battery-operated dog on a table (Green, 1958; Sullivan, Miller, and Polisar, 1962), pop-up toys (Knox, 1960), and a merry-go-round (Denmark, 1950).

My disappointment and dissatisfaction with such consequating procedures is that the advancement of procedural technology since the toy train or the "peep show" has been limited to the theme of "my reinforcer is better than yours." Other than the use of earphones instead of sound field, these procedures have advanced little in three decades. In fact, Statten and Wishart's (1956) contingencies were more advanced than most procedures commonly in use today. Statten and Wishart made provisions for pairing a visual cue with the auditory signal, if needed, in the training phase. They also based their procedure on a "free operant" technique that allows a child to investigate his environment before the contingencies are introduced.

Behavioral Observation and Other Localization Procedures. Behavioral observation audiometry (BOA) procedures are similar in principle to the COR procedure, but do not necessarily include response consequation. Various stimuli are presented through speakers placed at an angle to the subject, and responses are observed by the examiners. DiCarlo and Bradley (1961) used music, white noise, and recorded pure-tones from four speakers with 50 children of ages 10 months to 3 years and found 31 had normal hearing and 19 had hearing losses.

Thompson and Weber (1974) used both BOA and "play" audiometry with 190 children 3 to 59 months (164 over 12 months) of age. Children over 18 months of age were tested with play procedures. The BOA procedures used two observers and noise and speech stimuli. Their results indicated that response levels were related to age until approximately 2 years of age and then plateaued (these results are similar to those previously discussed with COR). The investigators indicated, however, that these responses were arousal levels, and thus were high. They concluded that BOA is best suited as a screening assessment procedure. Only 2% of the children under 24 months of age responded to play audiometry.

From my own clinical experience, I concur with Thompson and Weber's statement that BOA, or any localization procedure, is a screening procedure or a procedure for obtaining reference data for other procedures. Unfortunately, many clinicians use BOA procedures as the sole measure of auditory sensitivity and make diagnoses based on this information.

Moore, Thompson, and Thompson (1975) used "complex visual" (animated toy), "simple visual" (blinking light), "social" and "no" consequations with 12- to 18-month-old children ($N = 12$ each consequence) and found that the "complex visual" consequence was the best and the "no" consequence the poorest (30 stimuli per condition). They claimed 99% interjudge reliability for observations of both stimulus and control trials. A response was defined as a head turn in the direction of the loudspeaker during or immediately after each presentation. The children responded to only 4.8% of the control trials. Lloyd and Wilson (1974) also reported that 3- to 6-month-old children responded better to the "complex visual" than to the "no" consequence condition.

BOA responses are highly unreliable measures. This opinion is borne out by Bench et al. (1976a, b) and Moncur (1968). Bench et al. (1976a), in an extensive analysis using a signal detection model and prestimulus analysis of videotaped BOA responses in neonates, stated, "This implies either that the behavioral responses occur sometimes in one part of the body and at other times in other parts, even for the same stimulus. Certainly, we found no specific behavioral acoustic reflex pattern." In a six-week follow-up study of essentially the same group of babies, they concluded:

> ... it is probably easier to obtain responses to most of the stimuli described at 6 weeks rather than during the first few days of life, but not markedly so. This difference between the two ages is probably largely due to the fact that neonates tend to fall into deep sleep over a period of testing more readily than do six-week-old infants. It is thus not necessarily the case that the older infants have lower auditory "thresholds" than the newborn .... Many observations indicate that audiometric behavioral testing of six-week-old infants is no easy task. (Bench et al. 1976b, p. 313)

Even though these studies were conducted with neonates and 6-week-old infants, the point is that it is very difficult to attain any reliability with this procedure.

Moncur's (1968) study of test-retest judgments of videotaped BOA responses in 8-month-olds further supports this point. Experienced pediatric audiologists, nonpediatric audiologists, and lay persons were the judges; two judgment systems were used. The first system required a single judgment of what response occurred; response events were classed as localization, body movements, facial movements, cessation or diminution, and status quo (no activity). The second system required two judgments: first, did a response occur—yes or no; and second, what was the strength of the response, scaled mild to strong? It was found that experienced pediatric audiologists indicated only slightly better test-retest agreement than the lay persons (87.5% to 82.0%); nonpediatric audiologists scored lowest (79.0%). Some of the findings from Moncur's extensive analysis are worth note: (1) Judges reversed themselves (second test) on 18% of the events. (2) Of the reversals 9% occurred on "no-stimulus" trials. (3) Judges indicated a response to 39% of the "no stimulus" trials and did not improve their skill on the second judgment. (4) The experimenter felt that reliability would be even lower with lower-intensity stimulus trials (stimuli were presented at 40 and 60dB). (5) If lay persons are instructed, they make better judgments than nonpediatric audiologists and almost as accurate judgments as experienced pediatric audiologists. Some of Moncur's findings may be more revealing about our skills as observers of behavior (the basis of auditory assessment) than we care to admit.

Wilson[1] and the University of Washington group are attempting to bring the localization response under tighter control. Their procedural approach differs from BOA in that they limit the behavioral response to a definite head-turning (localization) response. Other behaviors such as eye movement, facial change, and such are not considered responses. In limiting the response criteria they are able to achieve greater observer reliability than noted by Bench et al. (1976a and b) and Moncur (1968). They have also indicated that the use of control trials (nonaudible stimulus trials) and observer reliability is standard practice in test applications. Finally, their use of mechanical dolls as reinforcers is a vast improvement over previously mentioned methods. In this procedure the test room is kept free of items that may be visually distracting or reinforcing. The mechanical dolls (reinforcers) are housed in smoked glass containers and are only visible (lighted) during appropriate consequation periods. The containers are portable and can be moved into the most advantageous proximity to the child under test. Because most of the current work by this group is concerned with suprathreshold measures of complex stimulus discriminations, they continued to present the stimuli via sound field. However, their procedures are also definite improvements over other sound-field procedures for gross binaural threshold measures.

Many of the procedures mentioned thus far, particularly BOA procedures, have used a variety of auditory stimuli. Noise and, more recently, filtered noise, have been commonly used. Whatever may be said about a child's ability to respond with greater ease to noise stimuli than to pure-tone stimuli, the physical properties of a noise stimulus must be considered. Even though a noise stimulus can be filtered to center at a specific point (for example, centered at 1000 Hz), this does not mean that the filtered noise stimulus can be equated to a 1000 Hz pure-tone. A good filter or narrow-band filter may "roll off" (attenuate) as much as 25dB per octave on each side of the center frequency. The responses obtained with such a stimulus can be misleading, particularly with persons having precipitous losses. For example, if a person indicates a response threshold to a filtered noise stimulus centered at 1000 Hz at 70dB, you do not know if that is the subject's response threshold for that particular stimulus or whether the response was to the ear being stimulated at 45dB at 500 Hz (an attenuation of 25dB per octave) or at 20dB at 250 Hz. Most commercial narrow-band masking generators attenuate around 7 to 10dB per octave. Therefore, the result would be even more deceiving than in the example presented. Orchik and Mosher (1975) demonstrate these effects in clinical application. In summary, noise, even filtered noise, can be a very deceptive stimulus for persons with precipitous losses.

Operant Audiometry. This generic term is truly a misnomer—all of the procedures thus far mentioned are based on measuring operant behavior. Lloyd

[1] Personal communication from Dr. W.R. Wilson, University of Washington, 1976.

(1966) discusses this point. The term evolved, or perhaps we should say caught on, from the strong influence of behavioral (operant) psychologists in the early days of adding more structure to the measurement of motor behavior responses in auditory assessment.

Meyerson and Michael (1960) and LaCrosse and Bidlake (1964) were among the early pioneers in this approach. In the mid-1960s, the Parsons Research Center and Parsons State Hospital and Training Center began to establish itself as a primary facility for advancing this approach. Lloyd, an audiologist, and Spradlin, a psychologist, with input from some of the earlier work began to structure an operant procedure for difficult-to-test (mentally retarded) persons (Lloyd, Spradlin, and Reid, 1968; Spradlin, et al., 1968). Although their stimulus-generation-and-response (button-press) instrumentation was not revolutionary, their procedures for conditioning were based on solid instrumental conditioning principles. They found that stimulus presentation, responses, and consequation could be controlled electromechanically. Also, they found that edible items or tokens that could be exchanged for other desired items usually served as reinforcing consequences and could be dispensed mechanically. This work led to the advent of the term TROCA (tangible reinforcement operant conditioning audiometry) (Lloyd, Spradlin, and Reid, 1968). Lloyd and Wilson (1974) have extended the TROCA procedure to young children (12–20 months).

Psychologists Bricker and Bricker (1969a, b) were also working on the problem of assessing retarded children at approximately the same time as the Parsons group. As might be expected from their psychology backgrounds, Bricker and Bricker concentrated on investigating training and generalization concepts, rather than stimulus properties. Their work demonstrated that procedures which pair a light with the auditory stimulus presentation require longer training sessions than procedures which train children to respond to the auditory stimulus alone.

It appeared at that time that the state of the art in the auditory assessment of difficult-to-test persons could be summarized as follows: (1) Some audiologists concentrated on manipulating the auditory stimulus (discriminative stimulus–S^D). This was based on their assumption that these populations could not respond to "abstract" and "meaningless" pure-tone signals; thus, they recommended noise, speech, and other complex signals. (Interestingly, pure-tone signals are processed peripherally, whereas complex signals are processed more centrally.) (2) A majority of the experimenters were manipulating the consequenting event and essentially were in a procedural conflict of demonstrating that "my reinforcer is better"—a fruitless contest at that, since examiners do not determine reinforcement. (3) There was unequal concern with the calibration of a stimulus (an easily quantifiable event) and the quantification of the behavioral response—a condition that is still prevalent. (4) Criteria for establishing a basis on which audiograms could be judged to be "successful" were significantly absent.

Although the initial work at Parsons did adhere to reinforcement principles, I felt, and still feel, that the acronym TROCA focuses attention on the reinforcement element of the paradigm and distracts from the primary goal of obtaining reliable responses to the auditory signal.

With a basically sound initial procedure that incorporated the principles of operant behavior and a compulsion for organization and test reliability, the question was, "Where do we go now?" The answer—refine and generalize, but never sacrifice reliability or principles.

The solution to further refinement lay in the interaction (arrangement) between the stimulus, response, and consequence events. (This was discussed earlier and is diagramed in Fig. 6-2). The refining process was one of repeated redesign and application to gain greater control over the variety of behaviors that emerged from the subjects. More accurately, the subjects taught us which procedures were successful—that is, which they would respond to reliably; we taught the subjects relatively little. Professionals learn slowly. It took several years to learn and to implement what the childrens' behavior was routinely telling us; yet these children learned to complete the task within minutes or at most a few hours.

The resulting procedural refinements are too lengthy and complex to address here, but they have been published (Fulton, 1974; Fulton and Spradlin, 1971, 1975; Spradlin, Locke, and Fulton, 1969) and presented on film (Fulton and Spradlin, 1973). The term "auditory stimulus–response control" has been used to title these procedures, drawing attention to what I feel is the critical issue—control of the stimulus, the response, and the stimulus-response interaction. The current procedures acknowledge the power of the reinforcement principle, adhere to its principles, and support its use. The primary issue, however, is behavioral management and control.

"Auditory stimulus–response control" (AS–RC) procedures (Fulton, 1974) use earphones for stimulus presentation, discrete button-press response, and reinforcement consequation, found in many procedures. However, emphasis is placed on provisions for other related factors which include:

1. The child becomes an active participant in the selection of a consequating event or agent.
2. The physical parameters of the signal and its presentation schedule are specified.
3. A button-press response with electronic programming arrangements to control its relation to the stimulus and the consequences is used. Attention is also given to the mechanical properties and topography of the response mechanism.
4. A programming arrangement makes provisions for reinforcing desired behavior and punishing undesired behavior.

5. The procedure has provisions for analyzing response behavior as discriminative or random.

6. The procedure is sequenced for training children in detection and generalization concepts.

Training children in detection and generalization concepts is one of the most significant features of the procedure. The AS–RC procedure trains subjects to detect acoustic changes in their auditory environment. This procedure also allows for generalization to the assessment of air- and bone-conduction thresholds, masked thresholds, the short-increment sensitivity index, the tone-decay test and psychoacoustic measurement—that is, frequency, intensity, and time (Fulton, 1974). Waryas and Brandt (1977) used the same model to study periodicity pitch perception. This AS–RC procedure was also shown to provide reliable repeated measures under varying reinforcement schedules and threshold-search techniques.

Since AS–RC procedures had been initially developed to assess severely retarded children, it was questioned whether the procedures were applicable to young children. Fulton, Gorzycki, and Hull (1975) extended a modified version of the procedure to children 9 to 25 months of age (mean = 13.8 months). Data were obtained on 7 of 12 subjects (2 were withdrawn as subjects and stimulus control criteria could not be established with 3). Of the test-retest threshold measures obtained, 73.9% were within ±5dB and only 7.6% were greater than ±10dB. Threshold validity was supported with impedance-tympanometry measures. Two of the subjects demonstrated ±5dB variability over six repeated measures (1000 Hz, right ear).

Nowles (1971) also found reliable (±5dB) test-retest results with 10 children from 18 to 30 months of age (mean = 26 months) using a modified version of the AS–RC procedure. All 10 children were conditioned within 2 to 9 (mean = 4.7) sessions of 15 to 30 minutes each.

Volkland (1972), using a modified version of the AS–RC procedure, obtained ±5dB test-retest threshold with five of six hard-of-hearing children (3 years 4 months to 7 years 10 months; mean age = 5 years 8 months). The procedure was also found applicable in obtaining sound-field responses from children wearing aids.

As should be expected, the AS–RC procedures could be generalized across populations. Generalization should be expected because behavior is not limited by etiological nor chronological boundaries. Hyperactivity, motivation, or any other behavioral variable may be found in all populations.

Masking

Most of the procedures discussed in this chapter make no provisions for obtaining masked thresholds when the need for such a measure is indicated. For those children who can follow conventional hand-raising or verbal-response procedure instructions, the introduction of a masking stimulus is not a major problem. The child is instructed to continue to listen for the "coded message" despite the noise.

Lloyd, Spradlin, and Reid (1968) recommended a technique in which the masking stimulus was gradually increased in intensity as stimulus control was maintained with the TROCA procedure.

Fulton's (1974) AS–RC procedures include provisions for training children to detect any acoustic change in their auditory environment. In completing the training sequence, the child is trained to detect a discriminative stimulus from a background of various noise and pure-tone stimulus conditions. With this training sequence, the child is trained to respond to any noise condition, including the absence of noise as found in unmasked thresholds. These same procedures permit the assessment of masked thresholds (air and bone), the short-increment sensitivity index, the tone-decay test, and psychoacoustic measures such as frequency-and intensity-difference limens.

Fulton (1974) and Lloyd, Spradlin, and Reid (1968) refer to Studebaker's (1964) procedures for applying masking levels. Other masking level procedures are also adaptable to either the AS–RC or TROCA procedures. Martin's (1972 and 1975) masking procedures are also recommended for their simplicity and ease of application.

Bone Conduction

Other than the AS–RC and TROCA procedures, bone-conduction responses are not discussed. However, any procedure that presents the discriminative stimulus through earphones also can be adapted to obtain bone-conduction measures. These measures are obtained in the same manner as air-conduction measures, except that the type of transducer delivering the signal and the level of masking needed differ. Again, Martin (1972 and 1975) and Studebaker (1964) are recommended for masking-level procedures.

Presenting the discriminative stimulus via a bone transducer also can often be an asset in developing auditory stimulus–response control with children having a profound hearing impairment. That is, when a child's estimated thresholds are near the limits of the audiometer, it is better to develop auditory stimulus–response control with a more intense signal, such as a bone response, then assess air-conduction thresholds after stimulus–response control has been established.

The Future of Behavioral Measurement

The future of behavioral auditory measurement with young children depends upon the philosophic stance and attitude of audiologists. Most audiologists can deal with routine hearing assessments and may never be confronted with the problems of assessing the difficult-to-test person. The bulk of the population is over 5 years of age; such subjects pose few problems in auditory measurement because they can follow complex procedural instructions If, however, audiologists believe that it is of utmost importance to identify auditory pathologies and provide corrective measures—either treatment or educational programming—at the earliest possible age, the problem of obtaining reliable auditory responses from young children must be squarely faced.

First, the principles for managing and analyzing behavior and for developing assessment and training procedures must be clearly understood. Second, quality of the measurement must assume priority over test-time expediency. These and other issues are not independent of each other. A review of currently available procedures clearly supports the need for more affirmative approaches and attitudes to the problem. Most procedures currently in use do not adhere to the principles of behavior management and auditory measurement; rather, they are designed to provide information quickly, without provisions for quality control of measurement. Over the years the most frequent reaction to the AS–RC procedures is that practicing audiologists and the facilities in which they work do not have time to use such a procedure. Seldom is there any reference to the procedure's reliability. Most audiologists are incensed by the accusation that the techniques they use provide low-quality service. But it is a fact that the overwhelming majority of difficult-to-test persons—including the pediatric population—are assessed with subjective observation techniques taking just a few minutes, and on this basis a diagnostic judgment is made.

The need for quality measurement is there. Children with deafness, hearing impairment, otologic pathologies, and detracting behaviors are waiting for quality attention. The principles for designing procedures are there. The technology for quantifying and qualifying behavior is there. The electronic and mechanical technology for implementing procedures is there. The question is, is the desire and philosophy to challenge the problem there? I think so. It just needs to be aroused. After all, we are contributing professionals, not technicians.

Behavioral measurement is becoming more and more important. It not only reflects how an organism's biologic system processes an incoming signal but also how that organism interrelates that event with all other impinging events and conditions.

CASE HISTORIES

The interpretation of test results and diagnosis for young children should not differ from that for persons of any other age range, even though the recommended treatment or training may vary with the age of the individual. Reliable results should reflect the capabilities of that particular individual's sensory system. The presence of disruptive behavior or the inability to establish stimulus-response control should not be confused with the pathologic state of the auditory system. More often than not, a description of a child's auditory capabilities is confounded by an analysis based on his behavioral skills.

Following are a few examples of interesting behaviors that have been observed over the years during the auditory assessment of difficult-to-test children.

One child could never be trained to make a button-press motor response. Instead, he made a vocal utterance which matched the pitch of the test signal each time the signal was presented. The reinforcement apparatus was controlled from the control room since the subject would not make a button-press response. The child never failed to make the vocal imitation when the signal was above threshold (demonstrated by repeated measurement) and never was noted to make the vocalization during a nonstimulus period.

Most children I have seen are unable to last in test sessions for more than 30 minutes. However, one schizophrenic child required an hour of withdrawal (hiding her head, etc.) and random play with the apparatus. Then, with only a short break for water during the session, she would settle down to another full hour of discriminative responding.

One child was reinforced by being allowed to show his anger and throw the candy that was dispensed for a correct response. This child was under excellent stimulus-response control. The consequence provided him with an item to be thrown and the opportunity to vocalize his displeasure. This increased and maintained his response behavior and thus was his reinforcer.

One little girl understood the concept that a button-press response in the presence of a signal generated a consequence, because she demonstrated correct behavior. During two sessions she "teased" the button with her finger and talked to it, trying to get the response button to activate upon her command. Another child pushed the button discriminatively with everything but his hand. Instead he used his nose, foot, elbow, or chin.

A 12-year-old retarded schizophrenic child had to be kept in psychiatric isolation (without even furniture) because of her destructive behavior, yet she was one of the most precise, accurate, and reliable responders I have ever seen. She would respond only for candy mints. If any other item was used as a consequence, she would try to destroy the apparatus.

A parent told us that her child did not like M&M candies and this statement appeared accurate during initial reinforcer selection periods. Yet, as training began and experimentation for effective reinforcers continued, M&Ms were reintroduced and accepted. In fact, not only did the child accept them, but he would work for 50 to 60 M&Ms per session for many sessions. The child is continuing to work for M&Ms in subsequent language training programs, and the mother continues to state that the child does not like M&Ms.

It is very common for clinicians to become very impatient because behavior cannot be shaped immediately. In most of these cases, behavior has been shaped—the clinician fails to recognize that he has been shaped by the child!

SUMMARY

A brief but emphatic discussion of the need for accurate pure-tone thresholds has been presented with no attempt to provide a list of procedures that are presumably designed for specific age levels, etiologies, or pathologies. Nor was an attempt made to relate developmental behavior to various auditory stimuli. Instead, the chapter took the position that the auditory system is intact at birth and that given behaviors can be exhibited and/or controlled at any age. The point, then, was not to present prescriptive techniques, but rather to present basic principles of behavior, behavioral control, and measurement integrity. Within this framework, example procedures were presented and their relation to the basic principles discussed. For the most part, the example procedures indicate that most current procedures did not adhere to the principles of behavioral control and reliable auditory measurement.

The purpose of this format was not to provide the audiologist with procedures and techniques that he can immediately implement. Simple reliance on implementing prescriptive techniques presumes that the audiologist, or, "consumer," takes on a technician's role. On the other hand, the audiologist's professionalism presumes him to be analytic and generative. The state of the art in auditorially assessing young children is neither adequate nor stable. Therefore, the purpose of the chapter is to present the reader with information that would challenge him, encourage him to be analytical, and, I would hope, encourage him to generate effective procedures based on sound principles.

RESEARCH NEEDS

It is tempting to develop a list of specific research questions that should be investigated. Such a list, however, is not consistent with this chapter's intent of attempting to make the reader analytical and generative. It does not appear too structured, however, to indicate the obvious. *Quality* procedures that incorporate efficiency need to be developed, or existing procedures need to be refined to provide quality measurements efficiently. To do so, we must investigate the parameters of response behavior with the same degree of specificity that we investigate the effects of the acoustic signal on the auditory system. The many auditory differential diagnostic tests currently available could provide us with valuable information about a developing individual; however, we have not yet developed sufficient skill in applying them to the behaviorally difficult. I would hope that, through research, we can become as knowledgeable about behavioral management as we are about the functioning of the auditory system.

REFERENCES

Aldrich, C.A., "A New Test for Hearing in the New-Born," *American Journal Diseases of Children, 35* (1928), 36–37.

Atkinson, C.J., "Perceptive and Responsive Abilities of Mentally Retarded Children as Measured by Several Auditory Threshold Tests," U.S. Office of Education, Cooperative Research Project No. 176 (6471), Southern Illinois University, Carbondale, Illinois, 1960.

Atkinson, C.J., "The Use of the Eyelid Reflex as an Operant in Audiometric Testing," *Journal of Experimental Analysis of Behavior, 2* (1959), 212.

Barr, B., "Pure Tone Audiometry for Pre-school Children," *Acta Oto-laryngologica Supp. 121,* 1955.

Bench, J., Y. Collyer, L. Mentz, and I. Wilson, "Studies in Infant Behavioral Audiometry: I. Neonates," *Audiology,* 15 (1976a), 85–105.

Bench, J., Y. Collyer, L. Mentz and I. Wilson, "Studies in Infant Behavioral Audiometry. II. Six-Week-Old Infants," *Audiology,* 15 (1976b), 302–314.

Bricker, D., and W.A. Bricker, "A Programmed Approach to Operant Audiometry for Low Functioning Children," *Journal of Speech and Hearing Disorders,* 34 (1969a), 312–320.

Bricker, W.A., and D.D. Bricker, "Four Operant Procedures for Establishing Auditory Stimulus Control with Low-Functioning Children." *American Journal of Mental Deficiency,* 73 (1969b), 981–987.

Curry, E.T., and G.H. Kurtzrock, "A Preliminary Investigation of the Ear-Choice Technique in Threshold Audiometry," *Journal of Speech and Hearing Disorders,* 16 (1951), 340–345.

Denmark, F.G.W., "A Development of the Peep-Show Audiometer," *Journal of Laryngology and Otology,* 64 (1950), 357–360.

DiCarlo, L.M., and W.H. Bradley, "A Simplified Auditory Test for Infants and Young Children," *Laryngoscope,* 71 (1961), 628–646.

Dix, M.R., and C.S. Hallpike, "The Peep Show: A New Technique for Pure-Tone Audiometry in Young Children," *British Medical Journal,* 2 (1947), 719–723.

Eagles, E.L., and S.M. Wishik, "A Study of Hearing in Children," *Transactions of the American Academy of Opthalmology and Otology,* 65 (1961), 261–282.

Ewing, A.W.G., *Aphasia in Children.* London: Oxford Medical Publications, 1930.

Fulton, R.T., editor, *Auditory Stimulus-Response Control.* Baltimore: University Park Press, 1974.

Fulton, R.T., P. Gorzycki, and W. Hull, "Hearing Assessment with Young Children," *Journal of Speech and Hearing Disorders,* 40 (1975), 397-404.

Fulton, R.T., and J.T. Graham, "Conditioned Orientation Reflex Audiometry with the Mentally Retarded," *American Journal of Mental Deficiency,* 70 (1966), 703-708.

Fulton, R.T., and J.E. Spradlin, "Conditioning and Audiologic Assessment," in *Auditory Assessment of the Difficult-To-Test,* edited by R.T. Fulton and L.L. Lloyd. Baltimore: Williams and Wilkins Co., 1975, pp. 154-178.

Fulton, R.T., and J.E. Spradlin, "Operant Audiometry with Severely Retarded Children," *Audiology,* 10 (1971), 203-211.

Fulton, R.T., and J.E. Spradlin, "The Temporal Parameters of Auditory Stimulus-Response Control." Bureau of Child Research, University of Kansas, and Parsons State Hospital and Training Center, 16mm film, 1973 (color, 9 min.).

Green, D.S., "The Pup Show: A Simple, Inexpensive Modification of the Peep Show," *Journal of Speech and Hearing Disorders,* 23 (1958), 118-120.

Guilford, F.R., and C.O. Haug, "Diagnosis of Deafness in the Very Young Child," *Archives of Otolaryngology,* 55 (1952), 101-106.

Haug, O., P. Bacarro, and F.R. Guilford, "A Pure-Tone Audiogram on the Infant: The PIWI Technique," *Archives of Otolaryngology,* 86 (1967), 101-106.

Hogan, D.D., "Autonomic Correlates of Audition," in *Auditory Measurements of the Difficult-to-Test,* edited by R. T. Fulton and L.L. Lloyd. Baltimore: Williams and Wilkins Co., 1975, pp. 262-290.

Hogan, D.D., "Some Physiological Determinants of Autonomic Responsivity to Sound," *Journal of Speech and Hearing Research,* 13 (1970), 130-146.

Horton, E.R., "An Experimental Investigation into the Reliability of Psychogalvanic Skin Resistance Audiometry with Two-, Three- and Four-Year-Old Children." Unpublished Master's thesis, University of Wisconsin, 1952.

Knox, E.C., "A Method of Obtaining Pure-Tone Audiograms in Young Children," *Journal of Laryngology and Otology,* 74 (1960), 475-479.

LaCrosse, E.L., and H. Bidlake, "A Method to Test the Hearing of Mentally Retarded Children," *Volta Review,* 66 (1964), 27-30.

Liden, G., and A. Kankkumen, "Visual Reinforcement Audiometry," *Acta Otolaryngologica* (Stockholm), 67 (1969a), 281-292.

Liden, G., and A. Kankkumen, "Visual Reinforcement Audiometry," *Archives of Otolaryngology,* 89 (1969b), 865-872.

Lloyd, L.L., "Use of the Slide Show Audiometric Technique with Mentally Retarded Children," *Exceptional Children,* 32 (1965), 93-98.

Lloyd, L.L., "Behavioral Audiometry Viewed as an Operant Procedure," *Journal of Speech and Hearing Disorders,* 31 (1966) 128–136.

Lloyd, L.L., "Puretone Audiometry," in *Auditory Assessment of the Difficult-to-Test,* edited by R.T. Fulton and L.L. Lloyd. Baltimore: Williams and Wilkins Co., 1975, pp. 1–36.

Lloyd, L.L., J.E. Spradlin, and M.J. Reid, "An Operant Audiometric Procedure for Difficult-To-Test Patients," *Journal of Speech and Hearing Disorders,* 33 (1968), 236–245.

Lloyd, L.L., and W.R. Wilson, "Recent Developments in the Behavioral Assessment of the Infant's Response to Auditory Stimulation." Paper presented at the XVI World Congress for Logopedics and Phoniatrics, August 26, 1974, Interlaken, Switzerland.

Luria, A.R., "Psychological Studies in Mental Deficiency in the Soviet Union," in *Handbook of Mental Deficiency,* edited by N.R. Ellis. New York: McGraw-Hill, 1963.

Maietta, F., "A Study of Generalization and Extinction in Eyelid Conditioning to Pure Tone Auditory Stimuli." Unpublished doctoral dissertation, University of Pittsburgh, 1955.

Martin, F.N., *Clinical Audiometry & Masking.* New York: Bobbs-Merrill, 1972.

Martin, F.N., *Introduction to Audiology.* Englewood Cliffs, N.J.: Prentice-Hall, 1975, pp. 97–108.

Matkin, N.D., and J. Thomas, "A Longitudinal Study of Visual Reinforcement Audiometry." Paper presented at ASHA Convention, Las Vegas, 1974.

Meyerson, L., and J.L. Michael, "The Measurement of Sensory Thresholds in Exceptional Children: An Experimental Approach to Some Problems of Differential Diagnosis and Education with Special Reference to Hearing," Cooperative Research Project No. 418, U.S. Office of Education, 1960.

Miller, A.L., "The Use of Slide Projectors in Pure-Tone Audiometric Testing," *Journal of Speech and Hearing Disorders,* 28 (1963), 94–96.

Moncur, J.P., "Judge Reliability in Infant Testing," *Journal of Speech and Hearing Research,* 11 (1968), 348–357.

Moore, J.M., G. Thompson, and M. Thompson, "Auditory Localization of Infants as a Function of Reinforcement Conditions," *Journal of Speech and Hearing Disorders,* 40 (1975), 29–34.

Nowles, M.M., "Operant Audiometry with Two-Year-Olds," Unpublished Master's thesis, Kansas State University, 1971.

O'Neill, J., H.J. Oyer, and J.W. Hillis, "Audiometric Procedures Used with Children," *Journal of Speech and Hearing Disorders,* 26 (1961), 61–66.

Orchik, D.J., and N.L. Mosher, "Narrow Band Noise Audiometry: The Effect of Filter Slope," *Journal of the American Audiology Society,* 1 (1975), 50–53.

Rosenberg, P.E., "Misdiagnosis of Children with Auditory Problems," *Journal of Speech and Hearing Disorders,* 31 (1966), 279–283.

St. James-Roberts, I., "Why Operant Audiometry—A Consideration of Some

Shortcomings Fundamental to the Audiological Testing of Children," *Journal of Speech and Hearing Disorders,* 37 (1972), 47–54.

Shimizu, H., and F. Nakamura, "Pure-Tone Audiometry in Children Lantern-Slides Test," *Annals of Otology, Rhinology, and Laryngology,* 66 (1957), 392–398.

Skinner, B.F., *Contingencies of Reinforcement: A Theoretical Analysis.* New York: Appleton-Century-Crofts, 1969.

Skinner, B.F., *Science and Human Behavior.* New York: Macmillan Co., 1953.

Spradlin, J.E., B.J. Locke, and R.T. Fulton, "Conditioning and Audiological Assessment," in *Audiometry for the Retarded: With Implications for the Difficult-To-Test,* edited by R.T. Fulton and L.L. Lloyd. Baltimore: Williams and Wilkins Co., 1969, pp. 125–163.

Spradlin, J.E., L.L. Lloyd, H.L. Hom, and M.J. Reid, "Establishing Tone Control and Evaluating the Hearing of Severely Retarded Children," in *Expanding Concepts in Mental Retardation: A Symposium from the Joseph P. Kennedy, Jr., Foundation,* edited by G.A. Jervis. Springfield, Ill.: Charles C. Thomas, 1968, pp. 170–180.

Statten, P., and D.E.S. Wishart, "Pure-Tone Audiometry in Young Children: Psychogalvanic-Skin-Resistance and Peep-Show," *Annals of Otology, Rhinology, and Laryngology,* 65 (1956), 511–534.

Sullivan, R.F., M.H. Miller, and I.A. Polisar, "The Portable Peep Show," *Archives of Otolaryngology,* 76 (1962), 61–63.

Studebaker, G.A., "Clinical Masking of Air- and Bone-Conducted Stimuli," *Journal of Speech and Hearing Disorders,* 29 (1964) 23–35.

Suzuki, T., and Y. Ogiba, "A Technique of Puretone Audiometry for Children Under Three Years of Age: Conditioned Orientation Reflex (C.O.R.) Audiometry," *Revue de Laryngologie,* 1 (1960), 33–45.

Suzuki, T., and Y. Ogiba, "Conditioned Orientation Reflex Audiometry," *Archives of Otolaryngology,* 74 (1961), 192–198.

Suzuki, T., Y. Ogiba, and T. Takei, "Basic Properties of Conditioned Orientation Reflex Audiometry," *Minerva Otorinolaringologica,* 22 (1972), 181–186.

Thompson, G., and B.A. Weber, "Responses of Infants and Young Children to Behavior Observation Audiometry (BOA)," *Journal of Speech and Hearing Disorders,* 39 (1974), 140–147.

Thompson, M., and G. Thompson, "Response of Infants and Young Children as a Function of Auditory Stimuli and Test Methods," *Journal of Speech and Hearing Research,* 15 (1972), 699–707.

Volkland, B.G., "Operant Audiometry with the Hard-of-Hearing Child." Unpublished Master's thesis, Kansas State University, 1972.

Waryas, P.A., and J.F. Brandt, "Periodicity Pitch Perception of Retarded Children," *Journal of the American Audiology Society,* 2 (1977), 142–150.

Weaver, R.M., "The Use of Filmstrip Stories in Slide Show Audiometry," in *The Audiologic Assessment of the Mentally Retarded: Proceedings of a National*

Conference, edited by L.L. Lloyd and D. Frisina. Parsons (Kansas) State Hospital and Training Center, 1965, pp. 71-88.

SUGGESTED READINGS

Ferster, C.B., and M.C. Perrott, *Behavior Principles.* New York: Appleton-Century-Crofts, 1968.

Fulton, R.T., *Auditory Stimulus-Response Control.* Baltimore: University Park Press, 1974.

Fulton, R.T., and J.E. Spradlin, "Conditioning and Audiologic Assessment," in *Auditory Assessment of the Difficult-to-Test,* edited by R.T. Fulton and L.L. Lloyd, Baltimore: Williams and Wilkins Co., 1975, pp. 154-178.

Hirsh, I.J. *The Measurement of Hearing.* New York: McGraw-Hill, 1952, pp. 255-275.

Hodgson, W.R., "Testing Infants and Young Children," in *Handbook of Clinical Audiology,* edited by J. Katz. Baltimore: Williams and Wilkins, Co., 1972, pp. 498-519.

Lloyd, L.L., "Pure-tone Audiometry," in *Auditory Assessment of the Difficult-to-Test,* edited by R.T. Fulton and L.L. Lloyd. Baltimore: Williams and Wilkins Co., 1975, pp. 1-36.

Northern, J.L., and M.P. Downs, *Hearing in Children.* Baltimore: Williams and Wilkins Co., 1974, pp. 135-170.

Whaley, D.L., and R.W. Malott, *Elementary Principles of Behavior.* Kalamazoo, Mich.: Behaviordelia, 1969.

CHAPTER SEVEN

Speech Tests of Hearing–
Age One Year through Five Years

FREDERICK N. MARTIN

INTRODUCTION

In the complete audiological evaluation of the adult patient, speech audiometry serves a number of useful and valuable purposes. Determination can be made of the extent to which a hearing handicap affects the ability to hear, discriminate, and tolerate speech. Through use of speech audiometry, diagnoses can be made regarding the type of hearing disorder and the general site of pathology. Speech audiometry also helps to determine the type of rehabilitative measures needed and their prognosis. In addition, it is an aid in verifying the reliability of pure-tone test results.

In many audiological settings speech audiometry is absent in the testing of small children for various reasons. In some cases its value is simply not recognized; in others, the facilities do not allow for the additional time and equipment required. Often speech tests with children require two clinicians, or an audiologist and a trained assistant—a price judged too dear to pay in some centers. At times speech audiometric procedures are not attempted because of an a priori decision that they will not work on a given child or that the results to be obtained do not justify the efforts involved.

While there is no doubt that in many cases speech audiometry with children may be arduous, the practical value obtained from these tests frequently makes the efforts worthwhile. Many children find speech audiometry easier and less abstract than pure-tone tests and are more willing participants. Often the results of speech tests verify or deny the clinical impressions of hearing disorders gleaned from subjective impressions or from other tests. At times, in fact, speech audiometry is the only procedure that can be successfully completed on a child. In such cases, although the child must, of course, be returned for further audiometric study, a valuable beginning will have been made.

To be sure, some children, because of their deficits in language skills, maturity, or mentation, cannot be tested using speech audiometry. The skilled examiner often recognizes this early in the evaluation. But when speech test results are obtainable, they should be pursued.

CHAPTER OBJECTIVES

This chapter will review the speech audiometric procedures that may be appropriate with small children. Specific tests to determine the different measurements of thresholds for speech and various measurements of speech discrimination will be mentioned. Although the literature will be reviewed objectively, my personal preferences for use in special situations will be stated. Some tests are intended for the mildly and moderately hearing-impaired child, others for the profoundly impaired. Mention will also be made of some of the specific problems in assessing the speech communication difficulties of children with central auditory processing disorders. While all pediatric audiologists may not agree with the recommendations made in this chapter, the information contained herein should allow the thinking clinician to arrange the tests that are presently available in a hierarchy of clinical feasibility for a given child. It is hoped that enough alternatives will be offered to cover the majority of eventualities.

HISTORICAL BACKGROUND

Speech signals are obvious selections as stimuli for the assessment of hearing deficiency in children. There is evidence that speech items were in use as early as 1883 (Meyerson, 1956) to determine hearing thresholds. Although the history of modern audiology is brief, it was pointed out over four decades ago (Bunch, 1934) that an important reason for performing speech audiometry in children is that speech items have higher face validity than do nonspeech items. Because children pay closer attention to verbal than to non-verbal stimuli (Hardy and Bordley, 1951), the probability of accurate responses is increased for those children whose language skills allow the use of speech as test stimuli. Clawson (1966) points out that mentally retarded children show an arousal to speech stimuli at significantly lower intensities than they do for pure-tones, resulting in a poorer correlation between these two measures than is normally seen in children with normal intelligence. He feels that speech tests, in addition to confirming pure-tone results, reveal insights into the difficulties that retarded children have in paying attention to sound.

Speech Detection Threshold

The speech detection threshold (SDT) may be defined as the level at which a listener may just detect the presence of an ongoing speech signal and identify it as speech (Martin, 1975, p. 156). While it is not known how frequently the SDT is used as a measurement of hearing in children, it is probably safe to assume that it is used with some regularity. It seems important to ask the reason why the SDT should be obtained.

238

The usual rationale for SDT is that it may be the only speech test obtainable from some children and that, while its usefulness is limited, there may be some predictability from the SDT to the speech *reception* threshold (SRT), in that studies have shown that it generally requires about 10 to 20 dB greater intensity to obtain the SRT than the SDT (Egan, 1948). Hirsh (1952, p. 127) correctly points out that the SDT provides about as much information as the threshold for a buzzer, a combination of pure-tones, or a number of different kinds of sounds. Since speech is a broad-band signal, it is impossible to predict audiometric configuration from SDT (Giolas, 1975, p. 51). The patient, if he is properly conditioned to respond, will do so to the portion of this broad band of frequencies at which his hearing is most sensitive. The spectrum of speech contains peaks and valleys, with most of the energy concentrated in the lower frequencies. Frisina (1962) found the SDT to be ±5dB of the 500 Hz threshold in cases of flat audiograms, or those which fall slightly or precipitously in the higher frequencies. When the audiometric curve rises in the higher frequencies, as it does in some cases of conductive hearing loss or some congenital sensorineural losses (Ross and Matkin, 1967), the SDT will be ±5dB of the pure-tone threshold revealing the best hearing sensitivity on the audiogram.

It must be remembered that some variability is to be expected when measuring the SDT, especially in children. Giolas (1975) points out that the data collected on a set of subjects under specific conditions of recording may not be the same with a different speaker or another set of variables. Giolas recommends finding the SDT by giving a child a set of instructions such as "Put the ring on the peg." The child is encouraged to perform this act and, once the concept is grasped, the intensity is lowered until the child can no longer follow the instructions. It seems to me that the level at which obedience to commands ceases may in some cases be above the SDT by a number of decibels and may, in fact, correlate highly with the threshold of intelligibility for sentence material.

Obviously the pure-tone audiogram may be a reasonably good predictor of the SDT, but the reverse does not hold true. In fact, if the audiometric configuration is irregular across frequency, the SDT may considerably underestimate the SRT, suggesting that it is lower than it truly is. Agreeing that the audiometric contour is not indicated by the SDT, Giolas (1975) nevertheless feels the procedure has advantages, especially for use in the sound field, but the spectrum of the speech signal must be kept in mind.

There may be times in the clinical evaluation of small children or other difficult-to-test patients when the SDT is the only measurement obtained on a given day. The experienced audiologist recognizes the limitation of this finding and should view it as he would view the threshold for a broad-band signal, recalling always the spectrum of speech. If the SDT is felt to be reliable and a hearing loss is indicated, the examiner is encouraged to test further and to begin considering remediative measures for the child. In such a case the extent of the hearing loss may be underestimated, but proper follow-up will have begun and the error will eventually be corrected. If the SDT suggests normal hearing or "hearing adequate for speech" (an expression commonly seen in the files of small children with language disorders) and no further audiometry is pursued, a tragic misdiagnosis may occur and the hearing loss may not be discovered until much later in the child's life when valuable therapy time will have been lost.

Speech Reception Threshold

Hirsh (1952, p. 127) points out that in proceeding from the concept of speech detectability to that of speech intelligibility it must be asked what level is required for speech to be just intelligible to a listener and, given a particular sample of speech, how intelligible the speech is. The definition for "just intelligible speech" is not entirely agreed upon, but we will say that the speech reception (intelligibility) threshold is the lowest hearing threshold level at which at least 50% of a list of spondaic words can be correctly identified (Martin, 1975, p. 156). Spondaic words, often called spondees, are two-syllable words pronounced with equal stress on both syllables.

Words alleged to be spondees are usually found to have at least slightly greater stress on one syllable than the other. Strictly speaking, therefore, a list of spondaic words cannot be printed or read, but only uttered, using a forced and unnatural stress pattern in English. Most two-syllable words are either trochaic (greater stress on the second syllable) or iambic (greater stress on the first syllable). Hudgins et al. (1947) found that two-syllable words uttered with spondaic stress are more uniform in their audibility than one-syllable words or two-syllable words uttered with trochaic or iambic stress. The increased homogeneity of spondees allows for measurement of SRT with a lesser number of test words. Whether the unusualness of artificial stress on two-syllable words has an effect on a child's ability or willingness to discriminate them has not been investigated. Until and unless this is shown to be a factor, audiologists will continue to use spondees in finding the SRTs of small children.

Most audiologists today appear to prefer SRT testing with monitored live voice to testing with prerecorded stimuli. This allows the freedom to substitute or eliminate words according to the apparent needs of the child being tested, to alter the speed of the test, and generally to tailor the procedure to the patient. While there is no doubt that stimulus control is usually better with recorded material, the flexibility of monitored live voice generally makes it preferable for small children.

In recent years the literature has shown a tendency towards standardization in SRT test procedure. The historic 50% criterion allowed for a good deal of variability in technique, with the consequent possibility of significant differences in SRT, depending on the procedure used. I feel that precise methods that allow the least subjective interpretation of SRT (Tillman and Olsen, 1973; Wilson, Morgan and Dirks, 1973; Martin and Stauffer, 1975) are preferable for adults, especially when the SRT is obtained without prior knowledge of the audiogram, thus objectifying the test even further (Martin and Stauffer, 1975). Obtaining such precision with children may prolong the test and prevent their completing it. Also, the use of 2-dB steps in measurement may yield slightly better precision than larger steps, if the test is completed, but their use may bore or tire the child so that he stops cooperating prematurely. Precision is the clinician's desire, not the child's. Monitored live voice testing using steps of 5 or sometimes even 10dB often yields rapid and acceptable results with children.

Although many young children give reliable test results on pure-tone tests (Eagles and Wishik, 1961; Frisina, 1973, p. 160), others show quite poor reliability on tests with pure-tone stimuli. In such cases the SRT lends valuable assistance in determining the extent of a hearing deficit (Keaster, 1947; Siegenthaler, Pearson, and Lezak, 1954). Children are likely to react more positively to familiar speech sounds than to abstract pure-tone stimuli, so long as they are free of any confounding linguistic deficits. Speech tests take considerably less time than do pure-tone tests, an important factor when the generally shorter attention span of young children is considered.

The SRT has a number of advantages in clinical audiology but not all audiologists agree upon the primary ones. To some, the SRT's greatest asset is that it describes the degree of a patient's handicap in his hearing of speech and the prognosis for rehabilitation (Hardy and Pauls, 1950). To others it serves predominantly as the reference point for a number of supra-threshold measurements, such as word discrimination. To still others it is a means of verifying the accuracy of the pure-tone audiogram, not only in adults (Carhart, 1946; Chaiklin, Ventry, and Dixon, 1971; Carhart and Tillman, 1972) but in children as well (Siegenthaler, Pearson, and Lezak, 1954). The SRT can best be predicted from the audiogram by averaging the pure-tone thresholds obtained at 500 and 1000 Hz and subtracting 2dB (Carhart, 1971), and only in patients with sharply rising or falling audiograms are cues from other frequencies effective in lowering the SRT below prediction (Carhart and Porter, 1971).

The high positive correlation between the SRT and the pure-tone average has encouraged some authorities (Davis, 1970, p. 208; Hirsh, 1962; Silverman and Hirsh, 1955) to argue that the determination of SRT is actually unnecessary. While it is true that the SRT does not provide the estimation of social efficiency for hearing that was once hoped (Silverman and Hirsh, 1955), the finding of a discrepancy between SRT and pure-tone average (PTA) is an important one in determination of the accuracy of both tests. The SRT therefore seems to be an indispensable test, expecially with children.

Many clinicians agree with Meyerson (1947) that the SRT is a reliable measurement on children with normal intelligence and even on some difficult-to-test children such as the retarded (Lloyd and Reid, 1966). While some children 3 years old and younger give reliable results on speech tests (Martin and Coombes, 1976; Siegenthaler, Pearson, and Lezak, 1954), many clinicians feel that the

SRT is an inconsistent measurement below the age of 4 years (Meyerson, 1956; Siegenthaler, Pearson, and Lezak, 1954). Generally, the success rate in testing children is greater for speech than for pure-tones (Hodgson, 1972a, p. 512). Although familiarizing the subjects with the test items usually improves the SRT test results (Tillman and Jerger, 1959), only about half the audiologists in a national survey (Martin and Pennington, 1971), actually do this. In using spondaic words to test SRTs in adults, Beattie, Svohovec, and Edgerton (1975) found that 17 of the 36 spondees from Central Institute for the Deaf (CID) Auditory Test W-1 gave greater precision and accuracy to the SRT procedure. Conn, Dancer, and Ventry (1975) found that by using 18 selected spondees, prior familiarization is unnecessary. Since 3 of those words fell outside of the recorded range of ±4dB acceptable by most clinicians, a final list of 15 words was recommended. No such lists have been designed for children and pretest conditioning is generally required to familiarize children, especially low-level retardates, with the words (DeWachter-Schaerlaekins, 1969).

Many children who have sufficient language skills and intelligible speech can take the speech reception threshold test rather easily, simply by repeating the words presented to them through an earphone or loudspeaker. Although special forms of encouragement and reward may be used, the procedure is essentially the same as for adults. Other children are simply not sufficiently motivated to go along with this kind of exercise; for them the SRT procedure must be modified into a form of game. Children often enjoy pointing to pictures or objects representing the stimulus word.

A number of point-to-the-picture tests have been described in the literature. Keaster (1947) used pictures of 25 nouns taken from a kindergarten-level word test. Commands such as "Put the rabbit on the floor" were given to the child. The level of the commands was progressively lowered until threshold was approximated. This test appeared to appeal to the child and required no verbal response, although the child was required to remember and understand not only the stimulus word but the entire command.

Lloyd, Reid, and McManis (1967) used pictures of standard spondaic words. These easily obtained pictures gave generally good results, despite the fact that the children were retarded. Other procedures utilizing colored pictures have resulted in frequently reliable results with children (MacFarlan, 1940; Siegenthaler and Haspiel, 1966; Siegenthaler et al., 1954).

Toys have been used as inducements to get SRTs from young children who are unwilling or unable to give verbal responses. Sortini and Flake (1953) used toys with two-syllable names, uttering the words with spondaic stress. Using different commands, they obtained results down to age 26 months. Northern and Downs (1974, p. 151) also suggest the use of toys in obtaining the SRT. They feel that the carrier phrase is important and recommend a procedure in which the phrase "Show me. . ." is uttered, then the hearing level is dropped quickly by 10 to 15dB. Naturally the carrier phrase is most important close to threshold, and Northern and Downs urge that the carrier phrase be audible even when the words themselves are at or slightly below threshold. Although research on adults should not be generalized to children, we have found (Martin and Weller, 1975) that neither the presence of a carrier phrase, nor its sensation level with reference to the spondaic word, has an effect on the SRT. Northern and Downs urge speed in testing, even at the sacrifice of accuracy. Since working with small children usually requires that the number of spondee pictures be limited, often to only three or four, the SRT thus measured may actually be closer to the SDT than many clinicians realize (Hodgson, 1972a, p. 512).

Agreeing with other authors that SRTs are frequently unreliable in children younger than 4, Griffing, Simonton, and Hedgecock (1967) developed a screening speech audiometric procedure for preschool children. The Verbal Auditory Screening Test for preschool Children (VASC) utilizes a board with pictures representing 12 spondaic words. Griffing, Simonton, and Hedgecock found that the procedure worked particularly well with 4- and 5-year-olds. Mencher and McCulloch (1970) tested kindergarten children with the VASC and compared the results to an audiometric screening with pure-tones at 20dB (ANSI 1969). They concluded that the test may miss children in the mild hearing loss range of 30 to 40dB. Ritchie and Merklein (1972) also found the VASC procedure to have less than the desired efficiency in identifying hearing loss in children, being less accurate than pure-tone tests. Hasegawa et al. (1974) did find the VASC useful in the auditory screening of a group of 2,564 children aged 3 through 6 years. Identifying pictures, particularly spondee pictures, can be accomplished with hearing sensitivity up to 1000 Hz, considering that the task requires a closed-set response.

Keaster (1947) outlines a number of problems in accurately determining SRTs in children:

1. The test must have sufficient appeal to maintain the child's attention long enough for threshold to be determined.
2. Most young children have a brief attention span, requiring a rapid procedure.
3. Since verbal comprehension is more highly developed than verbal production in small chiildren, nonverbal responses are preferred.
4. Neither the child's short memory span nor his ability to understand the task must be exceeded.
5. Test words must be within the child's vocabulary.

While a variety of reinforcers has been used to encourage responses to pure-tone stimuli, with speech tests the reinforcement has been mostly social. A smile, pat on the head, nod, or word of praise is sufficient reinforcement with many young children, but others find such intangibles insufficiently motivating to continue repeating words or pointing to pictures or objects. With this in mind we (Martin and Coombes, 1976) developed a procedure for immediate tangible reinforcement of appropriate responses to speech items. The child is instructed to touch a part of a brightly colored clown. If the response is correct he is immediately rewarded with a small piece of chocolate candy, which falls into a cup held in the clown's hand. Parts of the clown are wired in series with a programming unit in the control room of a two-room audiometric environment. More than one response or an incorrect response locks out a possible reward.

We found the procedure to be extremely rapid and accurate with children as young as age 2½ years with normal hearing. As a matter of fact, the children enjoyed it so much that they finished in a good humor and other tests could be completed with little difficulty. We are now investigating the efficacy of this device for use with mentally retarded subjects.

Most modern diagnostic audiometers are capable of delivering speech stimuli to a bone-conduction vibrator. While the manufacturer provides no normal hearing standards for speech by bone conduction, most clinicians find that a correction factor of about -30 to -40dB is necessary because the speech circuit is designed to drive the small diaphragm in the earphone. Speech can be routed to the bone-conduction vibrator, which can be placed on the mastoid or forehead of the child. Comparing SRTs obtained by bone conduction to those obtained by air conduction reveals the presence of a conductive component. Goetzinger and Proud (1955) and Merrell, Wolfe, and McLemore (1973) found a high correlation between the average bone-conduction thresholds at 500, 1000, and 2000 Hz and the bone-conduction speech reception threshold. Bone-conducted speech results may serve not only as a diagnostic tool but also as a rehabilitation guide (Stockdell, 1974). When speech discrimination scores by bone conduction are superior to those by air conduction, it may, for example, suggest that a bone-conduction transducer on a hearing aid is preferable for that particular child.

Regardless of the procedure, the SRT is only as useful as the pediatric audiologist makes it. The SRT is never a goal in itself. Recognizing the possibility of missing high-frequency hearing losses, Meyerson (1956) used high-pass filters with spondaic words. This idea has great merit, but the extent to which it is practiced today is not known. However, the idea of frequency splitting with the VASC is attractive, in that both the upper- and lower-frequency bands may be screened.

In Chapter 6 Dr. Fulton repeatedly cautions the reader regarding the importance of stimulus–response control in the measurement of pure-tone thresholds. This admonition is equally applicable to speech audiometry. Details of recommended methods of finding the SRTs of small children will follow later in this chapter.

Speech Discrimination

A question of their hearing-impaired patients that all audiologists want answered is how well they hear and understand speech. Some information about the ability to hear speech may be gleaned from the SRT, but information about how well speech is processed and discriminated has required other special tests. Such information is useful not only to diagnose the type and severity of the hearing disorder but also to determine the best approach to and prognosis for aural rehabilitation.

The development of speech discrimination tests, such as PB word lists, for adults has been well documented and is familiar to the readers of this book (Egan, 1948; Hirsh et al., 1952; Lehiste and Peterson, 1962, 1959; Tillman and Carhart, 1966; Tillman, Carhart and Wilber, 1963). Many children, even as young as age 4 and 5, can be tested using adult PB words, although it might be added that these are the children who present the least difficulty in testing in general and often who show the smallest problems in the way of auditory defects.

Common sense, as well as research data (Watson, 1957), has long shown that many words on PB word lists are not in the vocabularies of small children. This motivated Haskins (1949) to develop four PB-50 word lists for children of kindergarten age, often called the PBK lists. No commercial version of this test has been recorded so each clinician performing this test must do so using monitored live voice.

The child's reward for cooperation on a speech discrimination test is usually social: praise, a smile, or some other gesture of approval. Smith (1969) systematically reinforced correct responses to speech discrimination items using an operant conditioning method. Both normal-hearing and hearing-impaired children showed substantial improvements in their speech discrimination scores, illustrating that without proper reinforcement, the child may perform at a level which does not indicate his maximum discrimination ability.

Written responses on PB word tests are, of course, out of the question for most small children. Even verbal responses may be limited by the child's language disorder, articulation defect, motivation, or a number of other factors. To bypass these problems and still test the word discrimination of small children, Myatt and Landes (1963) developed a multiple-choice picture-identification test for use with 4- and 5-year-old children. The lists were standardized on normal and trainable mentally retarded children. Lerman, Ross, and McLaughlin (1965) performed the Myatt and Landes test on hearing-impaired children and found it less than completely effective. Subsequently Ross and Lerman (1970) developed the WIPI test, an acronym for word intelligibility by picture identification.

The WIPI test is simple to administer, but it does require two clinicians, or a clinician and an alert helper. Like other speech discrimination tests, it can be administered in the sound field or through earphones if the child permits. The helper shows the child a card with a matrix of six colored pictures. Four of the pictures have words that rhyme, the other two are presented as foils to decrease the probability of a correct guess. Through the speech audiometer set at a level above his speech threshold, the child is instructed to touch one of the pictures. If the response cannot be viewed by the examiner, it may be relayed by the assistant. For each correct identification of a picture, the child is credited with 4 percentage points. The total of 25 words in each test yields a possible maximum score of 100%.

There are differences between the PB-word and WIPI-type approaches to auditory discrimination testing besides the obvious fact that the latter is pictorially represented. PB words represent an open-response paradigm, in which the child is forced to select an answer from an unlimited set of possibilities. Like rhyme tests used on adults, the WIPI is a closed-response set, the child's response being a forced choice. Jones and Studebaker (1974) compared the two types of response systems on a group of hearing-impaired children. They found the closed response to be more productive with children evidencing very poor word-discrimination abilities, and that closed-response test scores were highly correlated to data which depended on hearing function. Jones and Studebaker concluded that closed-response-set data tend to demonstrate auditory speech discrimination difficulties in a more satisfactory way than do open-response-set data.

In a study comparing the word discrimination scores of normal-hearing children, Sanderson and Rintelmann (1971) found that higher scores were shown on the WIPI than on the PBKs, and that both tests revealed higher scores than the PB words of NU-6. These score differences tended to disappear with age. The conclusion drawn from this research is that the WIPI serves best for young children, and a combination of the WIPI and PBK lists works well for older children. NU-6 should be reserved for older children when a more discriminating test, such as a hearing-aid evaluation, is required. Hodgson's (1973) data agree with my own clinical observations that conventional WIPI scores are higher than PBKs or the WIPI presented as an open-message set.

The child with a sensorineural hearing loss usually shows signs of dysacusis—speech discrimination difficulties associated with the loss of sensitivity. Often this discrimination difficulty is so great that monosyllabic words cannot be discriminated at all or, at best, very poorly. Egan (1948) showed that the greater the acoustic redundancy in a speech signal, the easier it is discriminated. Such redundancy increases with increased numbers of phonemes and syllables.

To increase the chances of measuring word discrimination ability on hearing-impaired children over that obtained from monosyllabic word tests, Cramer and Erber (1974) used pictures of ten spondaic words recorded on Language Master cards and presented the words through a single, insert-type earphone. It took several sessions before all the children were familiar enough with the procedure to be tested reliably, but results were quite interesting. Scores were bimodally distributed, clustering in the 0 to 65% and 66 to 100% ranges. Pure-tone averages less than 93dB (ANSI 1969) showed the higher score groupings, pure-tone averages greater than 103dB showed the poorer scores. A close relationship did not exist between degree of hearing loss and spondee recognition scores for children with losses in the 93 to 103dB range. Those recognition scores varied as a function of repeated testing in three ways: stable performance, steadily improving scores, and inconsistent performance. In another study Erber (1974) also found that scores clustered in the high range (70 to 100%) for children with losses milder than 85dB (ANSI 1969) and in the low range (0 to 30%) for losses greater than 100dB. Scores for spondee recognition in children showing hearing losses between 86 and 100dB were difficult to predict. Similar data were reported much earlier by Hudgins (1954) and more recently by Erber and Alencewicz (1976).

Because word recognition so often appears very poor in children with sensorineural hearing impairments, the visual channel is sometimes added to improve overall discrimination. It has been known for some time that visual cues augment auditory cues in the discrimination of speech. Ross et al (1972) found that, using the WIPI test, combined auditory and visual scores are better than the sum of auditory and visual scores alone. The score sheet accompanying the commercial version of the WIPI test provides space for testing hearing alone, vision alone, and hearing and vision combined.

Erber (1972) illustrated that visual cues allow normal-hearing and severely and profoundly hearing-impaired children to discern information regarding the place of articulation of consonant sounds; they were able to separate bilabials from alveolar and velar consonants. The normal group had no problem recognizing auditory cues alone, the severely impaired group could recognize voiced and voiceless plosives and nasals, and the profound group showed poor overall hearing perception. In the combined mode, the profound-loss group showed only slight improvement over the visual mode alone, but the other two groups performed nearly perfectly. Monosyllabic, spondaic, and trochaic words were presented in the presence of a low-frequency noise. Several signal-to-noise ratios were used. Subjects were children who had normal hearing, were moderately hearing-impaired, or were profoundly hearing-impaired. Once again the profoundly impaired group was helped least by the audio-visual channel.

The testing of speech discrimination on children with severe hearing disorders and the consequent language limitations is often not attempted because the difficulties to be encountered are predictable, and often the clinician feels that the efforts will not be justified. Erber and Alencewicz (1976) discuss their approach to a complete audiologic evaluation of these severely hearing-impaired children, including a new speech perception test. They use 12 picture cards illustrating 4 nouns in each of 3 stress categories—monosyllables, trochees, and spondees. The child is first shown all the cards and asked to name each one, to insure that the word is in his vocabulary. He then identifies each picture as it is presented audio-visually. Any word not in the child's vocabulary is replaced with one that is. These words are used to determine the speech-detection threshold as well as the levels of most comfortable and uncomfortable loudness. For the discrimination portion of the test, each word is presented twice at the most comfortable listening level with no visual cues. Scoring is accomplished in two ways:

according to the percent of the words correct and the percent categorized correctly by stress pattern. The procedure is appropriate for children over 5 years of age. Perhaps the greatest value of this test is that it assists in selecting the appropriate ear for a hearing aid and in deciding if binaural hearing aids would be appropriate.

Certain basic assumptions of many audiologists may be incorrect. For example, Giolas (1975, pp. 48–49) points out that data collected on a subject under specific conditions of recording will not be the same with a different talker. Kruel, Bell, and Nixon (1969) have shown that test difficulty changes with different talkers and different carrier phrases, but it does not change with words uttered by the same speaker. They point out that the auditory test is not the list of words, but rather the recording of these words, or, in the case of children we see in the clinic, the manner in which the words are uttered using monitored live-voice. The use of a properly monitored carrier phrase before each test word has been shown to influence word discrimination scores significantly (Gladstone and Siegenthaler, 1971; Schwartz and Goldman, 1974).

At times no standardized test gives an appropriate measure of speech discrimination. In children this may be true because of the child's inadequate language or because the discrimination problem is very grave. If the child can be taught the concepts of "same" and "different," he may be tested with such gross speech sounds as sustained vowels. In this way it can be determined if he can make any auditory discriminations at all, assuming that the stimulus can be presented above threshold without reaching discomfort intensities.

Ling[1] has used a test for more than ten years with gratifying results. The test involves three vowels, *a, u,* and *i,* and two consonants, *s* and *ʃ*. Dr. Ling feels that the test taps the hearing for particular formants and is useful as a quick check of a child's potential speech discrimination. For example, if a hearing aid cuts the low frequency-sounds excessively *u* and *i* will be less audible than *a*. If hearing above 2000 Hz is poor, or if a hearing aid does not amplify well in the upper frequency range, the *i* will be inaudible for a child for whom no low-frequency information is provided. Audibility of *ʃ* indicates potential audibility of the second formant of the vowel *i*. This test can be performed under earphones or aided and unaided in the sound field. The test can be performed as the sole test of speech discrimination if necessary, or it can be used in conjunction with other tests, such as the WIPI. Dr. Ling informs me that he has used this test successfully with children as young as 6 months.

Earlier in this chapter the subject of the bone-conducted speech reception threshold was discussed briefly. Word discrimination can be measured by bone conduction (Goetzinger and Proud, 1955), and such measurements are of value in severe mixed-type losses to determine speech discrimination ability when the level for air conduction cannot be made high enough to determine the maximum

---

[1]Personal communication with Dr. Daniel Ling, 1976.

score. A high speech discrimination score by bone conduction also helps eliminate any doubt that the pure-tone bone-conduction thresholds may have been the result of tactile rather than auditory perception (Nober, 1970).

When testing can be performed properly, speech discrimination measurements are important aids to diagnosing the type and degree of hearing disorder in children and for determining appropriate remediation, proper ear for a hearing aid, and such. If, for whatever reason, no speech discrimination estimate is available, the audiologist may have to proceed with the data he has, based on the SRT and pure-tone audiogram. In such cases a general rule is that the greater the sensorineural loss, the greater the discrimination problem.

Central Auditory Disorders

At times the clinical audiologist will see a small child whose parents complain that he has either poor or inconsistent hearing. Many of these children are found to have fluctuant conductive hearing losses or high-frequency losses. Still others check out perfectly normal on pure-tone and speech tests. At such times the audiologist might advise the parents that the child's hearing is normal, that possibly a previous problem has resolved itself, or that the child suffers from parental anxiety. These explanations, however, may be too simplistic.

A variety of auditory tests has been developed for adults to assess the integrity of the central auditory system. To assume that such disorders are present in adults but not in children is unrealistic. Determining the presence of such difficulties as early as possible may show a specific learning disability and provide the opportunity for valuable therapy (Stubblefield and Young, 1975).

Most authorities agree that diagnosis of abnormalities in the central auditory system requires more than the routine test battery. Hodgson (1967) reported on a patient with a complete left cerebral hemispherectomy who showed normal hearing on pure-tone tests and on routine speech audiometry. It has been found necessary to develop new and refined speech tests to evaluate the central pathways. According to Hodgson (1972b) the following five effects may be observed in the presence of pathology of the central auditory system:

1. Pure-tone thresholds are essentially normal in both ears.
2. Supra-threshold pure-tone tests are essentially normal in both ears.
3. Speech discrimination scores may be reduced in the ear contralateral to the damaged portion of the brain. This becomes more evident if the speech is distorted.
4. Dichotic listening tasks are more difficult than for persons with intact central auditory nervous systems.
5. When speech is presented to one ear and a competing signal to the other ear, poorer discrimination may be evidenced in the ear contralateral to the lesion.

The argument for new tests for central disorders in adults has been amply made for some time (Berlin and Lowe, 1972; Bocca and Calearo, 1963; Bocca, Calearo, and Cassinari, 1954; Goetzinger, 1972; Hodgson, 1972b; Jerger, 1964; Katz, 1968; Kimura, 1961; Matzker, 1959). Only recently have some audiologists, such as Katz and Illmer (1972), pointed out the need for the audiologist to evaluate the central auditory system of children, a need that will necessitate the development of new procedures or the adaptation and modification of traditional speech audiometric procedures.

The use of PB words with children has been described earlier in this chapter. If the child has the maturity, patience, and motivation to participate in a number of PB word tests, a performance intensity (PB-PI) function may be constructed. Since Jerger and Jerger (1971) found discrimination scores to decrease beyond a certain intensity in one ear of centrally disordered patients, this "rollover" phenomenon suggested the inclusion of PB word tests as part of a battery of tests for central disorders in adults. This notion can be carried to children where practicable.

While Hodgson (1966) found that tests using speech passed through a single low-pass filter did not separate normal children from those with learning problems or the probability of learning problems, Stubblefield and Young (1975) found that children with learning disabilities consistently made more errors on the Staggered Spondaic Word test (Katz, 1962, 1968) than did normal children. Other recent work holds out promise for diagnostic speech tests for children with central auditory disorders by using filtered speech, competing sentences, and binaural fusion (Willeford, 1976), or time-compressed speech signals (Beasley, Maki, and Orchic, 1976).

The average audiologist is not a specialist in language disorders in children, nor is he likely to become one. He requires methods for screening out those children who should be referred to language specialists. It is hoped, for the sake of the children involved, that such tests will not be long in coming.

CLINICAL METHODS AND INTERPRETATIONS

As a general rule there is a positive correlation between a child's age and the level of cooperation that can be expected on audiometric procedures. To be sure, there are some notable exceptions to this rule. Expecting full cooperation from an older child is less realistic than predicting a lack of cooperation and attention from a younger one.

The pediatric audiologist budgets his time carefully. He asks himself which procedures will give him the most information about an individual child in the least time, and he always works on the assumption that the child may discontinue the procedure at any moment. If the child has adequate speech and language, determining the SRT is a good place to begin.

Speech Reception Threshold

Before a formal SRT procedure is attempted, the clinician should speak with the child, however briefly, to get an estimate of the severity of any problem. If the child answers questions posed in a normal conversational voice, the SRT should not show any more than a mild hearing loss, at least in the better ear (assuming, of course, that the clinician has been careful to avoid lipreading cues). From his observations the audiologist also determines the formality of the tests to be used.

For an older child with adequate speech and language, a traditional SRT procedure may be used. The child may be instructed to repeat words into a microphone. The suggestion that this is an "airplane game," with the child the pilot often makes the procedure more fun. The clinician should initially set the talk-back gain at a low level, since many children will feel compelled to shout their responses. This is especially true if the clinician is wearing a headset. (Wearing a headset is often a good idea, since the child will enjoy having these accoutrements in common with his older game player).

Although earphone SRTs are preferable, the child may fear these or find them uncomfortable. Realizing that even very young children like to talk on the telephone, Dr. Dean Harris[2] arranged with the Dallas telephone company to mount a TDA-39 earphone in place of a standard telephone receiver. The phone was wired with standard telephone plugs coming from the base, which led to the jack panel of a two-room audiometric suite, replacing the earphone and talk-back microphone. SRTs on normal-hearing subjects showed a high correlation (±4dB) between standard earphones and the telephone-mounted earphone.

With some children the clinician may successfully insist that the test continue under earphones; with others he may wish to go to a less valuable but more feasible procedure. Testing in the sound field does determine the level at which the child is receiving speech, at least in his better ear. Sound field audiometry requires careful adjustment of the gain of an auxiliary amplifier, which must be interposed between the output of the audiometer and sound field loudspeaker. Such calibration may be accomplished psychoacoustically, finding the sound-field SRTs of a group of normal-hearing subjects, or electroacoustically, using a sound-level meter.

After calibration for sound-field audiometry has been carried out, a heavy, relatively immovable chair should be set 3 to 4 feet in front of and facing the loudspeaker. The child should be seated in this chair and encouraged to look toward the speaker. Sometimes an assistant can help direct the child's attention. It seems almost silly to calibrate the system carefully, then allow the child to roam about the room, allowing no knowledge of the intensity of the sound at the child's ear at a given time. At times some compromises are necessary, but the

[2]Personal communication with Dr. Dean Harris, 1976.

clinician should note this in his report for proper interpretation of the test results. A feeding table can be extremely useful for positioning the small child appropriately and providing space for toys and test objects.

Ideally, the child should repeat the spondees. If he will not or cannot, he may point to pictures or items. If spondees are not usable then body parts, items of clothing or furniture, or other persons in the room may be used. The simple instruction, "Show me the ——," is often very useful. When response to stimulus words is judged to be too "test-like" for the child, the clinician may engage him in conversation, asking questions and hoping for either a verbal or nonverbal indication that the child has heard the words at a particular hearing level.

The sound level to begin the test at should be considered carefully, regardless of whether the test is formal or informal, under earphones, in the sound field, or with a bone-conduction vibrator. If no evidence of a significant problem appears, a good starting level is 50dB HL: loud enough to elicit responses from children with mild losses without being alarmingly loud for normal hearers. If no reaction is observed at 50dB, the level may be increased in 15 or 20dB steps.

With a cooperative child, the SRT may be obtained in 5-dB steps. My personal view is that the additional accuracy gleaned from 2-dB steps does not warrant the time spent or the increased danger that the child will lose interest. The child will look occasionally to the window of the two-room suite for some sign from the clinician. Most often the reward received for cooperation is a smile, a nod, clapping of hands, or words of encouragement. Monitored live voice is the most flexible approach to testing.

As mentioned earlier, the question of the carrier phrase in SRT testing with children has not been resolved. From my own experience I would suggest that using the carrier phrase for the first few stimulus words like "Say the word . . ." or "Show me . . ." gives the child the idea of what he is to do and further repetition of the phrase is often unnecessary. Apparently Northern and Downs (1974, p. 151) have found the carrier phrase to be of greater importance, especially near threshold, and recommend that the carrier phrase be spoken 10 or 15dB above the test level of the word, turning the dial down quickly 10 or 15dB just before the test word is spoken. I find this awkward. When the carrier phrase is deemed necessary I use a two-channel speech audiometer, presenting both channels to the same earphone or loudspeaker, with the hearing-level dial set about 10dB higher in one channel than the other. After the carrier phrase is spoken, depression of the tone-interrupter bar defeats the channel transmitting the phrase and allows only the test word to be heard at the lower level.

If pictures are to be used as stimuli it should be determined in advance that the word is in the child's vocabulary. Often the parents may provide this information. Showing pictures on a flannelboard allows for rapid elimination of unfamiliar test words or substitutions of new ones. Some children will point to the picture, others will touch it with a finger or pointer, others will hit at it. Sometimes you have to tolerate anything short of violence in the interest of diagnosis.

Tangible reward is often necessary when testing the SRTs of some children. An assistant hands the item, either candy or cereal, to the child on a fixed ratio basis, usually averaging one reward for three correct responses. We also use an automatic token and candy-pellet dispenser mounted on the wall above a child-sized table and chairs. The stimulus items are placed on the table where the clinician and child sit facing each other. When the child makes the appropriate response, it is conveyed to the clinician in the control room delivering the stimuli, who then releases the reward by activating a relay.

With some small children we resort to the clown device described earlier. Children usually sit or stand before the device and are shown how to depress a body part when they hear that part named. Since the microswitch behind the movable part is wired in series with the programmer in the control room, the reward is delivered as soon as the correct response is made, resulting in more rapid conditioning and slower extinction.

If children are wearing hearing aids it is often a good idea to condition them to respond to the speech items in the sound field with their aids on. After an SRT is determined, another measurement with the aid off gives an estimate of the gain provided for speech. After sound-field testing, the child will often have learned, because of his repeated visits to the audiology center, to be unafraid and will by then tolerate the earphones.

Children who wear hearing aids and will not accept earphones may be tested by using an insert-type receiver. The receiver cord may be attached to the auxiliary output of the audiometer and the receiver itself coupled to the child's ear with his own ear mold. Naturally, some recalibration is necessary, and a slight correction factor must be applied. I have found this most useful in obtaining not only speech results but pure-tone thresholds as well, with very little objection from even small children. The size and weight of the headset is just too formidable for some children.

Masking in SRT Tests. Conductive and unilateral hearing losses are not uncommon in children. Contralateralization of speech stimuli, therefore, is a frequent complication in speech reception threshold tests. While audiologists should never rely on their patients to call test artifacts to their attention, an adult is more apt to mention, for example, that he is hearing all the words in one ear than a child is. When the SRT is more than 40dB above the bone-conduction thresholds of the opposite ear, the clinician should suspect that crossover may have taken place. The frequencies by bone-conduction at the nontest ear that should be compared to the SRT in the test ear have not yet been established, although we are presently engaged in research along these lines. How to mask is a matter of personal preference, although some standardization of masking level should be used (Martin, 1975, p. 136).

Children seem to have less difficulty in taking masked speech threshold tests than in taking masked pure-tone tests. It is hard to convince a young mind to ignore a loud uninteresting signal (masking noise) and to put attention to a soft uninteresting sound (pure-tone). If the noise is explained away as a part of the listening game and the child is interested by, or sufficiently rewarded for, responses to speech stimuli, the masked SRT should not be difficult to obtain.

Speech Detection Threshold

The SDT is a measurement I make only as a last resort, when all attempts at pure-tone thresholds and SRT have failed. Since the SDT can be very misleading, especially in the often-seen cases of high-frequency hearing loss, these results must be interpreted with the greatest care. I have not personally had good luck with band-pass filtering of speech stimuli in attempts to get frequency-related information. I have seen cases where the SDT was in the normal range with the 1000 Hz threshold 50dB HL or greater when hearing sensitivity in the low frequencies was normal.

One of our larger sound suites has been set up with a special output from our diagnostic audiometer so that speech, pure-tones, or a variety of noises can be directed to any one of six loudspeakers mounted near the ceiling in the child's room. A small console contains six buttons labeled to correspond to the speakers. Since most children over 6 months of age can localize sound, unless thay have unilateral losses or central disorders, we use a variety of speech signals—for example, calling the child's name, and asking "Where's mommy?" We are able to observe startle responses at times when the level is above threshold but also, if the child can be kept interested in the game, we can approximate the sound-field SDT.

The kind of material used for SDT with adults, usually cold running speech, is not appropriate for children. The determination of SDT is often made on a clinical-hunch basis, with very little objectivity. The SDT can easily overestimate or underestimate the degree of hearing loss in a child, resulting in considerable misdiagnosis unless the SDT is verified by other, more valid tests of hearing sensitivity.

Speech Discrimination Testing

Frequently, tests of speech discrimination in children are performed following SRT and pure-tone tests. These tests are usually considered the capstone of the routine test battery and, with adults, are performed on a routine basis. With children, the speech discrimination tests are sometimes not performed because the child has stopped cooperating, because there are no tests appropriate to the child's age or language skills, or because the clinician feels that estimates of speech discrimination ability can be inferred from other tests. While the first two reasons may be acceptable, the third one is not, at least to me. Speech discrimination tests should be used whenever possible, despite their various limitations.

After speech reception testing and pure-tone testing (if feasible), the speech discrimination test should be administered. The child should take the most difficult test he can handle. If vocabulary permits, adult PB word lists may be used. Kindergarten PBs may be substituted if necessary. If the child's language, articulation of speech, or reticence proscribes vocal responses, the WIPI test is my next choice.

The WIPI test has been in constant use in audiology centers that I have been associated with, although it is not without its difficulties and limitations. While the test is easy to administer and often fun for the child to take, scores sometimes fall short of prediction. At times a child fails to point to the appropriate picture because he has misunderstood the auditory signal, but at other times the child fails because the word is simply not in his vocabulary. The authors of this test recognized this and recommended that the child be queried over the incorrect items, but I believe that this is not done as frequently as it should be. The WIPI is useful in checking the gain of hearing aids by testing in the sound field, unaided and aided. It is also useful in checking the synergistic effect of combining visual and auditory cues. If there are objections to the WIPI, they may be that the test is perhaps too easy to tax the mildly impaired auditory system where speech discrimination problems exist. The WIPI was designed, however, for the more severely impaired child with unintelligible speech and virtually no writing ability. Furthermore, the standardization that can be accomplished with prerecorded materials is absent in this test as it is in all tests delivered by monitored live voice.

Testing the discrimination of the severely or profoundly hearing-impaired child is limited by a combination of his linguistic and vocabulary deficits, motivation, and dysacusis. Some of the tests mentioned earlier in this chapter for use with profoundly hearing-impaired children are new, and thus have not come into popular use. Using the concepts of "same" and "different" can provide some information about such a child's discrimination. This is useful with children who can be communicated with by sign language. The clinician may utter two or three different vowels at a comfortable listening level into one ear. The child may compare the different sounds for similarity and difference and report this manually. Some children with severe or profound hearing losses evidence audiograms that are very similar in both ears, but show a lack of discrimination in one ear and some abilities in the other. In such a case I would opt for a monaural aid rather than binaural hearing aids.

When children are seen because parents or teachers are concerned about a hearing disorder, yet results on all auditory tests are normal, there is good reason to be concerned about the testing. At the University of Texas Speech and Hearing Center, we are now working on several approaches using speech discrimination tasks to screen for central auditory disorders in children. Obviously we cannot refer every child who is seen because of such a complaint to a language pathologist, although we do make such referrals when the patient's history suggests a central disorder, even though our tests may deny it. Audiologists are not specialists in language disorders in the traditional sense, although educational audiologists are beginning to look, appropriately, at hearing loss as a language disorder. We need simply administered tests of speech discrimination as screening instruments to identify the probability of a processing disorder so that appropriate referral can be made.

Masking in Speech Discrimination Tests. Because so many children have conductive or unilateral hearing losses, the problem of crossover is even greater for speech discrimination tests than for SRT or pure-tone tests. It is difficult to know just when the nontest ear is augmenting the discrimination score of the test ear, but crossover should be suspected whenever the test hearing level minus about 40dB (for the loss of speech energy as it travels around, across, and through the skull) exceeds any of the bone-conduction thresholds of the nontest ear. In such cases, appropriate levels of masking should be used. Each clinician has his own system for masking and mine has been set forth elsewhere (Martin, 1975, pp. 145–146). Masking cannot be ignored in speech discrimination tests of children any more than it can for adults. However, the approach for the two groups may have to be different.

Adults requiring masking for speech discrimination tests are simply told to ignore the noise in one ear while they repeat, or otherwise indicate, the words they hear in the other ear. The child may be told the same thing or he may be told that the noise comes from the airplane engine and he has to make believe it isn't there. Actually, and fortunately, masking for speech discrimination is less distracting than for threshold tests since the loudness of the speech signal is not affected to any significant degree by the noise, and any drop in discrimination score below the unmasked condition will have to be attributed to elimination of the contribution of the nontest ear.

CASE HISTORIES

Every clinician has had experiences that he can use to prove or disprove his biases. Some are amusing, others shocking. All are illuminating.

Disagreement between results obtained with speech audiometry and those obtained with pure-tones have long been recognized as an indication of pseudohypacusis. I remember Zachary, a little boy 4 years old who obviously had a nonorganic problem and was having the hardest time convincing me that he could not hear. He simply refused to repeat spondees or raise his hand for pure-tones at even the highest intensities. When I asked him why (in a normal conversational voice) he answered that he couldn't hear. I instructed him to guess at the words and that it was all right if he was incorrect. In the first two responses, he substituted "hamburger" for "hot dog" and "submarine" for "airplane" at about 20dB HL. What started out to be a speech reception threshold test wound up as a word association game, but we were nevertheless able to determine that his hearing was normal.

A small girl, Erica, had failed the hearing screening test in kindergarten. Parental anxiety over a possible hearing loss had obviously netted her significant secondary gains, and she played the role in the audiology clinic by showing a 100dB hearing loss on the pure-tone audiogram. The test was completed by presenting the tones through one channel and speech through a second channel of the audiometer to the same earphone. Each time the tone was presented the child was asked (at 25dB HL) whether she heard it. In each case she responded "no." She gave no responses below 15dB HL. These negative responses were tracked down to show pure-tone thresholds well within the normal range.

The final case to be reported here is that of Michael, a small boy with suspected hearing loss. Air-conduction thresholds agreed with the SRT, suggesting a hearing loss of about 35dB. Bone-conduction thresholds were normal. All results appeared reliable. When the speech discrimination score was poor, a bone-conduction SRT was performed and gave essentially the same results as the air-conduction SRT. Retesting of bone conduction revealed that I had accepted false positive responses for bone conduction. The loss was sensorineural, which was borne out by acoustic impedance measurements. In this case the values of the speech discrimination test and of the bone conduction SRT are self-evident.

SUMMARY

The principles of behavior outlined in Chapter 6 on pure-tones may be general-ized, in many instances, to speech and audiometry. Because speech audiometry requires at least some degree of language development, it is often limited to children older than those who can sometimes be tested with pure-tone audi-ometry. When speech audiometry is possible in any form, from the most rigidly controlled to the most "arty," it should be carried out, because it serves a number of useful and often irreplaceable functions. Speech audiometry includes measurements of speech detection, speech reception, speech discrimination, and special discrimination tests for central auditory disorders.

The speech detection threshold, although it has limited utility with children in predicting hearing loss, can be used if no other test can be performed. If other tests are available and considered reliable, an SDT adds little in the way of useful diagnostic information. It should, in my opinion, serve as a test of last choice, to be performed only when more definitive tests such as pure-tones or speech reception thresholds cannot be established at the time.

The speech reception threshold provides useful information regarding the accuracy of the pure-tone thresholds or as a stopgap measurement while the child is being conditioned to take the pure-tone tests. The SRT is never a substitute for the pure-tone audiogram and testing the former without the latter in no way indicates that testing has been completed, no matter what the results. The SRT can be used with children to indicate the gain of a hearing aid, to estimate—with a modicum of accuracy—the kinds of communication difficulties the child has, and to hazard a prognostic judgment for aural habilitative or rehabilitative measures. The SRT is also useful in determining the appropriate level for speech discrimination tests.

Speech discrimination measures give information that allows comparison of receptive aural communication of the child to normal children and of the child's right ear to his left. In this way, the diagnosis of conductive versus sensorineural hearing loss may be substantiated, the selection of the ear to aid with amplification can be made, and statements about probable future and present communicative problems may be ventured. No method of speech discrimination measurement is truly satisfactory for children, and future research is needed desperately in this area.

The diagnosis of auditory processing disorders is difficult and often inaccurate. At the present the average audiologist does little about this problem. Normal hearing on the audiogram and speech reception and discrimination tests do not necessarily eliminate the possibility of a deficit beyond the peripheral mechanism.

RESEARCH NEEDS

Imaginative minds are even now at work attempting to develop procedures and methodologies that will allow some determination of speech thresholds and discrimination ability in children who have been considered too young, too deaf, or too difficult to test. What is needed in speech audiometry is not a plethora of tests that are no more than additions to existing tests. New test instruments will have to show a departure from the traditional kinds of stimuli. Screening procedures using speech audiometry are sorely needed to identify auditory disorders at the processing level where losses of sensitivity are not in evidence. We are at the threshold of such innovations.

REFERENCES

Beasley, D.S., J.E. Maki, and D.J. Orchik, "Children's Perception of Time-Compressed Speech on Two Measures of Speech Discrimination," *Journal of Speech and Hearing Disorders*, 41 (1976), 216–225.

Beattie, R.C., D.V. Svihovec, and B.J. Edgerton, "Relative Intelligibility of the CID Spondees as Presented Via Monitored Live Voice," *Journal of Speech and Hearing Disorders*, 40 (1975), 84–91.

Berlin, C.I., and S.S. Lowe, "Temporal and Dichotic Factors in Central Auditory Testing," in *Handbook of Clinical Audiology*, edited by J. Katz. Baltimore: Williams and Wilkins Co., 1972, pp. 280–312.

Bocca, E., and C. Calearo, "Central Hearing Processes," in *Modern Developments in Audiology*, edited by J. Jerger. New York: Academic Press, 1963, pp. 337–370.

Bocca, E., C. Calearo, and V. Cassinari, "A New Method for Testing Hearing in Temporal Lobe Tumors," *Acta Oto-laryngologica*, 44 (1954), 219–221.

Bunch, C., "Methods of Testing the Hearing in Infants and Young Children," *Journal of Pediatrics*, 5 (1934), 535–544.

Carhart, R., "Monitored Live Voice as a Test of Hearing Acuity," *Journal of the Acoustical Society of America*, 17 (1946), 339–349.

Carhart, R., "Observations on Relations Between Thresholds for Pure Tones and for Speech," *Journal of Speech and Hearing Disorders*, 36 (1971), 476–483.

Carhart, R., and L.S. Porter, "Audiometric Configurations and Prediction of Threshold for Spondees," *Journal of Speech and Hearing Research*, 14 (1971), 486–495.

Carhart, R., and T.W. Tillman, "Individual Consistency of Hearing for Speech Across Diverse Listening Conditions," *Journal of Speech and Hearing Disorders*, 15 (1972), 105–115.

Chaiklin, J., I.M. Ventry, and R. Dixon, *Hearing Measurement*, New York: Appleton-Century-Crofts, 1971, p. 207.

Clawsen, J., "Threshold for Pure Tone and Speech in Retardates," *American Journal of Mental Deficiency*, 70 (1966), 556–562.

Conn, M., J. Dancer, and I.M. Ventry, "A Spondee List for Determining Speech Reception Threshold Without Prior Familiarization," *Journal of Speech and Hearing Disorders*, 40 (1975), 380–396.

Cramer, K.D., and N.P. Erber, "A Spondee Recognition Test for Young Hearing-Impaired Children," *Journal of Speech and Hearing Disorders*, 39 (1974), 304–311.

Davis, H., "Audiometry: Pure Tone and Simple Speech Tests, in *Hearing and Deafness*, 3rd ed., edited by H. Davis and S.R. Silverman. New York: Holt, Rinehart and Winston, 1970, pp. 179–220.

Dewachter-Schaerlaekins, A.M., "The Influence of Intelligence on Speech Audiometry Test," *Acta Oto-laryngologica*, 23 (1969), 497–503.

259

Eagles, E., and S. Wishik, "A Study of Hearing in Children," *Transactions of the American Academy of Ophthalmology and Otology*, 65 (1961), 261–282.

Egan, J.P., "Articulation Testing Methods," *Laryngoscope*, 58 (1948), 955–991.

Erber, N.P., "Auditory, Visual, and Auditory-Visual Recognition of Consonants by Children with Normal and Impaired Hearing," *Journal of Speech and Hearing Research*, 15 (1972), 413–422.

Erber, N.P., "Pure-Tone Thresholds and Word-Recognition Abilities of Hearing-Impaired Children," *Journal of Speech and Hearing Research*, 17 (1974), 194–202.

Erber, N.P., and C.M. Alencewicz, "Audiologic Evaluation of Deaf Children," *Journal of Speech and Hearing Disorders*, 41 (1976), 256–267.

Frisina, R.D., "Audiometric Evaluation and Its Relation to Habilitation and Rehabilitation of the Deaf," *American Annals of the Deaf*, 107 (1962), 478–481.

Frisina, R., "Measurement of Hearing in Children," in *Modern Developments in Audiology*, 2nd ed., edited by J. Jerger. New York: Academic Press, 1973, pp. 155–174.

Giolas, T.G., "Speech Audiometry," in *Auditory Assessment of the Difficult-to-Test*, edited by R.T. Fulton and L.L. Lloyd. Baltimore: Williams and Wilkins Co., 1975, pp. 37–70.

Gladstone, V., and B. Siegenthaler, "Carrier Phrase and Speech Intelligibility Test Score," *Journal of Auditory Research*, 4 (1971), 101–103.

Goetzinger, C.P., "Rush Hughes Test in Auditory Diagnosis," in *Handbook of Clinical Audiology*, edited by J. Katz. Baltimore: Williams and Wilkins Co., 1972, pp. 325–333.

Goetzinger, C.P., and G.O. Proud, "Speech Audiometry by Bone Conduction," *Archives of Otolaryngology*, 62 (1955), 632–635.

Griffing, T., K. Simonton, and L. Hedgecock, "Verbal Auditory Screening for Preschool Children," *Transactions of the American Academy of Ophthalmology and Otolaryngology*, 71 (1967), 105–110.

Hardy, W., and J. Bordley, "Special Techniques in Testing the Hearing of Children," *Journal of Speech and Hearing Disorders*, 16 (1951), 122–131.

Hardy, W., and M. Pauls, "So That Children May Hear Better," *The Child*, 15 (1950), 18–22.

Hasegawa, S., T. Yoshida, I. Ohashi, T. Manage, and E. Itami, "The Verbal Auditory Screening Test for Children," *Audiology Japan*, 17 (1974), 148–155.

Haskins, H., "A Phonetically Balanced Test of Speech Discrimination for Children." Unpublished Master's thesis. Northwestern University, 1949.

Hirsh, I.J., *The Measurement of Hearing*. Highstown, N.J.: McGraw-Hill Book Co., 1952.

Hirsh, I.J., "Speech Audiometry—Special Remarks," *International Audiology*, 1 (1962), 183–185.

Hirsh, I., H. Davis, S.R. Silverman, E. Reynolds, E. Eldert, and R.W. Benson, "Development of Materials for Speech Audiometry," *Journal of Speech and Hearing Disorders*, 17 (1952), 321–337.

Hodgson, W.R., "Audiological Report of a Patient With Left Hemispherectomy," *Journal of Speech and Hearing Disorders*, 32 (1967), 39–45.

Hodgson, W.R., "A Comparison of WIPI and PB-K Discrimination Test Scores." Paper presented at the Annual Convention of the American Speech and Hearing Association, Detroit, 1973.

Hodgson, W.R., "Filtered Speech Tests," in *Handbook of Clinical Audiology*, edited by J. Katz. Baltimore: Williams and Wilkins Co., 1972b, pp. 313–324.

Hodgson, W.R., "Speech Discrimination of Children With Suspected Central Nervous System Impairments." Paper presented at the annual Hearing and Speech Seminar, Kansas University Medical Center, 1966.

Hodgson, W.R., "Testing Infants and Young Children," in *Handbook of Clinical Audiology*, edited by J. Katz. Baltimore: Williams and Wilkins Co., 1972a, pp. 498–519.

Hudgins, C.V., "Auditory Training: Its Possibilities and Limitations," *Volta Review*, 56 (1954), 339–349.

Hudgins, C.V., J.E. Hawkins, J.E. Karlin, and S.S. Stevens, "The Development of Recorded Auditory Tests for Measuring Hearing Loss for Speech," *Laryngoscope*, 57 (1947), 57–89.

Jerger, J., "Auditory Tests for Disorders of the Central Auditory Mechanism," in *Neurological Aspects of Auditory and Vestibular Disorders*, edited by W.S. Fields and B.R. Alford. Springfield, Ill.: Charles C. Thomas, 1964, pp. 77–93.

Jerger, J., and S. Jerger, "Diagnostic Significance of PB Word Functions," *Archives of Otolaryngology*, 93 (1971), 573–580.

Jones, K.O., and G.A. Studebaker, "Performance of Severely Hearing-Impaired Children On A Closed-Response, Auditory Speech Discrimination Test," *Journal of Speech and Hearing Research*, 17 (1974), 531–540.

Katz, J., "The SSW Test—An Interim Report," *Journal of Speech and Hearing Disorders*, 33 (1968), 132–146.

Katz, J., "The Use of Staggered Spondaic Words for Assessing the Integrity of the Central Auditory Nervous System," *Journal of Auditory Research*, 2 (1962), 327–337.

Katz, J., and R. Illmer, "Auditory Perception in Children with Learning Disabilities," in *Handbook of Clinical Audiology*, edited by J. Katz. Baltimore: Williams and Wilkins Co., 1972, pp. 540–563.

Keaster, J.A., "A Quantitative Method of Testing the Hearing of Young Children," *Journal of Speech and Hearing Disorders*, 12 (1947), 159–160.

Kimura, D., "Some Effects of Temporal-Lobe Damage on Auditory Perception," *Canadian Journal of Psychology*, 15 (1961), 156–165.

Kreul, E.J., D.W. Bell, and J.C. Nixon, "Factors Affecting Speech Discrimination

Test Difficulty," *Journal of Speech and Hearing Research*, 12 (1969), 281–287.

Lehiste, I., and G.E. Peterson, "Linguistic Considerations in the Study of Speech Intelligibility," *Journal of the Acoustical Society of America*, 31 (1959), 280–286.

Lehiste, I., and G.E. Peterson, "Revised CNC Lists for Auditory Tests," *Journal of Speech and Hearing Disorders*, 27 (1962), 62–70.

Lerman, J.W., M. Ross, and R.M. McLaughlin, "A Picture-Identification Test for Hearing-Impaired Children," *Journal of Auditory Research*, 5 (1965), 273–278.

Lloyd, L.L., and M.J. Reid, "The Reliability of Speech Audiometry with Institutionalized Retarded Children," *Journal of Speech and Hearing Research*, 9 (1966), 450–455.

Lloyd, L.L., M.J. Reid, and McManis, D.L., "The Effects of Response Mode on the SRTs Obtained from Retarded Children," *Journal of Auditory Research*, 7 (1967), 219–222.

McFarlan, D., "Speech Hearing and Speech Interpretation Testing," *Archives of Otolaryngology*, 31(1940), 517–528.

Martin, F.N., *Introduction to Audiology*. Englewood Cliffs, N.J.: Prentice-Hall, 1975.

Martin, F.N., and S. Coombes, "A Tangibly Reinforced Speech Reception Threshold Procedure for Use with Small Children," *Journal of Speech and Hearing Disorders*, 41 (1967), 333–338.

Martin, F.N., and C.D. Pennington, "Current Trends in Audiometric Practices," *Asha*, 13 (1971), 671–677.

Martin, F.N., and M.L. Stauffer, "A Modification of the Tillman-Olsen Method for Obtaining the Speech Reception Threshold," *Journal of Speech and Hearing Disorders*, 40 (1975), 25–28.

Martin, F.N., and S.M. Weller, "The Influence of the Carrier Phrase on the Speech Reception Threshold," *Journal of Communication Pathology*, 7 (1975), 39–44.

Matzker, J., "Two New Methods for the Assessment of Central Auditory Functions in Cases of Brain Disease," *Annals of Otology, Rhinology and Laryngology*, 68 (1959), 1185–1197.

Mencher, G.T., and B.F. McCulloch, "Auditory Screening of Kindergarten Children Using the VASC," *Journal of Speech and Hearing Disorders*, 35 (1970), 241–247.

Merrell, H.B., D.L. Wolfe, and D.C. McLemore, "Air and Bone Conducted Speech Reception Thresholds," *Laryngoscope*, 83 (1973), 1929–1939.

Meyerson, L., "Hearing for Speech in Children: A Verbal Audiometric Test," *Acta Oto-laryngologica Supplement 128*, 1956.

Meyerson, L., "A Verbal Audiometric Test for Young Children," *American Psychologist*, 2 (1947), 291–295.

Myatt, B., and B. Landes, "Assessing Discrimination Loss in Children," *Archives of Otolaryngology*, 77 (1963), 359–362.

Nober, E.H., "Cutile Air and Bone Conduction Thresholds of the Deaf," *Exceptional Children*, 36 (1970), 571–579.

Northern, J.L., and M.P. Downs, *Hearing in Children*. Baltimore: Williams and Wilkins Co., 1974, p. 151.

Ritchie, B.C., and R.A. Merklein, "An Evaluation of the Efficiency of the Verbal Auditory Screening Test for Children (VASC)," *Journal of Speech and Hearing Research*, 15 (1972), 280–286.

Ross, M., and J. Lerman, "A Picture Identification Test for Hearing-Impaired Children," *Journal of Speech and Hearing Research*, 13 (1970), 44–53.

Ross, M., M. Kessler, M. Phillips, and J. Lerman, "Visual, Auditory and Combined Mode of Presentations of the WIPI Test to Hearing Impaired Children," *Volta Review*, (1972), 90–96.

Ross, M., and N. Matkin, "The Rising Audiometric Configuration," *Journal of Speech and Hearing Disorders*, 32 (1967), 377–382.

Sanderson, M., and W. Rintelmann, "Performance of Normal-Hearing Children on Three Speech Discrimination Tests." Paper presented at the Annual Convention of the American Speech and Hearing Association, Chicago, 1971.

Schwartz, A., and R. Goldman, "Variables Influencing Performance on Speech-Sound Discrimination Tests," *Journal of Speech and Hearing Research*, 17 (1974), 26–32.

Siegenthaler, B., and G. Haspiel, "Development of Two Standardized Measures of Hearing for Speech by Children." Cooperative research program, Project #2372, U.S. Office of Education, 1966.

Siegenthaler, B., J. Pearson, and R. Lezak, "A Speech Reception Threshold Test for Children," *Journal of Speech and Hearing Disorders*, 19 (1954), 360–366.

Silverman, S.R., and I.J. Hirsh, "Problems Related to the Use of Speech in Clinical Audiometry," *Annals of Otology, Rhinology and Laryngology*, 64 (1955), 1234–1245.

Smith, K., "An Experimental Study of the Effects of Systematic Reinforcement on the Discrimination Responses of Normal and Hearing Impaired Children." Unpublished doctoral dissertation, University of Kansas (1969).

Sortini, A., and C. Flake, "Speech Audiometry Testing for Preschool Children," *Laryngoscope*, 63 (1953), 991–997.

Stockdell, K.G., "Speech by Bone Conduction in Diagnostic Audiometry," *Audecibel*, 23 (1974), 100–109.

Stubblefield, J.H., and C.E. Young, "Central Auditory Dysfunction in Learning Disabled Children," *Journal of Learning Disabilities*, 8 (1975), 89–94.

Tillman, T.W., and R. Carhart, "An Expanded Test for Speech Discrimination Utilizing CNC Mono-Syllabic Words." Northwestern University Auditory Test #6, Technical Report, SAM-TR-66-55. Brooks Air Force Base, Tex.:

USAF School of Aerospace Medicine, Aerospace Medical Division (AFSC), 1966.

Tillman, T.W., R. Carhart, and L. Wilber, "A Test for Speech Discrimination Composed of CNC Monosyllabic Words." Northwestern University Auditory Test No. 4, Technical Report, SAM-TDR-62-135. Brooks Air Force Base, Tex.: USAF School of Aerospace Medicine, Aerospace Medical Division (AFSC), 1963.

Tillman, T.W., and J.F. Jerger, "Some Factors Affecting the Spondee Threshold in Normal-Hearing Subjects," *Journal of Speech and Hearing Research*, 2 (1959), 141-146.

Tillman, T.W., and W.O. Olsen, "Speech Audiometry," in *Modern Developments in Audiology*, 2nd ed., edited by J. Jerger. New York: Academic Press, 1973, pp. 37-74.

Watson, T.J., "Speech Audiometry for Children," in *Educational Guidance and the Deaf Child*, edited by A.W.G. Ewing. Manchester, England: University Press, 1957, pp. 278-296.

Willeford, J.A., "Central Auditory Function in Children with Learning Disabilities," *Audiology and Hearing Education*, 2 (1976), 12-20.

Wilson, R.H., D.E. Morgan, and D.D. Dirks, "Proposed SRT Procedure and Its Statistical Precedent," *Journal of Speech and Hearing Disorders*, 38 (1973), 184-191.

CHAPTER EIGHT

Differential Diagnosis

PATRICIA R. COLE, MARY LOVEY WOOD

265

INTRODUCTION

Many children with abnormal verbal, social, or academic behavior experience difficulties in the utilization of information received auditorially. Children with normal hearing sensitivity may respond to sound abnormally and hence appear to have a hearing loss. Hard-of-hearing children may experience auditory problems in addition to those resulting from abnormal hearing sensitivity. Inappropriate or inconsistent responses to sound, failure to learn language normally, deviant social behavior, and academic difficulties may be symptoms of nonsensory auditory deficits.

Differential diagnosis is necessary to determine the nature and scope of auditory disorders so that proper treatment can be obtained. Other chapters in this book address identification of losses in hearing sensitivity. This chapter discusses auditory deficits resulting in children's failure to use sound appropriately for communication and learning. In this chapter, the terms auditory disorders, auditory impairments, auditory deficiencies, nonsensory auditory problems, or auditory reception deficits refer to abnormal utilization of auditory sensations, not to losses in hearing sensitivity.

Audiologists may be among the first professionals to see a child suspected of having an auditory deficit. Describing hearing sensitivity is a valuable part of the diagnosis of children with abnormal auditory functioning. However, the adequacy of other facets of audition cannot be inferred from pure-tone or speech-reception thresholds. As members of the differential diagnosis team, audiologists should be prepared to identify or rule out the presence of a hearing loss, to recognize symptoms of other auditory problems, to relate pertinent information to parents, and to refer patients to appropriate sources for further evaluation or remediation.

CHAPTER OBJECTIVES

The purpose of this chapter is to provide information to aid the audiologist, as a member of the differential diagnostic team, in recognizing auditory deficiencies

267

other than a loss in hearing sensitivity. The procedures described do not include all of the tasks or techniques necessary for making a definitive diagnosis. The intent is to assist diagnosticians in forming a tentative hypothesis about the nature of auditory functioning so that appropriate follow-up procedures can be recommended.

This chapter will describe (1) the purpose of differential diagnosis, (2) parameters of normal auditory functioning that contribute to effective communication and learning, (3) deficiencies in auditory functioning and their effects on behavior and development, (4) related nonauditory deficits, (5) acquisition and interpretation of pertinent background information, (6) etiological and other diagnostic categorization of children with auditory disorders, and (7) interpretation of diagnostic information to parents.

DIFFERENTIAL DIAGNOSIS

The purpose of differential diagnosis is to identify the nature and extent of a disorder and to describe behaviors in terms of deficient and normal learning processes. The diagnosis should provide accurate information on which to base treatment or therapy if it is to benefit parents, teachers, remediation specialists, and the child (Bangs, 1969; Hegrenes, Marshall, and Armas, 1970). A diagnosis can be made only after factors contributing to the problem have been differentiated from other conditions which might produce similar symptoms (Myklebust, 1954).

In evaluating behavior and learning, it is important to identify an individual's assets and weaknesses in many areas of functioning (Bangs, 1969). Children with a deficit in one area may be deficient in all other aspects of learning; so that their overall development is depressed, but progressing at a relatively even rate. Other children may have weaknesses in one or two areas but function significantly higher in others. Hasty judgments or predictions about general ability to learn, the nature or extent of the disorder, the cause of the deficit, or the appropriate treatment program can lead to errors of diagnosis harmful to the child.

An interdisciplinary team of professionals—audiologists, speech pathologists, psychologists, occupational therapists, teachers, and/or physicians— frequently is required for accurate diagnoses of auditory disorders. All members of such a team are responsible for performing those functions for which they are specifically trained as well as for recognizing observed or reported symptoms indicating the need for assistance from experts in another area, and for participating in an interchange of information with other team members. A single specialist should neither accept the responsibility for, nor afford himself the privilege of, making a differential diagnosis of auditory disorders without benefit of information from a variety of sources.

In evaluating auditory skills in children, certain types of errors often preclude a complete assessment and result in misdiagnosis. Misjudgments can occur if normal functioning of the total auditory system is inferred because hearing sensitivity has been identified as normal. Audiologists and other members of the diagnostic team must recognize hearing sensitivity as only one facet of auditory behavior. They must continue beyond evaluation of sensitivity and assess a child's ability to use audition in communication and learning (Myklebust, 1954). A second type of misjudgment can occur if examiners automatically assume that a child's failure to respond to sound is the result of a loss in hearing sensitivity. Other abnormalities can cause children to respond to sounds inconsistently, to ignore certain sounds but react to others, or to reject sound altogether (Johnson and Myklebust, 1967; Eisenson, 1968). A third type of diagnostic error can occur if assessment is halted as soon as one type of deficit has been identified. The high incidence of multiple handicaps demonstrates the importance of evaluating all aspects of behavior before making a diagnosis (Denhoff and Novack, 1967; Bangs, 1969; Berry, 1969).

Audiologists and other professionals must make judgments about the significance of reported or observed behaviors. Unfortunately, screening tests used to judge normalcy in development frequently examine an isolated aspect of behavior or are only gross measurements of developmental skills. In-depth assessment is time-consuming and requires skills generally not acquired in an audiologist's training. However, accurate judgments of normalcy of behavior and appropriate referrals may be possible if audiologists recognize common symptoms of abnormal auditory functioning. If audiologists are aware of components of auditory functioning that contribute to learning and of behaviors which suggest deficits in one or more aspects of audition, they will be able to interpret their observations appropriately. Audiologists who recognize symptoms of deviant auditory behavior and realize its significance should be able to make appropriate referrals and to explain to parents the need for additional assistance.

NORMAL PROCESSING AND USE OF AUDITORY INFORMATION

Normal children use hearing to scan and interpret their surroundings so that they can relate meaningfully to their environment. Appropriate use of sound is basic to the development of language and academic skills. Accurate interpretation of auditory information requires normal processes of sensation, perception, symbolization, and conceptualization.

Levels of Auditory Experience

Sensation refers to the activation of sensorineural structures; impairments at this level include peripheral auditory deficits (Johnson and Myklebust, 1967). As discussed in Chapters 2 and 3, auditory deficits that are sensory in nature interrupt normal developmental patterns of speech, language, and social behavior and restrict children's interactions with their environment. A sensory impairment may occur either as a solitary deficit in an otherwise intact auditory system or as one aspect of multiple auditory handicaps (Eisenson, 1968).

Perception is the process of distinguishing the characteristics of stimuli (Mecham, 1966a; Menyuk, 1974). Auditory perception permits a child to recognize and attend to differentiating properties of acoustic stimuli, to screen immediately pertinent sounds from incidental background noise, to discriminate among sounds and sound sequences, or to recognize a word after hearing only part of it. Auditory perceptual disorders may exist in children with certain types of sensory hearing impairments as they experience distortion of speech (Bangs, 1969). In some children with normal hearing sensitivity, the ability to perceive sounds appropriately is impaired (Eisenson, 1968). Deficits in auditory perception adversely affect children's ability to make maximum use of what they hear for communication and learning.

Verbal symbolization occurs in language development when particular sounds and sound combinations are assigned meanings and become symbols to represent objects, experiences, concepts, or ideas (Johnson and Myklebust, 1967; Bowerman, 1974). Adequate reception and perception of stimuli are necessary for development of symbolic behavior. Normally developing children hear what others say and perceive the characteristics of what they hear. By relating the speech they hear to what they see or do, they learn to interpret verbalizations (Bloom, 1974). Children who are unable to use sounds symbolically have deficits in understanding spoken language and in expressing information verbally. Symbolization is prerequisite to reasoning and concept formation.

Conceptualization, the most abstract level of language functioning, includes the ability to generalize and to perform abstract associations. Conceptual behavior is observable in simple categorization tasks as well as in more complex activities that call for drawing conclusions by recognizing relationships among experiences (Berko, 1966; Bruner, Goodnow, and Austin, 1967). A breakdown in sensation, perception, symbolization, or the integration of these processes interferes with conceptualization. Conceptual deficits may result in overly literal interpretation of verbal stimuli, in an inability to apply previously learned information in new situations, or in failures to predict consequences of behaviors. Interpretation and integration of auditory information is important for concept development. Efforts to define the nature and cause of conceptual deficits should include assessments of auditory functioning.

Integration of Information

Perception, symbolization, and conceptualization are interdependent processes influenced by the integration of auditory, visual, tactile, and proprioceptive information. Children learning to understand speech associate an auditory pattern with a visual stimulus in learning names for objects, letters, shapes, or actions. They learn to associate an auditory stimulus with a certain tactile sensation to understand the meaning of descriptive words such as *hot, smooth,* or *soft.* Integration of visual and tactile information permits a person to predict how something feels by looking at it. An example may help to clarify the use of intersensory integration in daily living.

A teenage boy, recently blinded in an accident, was explaining that he had been given demerits in his dormitory for failing to keep his floor shiny. When asked how he knew if the floor was shiny, he responded that he could tell by sliding his finger across the floor. If the floor was dull, his finger would stick. If the floor was shiny, his finger would glide smoothly across the surface. This young man's explanation provided evidence of his integration of tactile, verbal, and visual information.

A breakdown in sensory integration may result in abnormal verbal or nonverbal behavior. Persons attempting to understand or describe abnormal functioning should consider the interrelationship of information acquired through different channels of sensory input.

Manifestations of Auditory Proficiency

The adequacy of children's auditory perception, symbolization, or conceptualization processes can be described in the framework of reception, expression, and reasoning behaviors. Auditory receptive behaviors are observable in children's responses to linguistic and nonlinguistic auditory stimuli. In infants, auditory reception skills progress from simple awareness reactions to differentiated responses to such familiar noises as mother's voice, the sound of a spoon in a cup, or the opening of the refrigerator. At a later age, learning to understand what others say becomes a crucial component of auditory reception. In addition to recognizing the meaning of single word utterances, children must understand an infinite number of word combinations. They cannot depend on memory for learning all new sentences. They must learn to interpret meanings signaled by various grammatical and semantic constructions specific to their language (Bloom, 1974). Using information received auditorially is the primary means by which children learn language.

Expressive manifestations of auditory processing proceed from differentiated babbling in infancy to imitations of linguistic and nonlinguistic sounds. Young children learn to use words and sentences referentially and as a means of controlling their environment. Children's learning from auditory information may be evidenced in their pronunciation of words, vocabulary, or sentence construction and in their success in transmitting information through speaking. Abstract reasoning based on auditory or verbal information reflects certain information about children's interpretation of what they hear. Children's proficiency in reasoning may surface through their interpretation of what is heard, in the form and content of their speech, or in their social and academic adjustments.

Receptive, expressive, and reasoning abilities are evidenced in language development, in emotional and social behaviors, and in academic achievement. Evaluations of auditory proficiency should consider an individual's functioning within each of these parameters.

SYMPTOMS OF AUDITORY DISORDERS

Although recognition of aberrant behaviors and their implications is an important component in the diagnosis of auditory disorders (Myklebust, 1954; Eisenson, 1968), behavioral observations should not serve as the sole source of information in making a differential diagnosis. Rather, behavioral observation should provide valuable clues to the nature of the disorder and to the type of additional information needed. In the literature and in our clinical practice, several common behavioral patterns occur repeatedly in descriptions of children with auditory disorders. The following discussion describes some of the reported or observed characteristics we find useful in recognizing auditorially deficient children.

Auditory Receptive Behavior

Some children with normal hearing sensitivity do not give overt responses to sounds in their environment. If they cannot differentiate among or attach meaning to sounds received physically, such children may ignore sounds and give the false impression of peripheral deafness (Myklebust, 1954). This distinction between sensory and nonsensory deficits must be made before treatment is recommended. The fitting of a hearing aid, appropriate for some children with sensory hearing losses, can be devastating to children with normal sensory intake but impaired auditory perception (Johnson and Myklebust, 1967). In addition to the danger of acoustic trauma, those children might find the bombardment and additional distortion of amplified sound confusing, disorienting, and uncomfortable.

Auditory perceptual disorders can cause an overreaction to sound (Ornitz and Ritvo, 1976). Some children appear to be auditorially defensive and cover their ears or scream in noisy situations such as a circus, party, construction sites, or when music is playing. Parents and teachers often describe these children as having better-than-normal hearing or as being overly sensitive to noise. However, overreaction to sound may be symptomatic of defective auditory perception and should signal the need for additional investigation of auditory functioning.

Children with auditory disorders often respond inconsistently to sound (Johnson and Myklebust, 1967; Eisenson, 1968). Some are unable to listen selectively to one sound in the presence of competing noise and may not respond to a seemingly obvious auditory stimulus (F. Berko, 1966; Wepman, 1969). This type of deficit sometimes is called an auditory figure-ground problem. The following example demonstrates this type of auditory disorder.

A mother brought her 6-year-old son to our speech and hearing center because she suspected that he had a hearing loss. The audiologist found that the child had normal pure-tone and speech-reception thresholds and his speech discrimination scores were above 90%. The mother's answers to our questions revealed that she was concerned because her son did not respond if she spoke to him when he was watching TV or listening to his record player. She noted that if there was noise in the house while he was watching TV, he always turned the volume up. The child's teacher reported that the boy did not pay attention when she called him on the playground (obviously a noisy situation), and that he seemed to attend better and to enjoy stories more when he listened to recordings through headsets than when she read aloud to the whole class. In a subsequent conversation with the teacher, we learned that during the story hour, the classroom was quite noisy because another class had recess on the playground adjacent to the room. The mother's and teacher's reports led us to suspect that this child had auditory figure-ground deficits that made him unable to select and attend to certain auditory stimuli in the presence of other sound. Subsequent testing corroborated this suspicion.

Inconsistent responses to speech also may be evidence of a child's inability to predict a total auditory pattern after hearing only part of it (Kirk and Kirk, 1971). The ability to close—that is, to predict the missing part of an utterance or word—is crucial to understanding speech in many situations. Frequently a listener does not hear every sound, syllable, or word spoken to him, either because part was masked by other noise or because he was not attending to the speech signal. A child with normal hearing sensitivity and normal auditory closure skills could hear, "Get a drink of wa——", and comprehend the statement. Those with inadequate auditory closure abilities probably would be unable to interpret the utterance because they could not predict the missing word or sounds on the basis of the partial information provided. Children with auditory closure deficits may fail to understand simple speech in some situations, but comprehend much more difficult verbalizations in others. They frequently ask for repetitions of what is said, especially if there is competing environmental noise or if their full attention is not directed to the listening task. They may understand the speech of adults but have unusual difficulty interpreting the imperfect speech of young children or defective speakers. This discrepancy probably results from their inability to use auditory clues to figure out the appropriate interpretation of mispronounced words. Parents and teachers often describe children with auditory closure deficits as inattentive or hard-of-hearing.

Deficits in auditory memory may be reflected in numerous receptive and expressive behaviors (Bangs, 1969; Menyuk and Looney, 1976). Auditory memory affects the ability to recall the order of sounds and words and to store auditory signals and their meanings so that they can be retrieved when needed. Children with deficient memory may follow only one part of a series of directions; they may fail to complete assignments in school because they forget what they were told; they may speak in short utterances or have a limited vocabulary. Certain types of memory deficits are evidenced by a child's performance of a task one day followed by a seeming lack of recognition of the same task the next day. Children with deficient auditory memory frequently are described as inattentive or daydreamers because they do not remember what they are told. Their intelligence may be questioned because they forget factual information presented in school or the names of their classmates or neighbors.

Some children have auditory symbolization deficits, demonstrated by their failure to attach meaning to what they hear. In severe cases, they may show an awareness of the presence of sound but be unable to interpret anything they hear (Myklebust, 1954). Some children learn to attach meaning to nonlinguistic auditory stimuli but do not understand spoken linguistic symbols. They may run to the telephone when it rings or get their toy fire truck when they hear a siren, yet give no meaningful response to what is said.

Behaviors reflecting inadequate comprehension of verbal stimuli are numerous. Some children with auditory comprehension problems appear disinterested in any verbal activities and ignore what is said. Others give random responses to verbalizations, acting as if they realize that verbalizations directed to them require a response, but giving little indication that they understand the meaning of what is said. Auditory comprehension deficits are observable in some children when they are required to understand connected utterances or sentences. Their responses may indicate that they understood one or two words in a verbal sequence but did not comprehend the meaning of the total utterance. For example, they may give the same response to differing verbal stimuli which have one or two key words in common.

A 4-year-old we saw recently had limited comprehension of connected speech. He responded by giving his teacher's name when asked what his teacher had given him, what story his teacher had read, and where his teacher lived. The questions were asked at different points in the interview to decrease the probability of perseveration. The child's responses suggested that he was interpreting the word *teacher,* common to all three questions, but that he did not understand the meaning of the utterances as a whole.

Echolalia, which is the meaningless imitation of verbal stimuli, often is a symptom of failure to understand what was said (Johnson and Myklebust, 1967; Fay and Butler, 1968). Rote imitation of a verbal stimulus is normal in some stages of language learning. In normally developing children, echolalic speech usually occurs intermittently along with meaningful verbalizations; it gradually decreases as language skills improve (Nelson, 1973). Some children with auditory deficits continue to be echolalic, have little if any meaningful speech, and do not give appropriate nonverbal responses to verbal stimuli. While they do not understand the meaning of what is said, they may realize that a verbal stimulus requires a verbal response and simply repeat or echo what they hear. Aram and Nation (1975) stated that children whose repetition skills are superior to comprehension skills or to meaningful production seem to treat language as a sensory motor phenomenon, transferring auditory input to spoken output without attaching meaning to the verbal signals.

Steven was typical of an echolalic child with severe auditory deficits. When brought to therapy at 3 years of age, he had no speech except for echoed responses and memorized phrases. Steven and the diagnostician had the following verbal exchange:

Examiner:	Hello Steven.
Steven:	Hello Steven.
Examiner:	How old are you?
Steven:	How old are you?
Examiner:	Where do you live?
Steven:	You live?
Examiner:	Steven, take off your coat.
Steven:	Take off your coat.

Steven produced other rote verbalizations in addition to immediate echoing responses. While looking through a magazine, he saw a package of wieners and sang a song from a television commercial advertising this food. Steven's parents reported that he had learned to read from watching a children's TV program. His mother wrote the word *cat* on the chalkboard and Steven sounded it out phonetically and then pronounced the word. The examiner then verbally presented several sound sequences, such as *h-o-p* and *d-o-g*. Steven repeated the sequence and then said the word that resulted from synthesis of sounds. In no instance could he appropriately select an object or picture of an object represented by the word. He had accomplished tasks requiring memory, sequencing, and sound synthesis but the words were void of meaning for him.

Steven either ignored verbalizations directed to him or responded by screaming "No!," by throwing himself against the wall or on the floor, or by giving nonmeaningful repetitions. He made no effort to use speech to communicate with his parents, peers, or examiners. On formal tests, Steven demonstrated superior functioning in nonverbal tasks so long as success was not tied to his understanding verbal instructions. He was unable to accomplish any meaningful verbal tasks.

Problems in interpretation of abstract verbal information or in drawing conclusions may be symptomatic of deficiencies in the ability to reason verbally (M. Berko, 1966). These problems most often become apparent in school-age children who do not understand the intended or implied meanings of what is said. They may fail to understand idioms, jokes, or puns. If a literal interpretation of what is said will suffice, they may function adequately. If they are required to infer beyond what is actually said, they fail. Their peers as well as parents and teachers often consider them naive or slow learners. Overly literal interpretations may be viewed as obstinate or disrespectful behavior and a child may be reprimanded for failing to draw the intended conclusions.

Ann, a second-grader with a history of severe auditory reception problems, was told by her teacher to alphabetize the words *cat, house, tree, pig,* and *baby.* Ann was denied recess when her completed assignment read *abby, act, eert, ehosu, gip.* Before lunch one day, Ann's teacher instructed the class to take one bite of everything on the cafeteria tray before throwing the food away. In the cafeteria that day, Ann took one bite of each item on her tray, threw the remainder in the garbage can, then told her teacher that she was still hungry and asked for another tray of food. As punishment for what the teacher considered to be insolent behavior, Ann was not permitted to eat with the class for the remainder of the week. In these and many other instances, Ann interpreted literally what she was told. She always thought she had done what she was instructed to do and did not understand why she was punished until the differences in the intent of the instruction and her interpretation were explained to her.

The inability to manipulate verbal information for making inferences and drawing conclusions can be debilitating and often is not recognized as a problem in auditory or language learning. Diagnosticians should be alert to behaviors suggesting this type of deficit.

Many children with auditory disorders accomplish nonverbal tasks at least as well as their peers, but experience difficulty when required to learn or to respond to verbal stimuli (Peterson, 1967; Kirk and Kirk, 1971). This may confuse parents or teachers. They recognize that the child functions well on some activities but fails on others. Parents or teachers are likely to describe children with discrepancies between verbal and nonverbal functioning as interested in only a few things, as stubborn and unwilling to try on some tasks, or as having a mental block against certain activities.

Verbal Expressive Behavior

A disorder in auditory reception often affects verbal expression (Johnson and Myklebust, 1967). Unless there is evidence of motor impairment, verbal expressive deficits usually are associated with auditory inadequacies (Eisenson, 1968). Problems in verbal expression resulting from deficient auditory functioning range in severity and type.

The most common expressive disorder described by parents and other laypersons is mispronunciation or misarticulation of words. Articulation, the learned behavior of producing speech sounds, requires integrity of certain auditory functions. Failure to acquire adequate articulation skills within a normal time frame may be symptomatic of auditory dysfunctions. The relationship between speech-sound discrimination ability and articulation proficiency has been investigated repeatedly (Weiner, 1967; Winitz, 1969). Results of these studies indicate that some but not all persons with defective articulation have inferior auditory discrimination. Deficient speech-sound discrimination ability is one of the possible causes of inadequate articulation and should be evaluated in persons with defective articulation. Sound omissions are a common type of articulation error. Panagos (1974) suggested that children who omit medial and final consonant sounds and speak primarily in consonant-vowel syllables, probably have deficits in the phonological, syntactic, and semantic components of language. Such errors in sound production often reflect deficiencies in one or more aspects of audition.

Some children's expressive deviations result from intraword sequencing errors (Kirk and Kirk, 1971). Children whose speech is characterized by mispronunciations such as *deks* for *desk, cools* for *school,* or *buffertye* for *butterfly* may have an underlying receptive problem in sequencing. Those who exhibit extreme problems in pronouncing polysyllabic words may have deficits in processing complex phonological combinations.

Children who fail to comprehend the constructional aspects of language may not use words within appropriate word class boundaries and may use incorrect grammatical structures (Johnson and Myklebust, 1967). They may place words in the wrong sequence in sentences, misuse certain words, and fail to use grammatical forms to signal intended meanings.

Five-year-old Mark had expressive problems that included misordering of words within sentences, failure to observe appropriate word class restrictions, and inappropriate use of morphological markers. His unusual sentence construction sometimes made his speech difficult to understand, although he had few errors in articulation. Mark's defective sentence construction was evident in his statement, "The lawn man mower the grass cut," which was said as he looked at a picture of a man pushing the lawnmower across the grass. Although the structure was abnormal, the meaning of the utterance was obvious to the clinician as she looked at the picture with Mark and probably would have been interpretable to someone who did not see the picture. Additional assessment revealed that Mark had normal hearing sensitivity but experienced extreme problems in comprehension of grammatical forms and in memory for auditory sequences. His abnormal expressive abilities were the most immediately evident, but identification of the associated receptive deficits was crucial to understanding his problems and to planning appropriate remediation.

Some children use telegraphic speech, including in their utterances only words which carry the most meaning (Peterson, 1967; Berry, 1969). Their utterances may take the form of "Man go store," or "I cut finger knife." Other children fail to use grammatical markers to signal past tense, plurality, or possession. These production errors may be symptoms of disabilities in receptive language.

Children who have difficulty interpreting speech will be restricted in their use of words and word combinations (Johnson and Myklebust, 1967; Eisenson, 1968). Limitations in expressive vocabulary may be evidence of deficiencies in the ability to understand speech. Vocabulary deficits may be demonstrated in children's limited word use so that it is obvious they have not learned many of the common words to which they have been exposed. Some children fail to learn multiple meanings of words. For example, they may learn the words *paint* and *nail* as nouns but not as verbs. Other children learn one word to express a concept, but do not learn additional words to express the same idea. For example, they may continue to refer to all canines as *puppy,* not acquiring the word *dog,* or to describe things as *pretty,* but fail to learn that the word *beautiful* has a similar meaning. Children who fail to expand their expressive vocabulary may have receptive inabilities that interfere with language and learning.

If children do not understand abstractions in the language that they hear, the content of their utterances will be concrete. Analysis of their verbal output is likely to reveal the absence of comparative statements, idioms, or abstract ideas. They may attempt to tell jokes, yet show obvious difficulty in telling or interpreting them correctly. Their explanations of events, situations, or ideas may be restricted to reports of factual information and exclude abstract interpretations of causal conditions or speculative descriptions.

Disfluency or disorganization within an utterance or a series of utterances often reflects difficulties in organizing verbal information and may be related to auditory disorders (Johnson and Myklebust, 1967). Children may be diagnosed as stutterers because they frequently stop in the middle of a sentence, repeat words or phrases, or have other disruptions in the rhythm and fluency of speech. Before the child is labeled a stutterer and placed in a treatment program for this problem, diagnosticians should be certain that the nonfluencies noted in speech are not symptoms of an inability to organize language. Mislabeling a child as a stutterer can have an adverse effect on his speech and language. Treating a child with language organization problems as though he were a stutterer is unlikely to result in improvement in his basic communication problem.

Extensive evaluation is required to determine the adequacy of expressive language skills, and additional assessment is necessary to identify the relationship between expressive and receptive language. Because expressive deficits are frequently symptoms of auditory disorders, the diagnostician should be alert to expressive problems and their potential relationship with receptive functioning.

Social-Emotional Behavior

Children whose verbal communication is disrupted by nonsensory auditory deficits often have difficulties in social behavior and adjustment. The extent of their social or emotional problems varies from complete withdrawal to minor difficulties in interactions with family members or peers. They may react to communication failures by emotional and social isolation and become overly passive or withdrawn (Eisenson, 1968). Their parents and teachers sometimes describe them as loners or social isolates. Peers may shun them because they cannot engage in the symbolic play and verbal exchanges so important to social interaction.

Children with auditory disorders frequently are described as socially immature. They may prefer younger playmates instead of those their own age, possibly because their limited communication skills allow them to interact and compete more successfully with a younger age group. Children with receptive language disorders may select books, television programs, or games appropriate for younger children, and their emotional reactions may be immature. Delay in social development, because it may be the product of limited communication skills, should be considered as a possible indication of receptive language deficits.

Children with linguistic deficits often appear to be disoriented and their behavior may be described as undirected (deHirsch, 1967; de Ajuriaguerra et al., 1976). They may move randomly from one task to another, misjudge the general orientation of a situation, or act and react in an inappropriate manner. If they cannot use auditory clues and linguistic information to assist in interpreting the meaning of a situation, their general behavior may be disorganized.

Auditorially handicapped children often are described as overly aggressive (M. Berko, 1966). Their vain attempts to understand and respond to a verbal world may prod them into extreme physical aggression or emotional outbursts. Children with normal language argue verbally, but those with deficient receptive or expressive verbal skills resort to physical interchanges to settle disputes. Older children with auditory reception disorders may be considered overly aggressive because of their lack of tact. Their inability to synthesize information results in a failure to learn codes of acceptable social conduct. Parents, teachers, and peers may consider them to be insensitive, hostile, or sometimes cruel. An example may help to emphasize the socially handicapping effects of certain auditory deficits.

A 15-year-old girl with a history of severe auditory receptive disorders had extreme problems in social adjustment. With extensive therapy she was able to use speech as a tool for communication and learning, but she continued to be literal in most verbal activities. Although she made above-average academic progress and scored at a superior level on most intelligence tests, she had no friends and she could not understand why her behavior had a negative impact on those around her. Her teacher reported that within a two-day period, she overheard this girl tell a boy that his shirt was old and faded, tell one classmate that her shoes did not match her dress, tell another that she should diet because she was overweight, and suggest to a shy classmate that he would make better grades if he studied more. The teacher noted that each of these comments, although true, was offensive to the recipient. In a subsequent conversation with this 15-year-old, we learned that she did not realize that her statements would be considered rude or offensive and saw no relationship between her behavior and her classmates' rejection of her. She used language in a concrete manner, having failed to learn to make the abstract interpretations necessary for social success.

Parents frequently describe their children with auditory reception disorders as discipline problems. They tell of their frustration in vainly trying to explain to their children what they can and cannot do and the reasons for rules of conduct. Not realizing that the children may understand little of what they are told, the parents describe them as defiant, stubborn, or unable to learn.

Parents and teachers sometimes complain because a child persists in the same behavior, even when it is no longer functional, appropriate, or acceptable (Myklebust, 1954; M. Berko, 1966). This type of repetitive behavior, sometimes called perseveration, is common in children with auditory disorders or with other types of learning deficits. Perseveration may be noted in many facets of behavior.

A teacher reported that 7-year-old Billy often began writing his name and continued to write *B* until he had filled a line or sometimes a whole page. A mother stated that she could not let her 6-year-old son put toothpaste on his toothbrush because unless supervised, he continued to squeeze the tube until it was empty. A kindergarten teacher expressed concern because a 5-year-old girl often spent the morning doing nothing but pouring sand from one bucket to another. In art class, the same child intermittently colored the entire page with the same crayon unless the teacher handed her a different one. The child's mother and teacher reported that once she started laughing or crying, she seemed unable to stop, even though the precipitating event was no longer in evidence.

Unless those who interact with a perseverative child recognize when behaviors are involuntary and understand how to cope with them, the child is likely to be misunderstood and mishandled.

Abnormal auditory functioning certainly is not the only cause of social and behavioral problems in children. Because many children with auditory deficits have problems in adjustment, auditory functioning should be evaluated when behavior problems are being defined and treated. In the differential diagnosis of auditory disorders, a careful analysis of social interactions can provide information of value in assessing the adequacy of auditory functioning.

Academic Behavior

Inadequate auditory reception and verbal expression adversely affect academic performance (Johnson and Myklebust, 1967; Vogel, 1975). If children cannot predict the proper grammatical construction in a spoken utterance, they will not have the clues for prediction in reading. They may read *ran* as *run*, *two dogs* as *two dog*, or *jumping* as *jump*. Those who cannot perceive or remember a sequence of sounds and blend them into a word on the basis of auditory clues will not be able to sound out written words and synthesize the sounds into words. They may learn sound-letter associations, correctly identify each sound in a word, then be unable to put the sounds together to read the word. Some children with auditory processing problems rely on visual memory for sight reading. Their reading problems may not become evident until they reach a point when they no longer can memorize every word they must read or until they are expected to read words they have not seen previously. Understanding the meaning of what is read is as important as accomplishing the mechanics of reading. Children with auditory reception deficits and limited language comprehension often fail to find meaning in what they read. Any deficit in interpretation of spoken language will be carried over into comprehension of written language.

The tasks of phonics and spelling require the integration of auditory with visual information. Some children reach school age with fairly adequate auditory and visual processing, but have not learned to relate information received through these sensory channels. They may use spoken language appropriately, yet be unable to relate spoken to written symbols. For example, a child may recognize rhyming words when he hears them, but have difficulty learning that rhyming words usually have similar visual configurations when written. Children unable to relate written and spoken symbols may recognize the initial sound in a word and make a seemingly absurd guess at what the word is. For example if a word begins with *e,* they call it *egg* or *elephant,* not realizing that a three-letter word such as *egg* could not possibly be the appropriate spelling for a three-syllable word such as *elephant.* When children reach an academic level where they are required to express information in writing, their writing is likely to reflect their deficits in oral language. A language-deficient child may omit or misuse words or demonstrate poor organization of content in his written work.

Mark is typical of many children brought to an audiologist or other specialist by desperate parents who hope that a reversible hearing loss accounts for their child's academic failures. Mark, a child who had deficient language as a product of auditory disabilities, wrote the following sentences when he was in third grade: "Two boy eated undr. They going to hom." When he read his sentences, Mark said, "Two boys eated under the tree. They are going to home." When asked to correct any errors in the written sentences, he remarked that he saw no inaccuracies. Mark's academic achievement was hindered further by his difficulty in remembering the teacher's sequence of instructions; as a consequence, he often did not complete his assignments. If he was writing while the teacher was talking, or if the classroom was noisy, Mark could not comprehend what was said by his teacher or his classmates. His deficits in auditory reception, verbal expression, and integration of visual and auditory symbols adversely affected his academic performance.

If children have difficulties with schoolwork, diagnostic efforts should examine their auditory abilities as well as their skills in relating auditory and visual symbols. By examining the nature of academic performance, the diagnostician may obtain clues to the nature of deficits in audition.

Related Non-Auditory Behaviors

A child with processing deficits in one modality is likely to demonstrate impairments in another (Wyatt, 1969). Children with auditory disorders are high-risk subjects for visual, tactile, and proprioceptive deficiencies, and they often have motor problems.

Deficits in perceiving and interpreting visual information may be present in children with auditory deficiencies (Berry, 1969). They may be unable to see a total visual configuration because of their absorbing attention to insignificant detail or because they cannot distinguish between important and unimportant information in a visual field. For example, they might examine a spot on a ball instead of perceiving the ball as an object for play. Children with disturbances of visual perception may recognize visual configurations only when they are sufficiently outlined, simplified, and segregated from a conglomerate visual background. Deficits in visual memory may interfere with the ability to recall certain visual symbols or patterns.

Inadequate tactile reception can result in acute sensitivity or misinterpretation of touch (Ayres, 1972). A child may withdraw or overreact to physical contact. Tactually disordered children may be irritable as babies. They may cry when held, or may move frequently in an attempt to avoid unseen or prolonged physical contact. They often feel discomfort after sitting on a hard surface, even for short periods of time. They may change positions often, or may move around the classroom. They are sometimes described as hyperactive. A defective tactile memory may cause children to touch everything they see because they cannot remember how things feel. If tactile and visual integration of information does not occur, visual inspection alone does not give information about texture, weight, or temperature, so the child may have to touch an object to recognize certain characteristics.

Proprioceptive feedback may be impaired so that children do not receive proper information from joints and muscles and thus about body movement and position in space. These children may not know what their bodies are doing unless they have constant visual or tactile cues. They may not realize that they are falling from a chair until they hit the floor. When blindfolded so that visual clues do not inform them of their location in space, they may be unable to sit or stand steadily or to pretend to throw a ball.

Tommy, a child with inadequate proprioceptive feedback, was blindfolded and asked to walk forward across the room. He moved his legs up and down, marching in place but making no forward progress. He was allowed to continue in this motion for about 60 seconds before the blindfold was removed. Tommy was astonished that he had not moved from his original location. When denied visual clues, he had been unable to determine whether or not he was moving forward.

Children with impaired proprioceptive systems may have difficulty with motor planning, which is the ability to put together a voluntary sequence of motor movements to perform an action. They may not remember how to put their arms into a shirt, tie shoelaces, write letters or numbers, or move their mouth to make a sound or word. Although motor planning deficits have a surface resemblance to coordination problems, they do not result from paralysis or coordination difficulties. Children with poor motor planning abilities may involuntarily perform a sequence of motor acts that they cannot do voluntarily, indicating that the movements can be accomplished, but not at will or on command.

A child with visual-motor processing problems may exhibit poor integration of one side of the body with the other and may use his body as though it were composed of two unconnected halves rather than one unit (Ayres, 1972). He might read the left half of a line with the left eye and the right half with the right eye, or draw the left half of a circle with the left hand and the right half with the right hand. Some children disregard one side of their body and do not recognize or attend to anything happening on that side. These kinds of problems interfere with the many visual and motor activities that require the child's body to function as a unit, with a dominant side and a complementing side.

Visual or tactile deficits may cause children to be quite active, although their motor activity may not be directed toward any particular task or for any particular purpose. They may interact or examine objects briefly, merely coming in contact with them, then quickly move to something else. They may be unable to focus on one thing while ignoring other stimuli in their visual field. Some of their activity may result from a need to avoid certain physical contacts which might be uncomfortable for them.

Delayed acquisition of gross and fine motor skills and lack of motor coordination may reflect deficits in a child's interpretation and use of tactile and proprioceptive clues or in his integration of information from various sensory modalities. Observations or reports of unusual clumsiness or awkwardness should not be dismissed as insignificant.

The meaningful use of gestures requires interpretation of nonverbal symbols and may necessitate relating to others in a meaningful way. Unlike children whose only deficit is a sensory auditory impairment, those with generalized symbolic deficits may not use gestures to communicate (Myklebust, 1954). They also may be deficient in interpreting other people's nonverbal signals, such as hand signs or body movements. Inappropriate or immature play with toys may characterize the child with deficiencies in symbolic skills. Using toys in a representative or creative manner requires a child's understanding what the toy represents and his projection of himself into an imaginary experience. This behavior requires integration of information and the ability to use symbols to represent certain aspects of the world.

Deficits in the use of information received through any modality can affect language, social, and emotional development. Such deficits often occur in conjunction with auditory disorders. Recognition of deficient functioning and appropriate assessment of all aspects of learning should be a part of the differential diagnosis process.

Interpretation of Previous Test Information

Proper interpretation of test results can be of assistance in recognizing children with learning disorders. A prerequisite to accurate interpretation is knowledge of what a specific test measures; without this information, overgeneralizations or misinterpretations are likely to occur (Berry, 1969; Weiner, 1971; Spellacy and Black, 1972; Black, 1973). Measures of intelligence, language, visual-motor skills, and inventories of social and emotional development are among the assessment tools commonly used with children with auditory disorders. Tests of academic achievement are administered routinely to most school-age children.

Intelligence tests attempt to identify mental abilities by comparing an individual's performance on certain tasks with normative data (Wechsler, 1964). Intelligence test scores may serve a descriptive function in defining a child's present abilities and a prognostic function in predicting potential rate and capacity for learning. Presentation methods and tasks required of the child vary from test to test. Some intelligence measures are highly verbal and require the child to understand and to use speech. The most commonly used test of this nature is the Stanford-Binet Intelligence Scale, Form L–M (Terman and Merrill, 1960). Reputable though this instrument is, it may not reflect accurately the intellectual capacity of children with auditory disorders because it is heavily loaded with verbal items. The Merrill Palmer Intelligence Test (Stutsman, 1948), the Leiter International Performance Scale (Arthur, 1952), and the Columbia Mental Maturity Scale (1959) are primarily nonverbal, assessing learning abilities through visual and motor tasks. Auditorially handicapped children typically score significantly higher on nonverbal tests than on those containing numerous verbal items.

The Wechsler Intelligence Scale for Children (Wechsler, 1974) and the Wechsler Preschool and Primary Scale of Intelligence (Wechsler, 1967) are divided into verbal and performance subtests. Verbal, performance, and full scale IQ scores can be derived. If significant discrepancies exist between verbal and performance scores, it is likely that the child has abnormal patterns of learning. Auditorially disordered children usually score significantly lower on the verbal than on the performance portions of these tests.

The Illinois Test of Psycholinguistic Abilities (ITPA) assesses children's functioning in verbal and nonverbal skills (Kirk, McCarthy, and Kirk, 1969). The ITPA is not an intelligence test, but is intended to provide a profile of a child's strengths and weaknesses in areas related to academic success. It contains subtests categorized as visual–motor or auditory–vocal, and comparison of a child's scores on various tests may reveal specific assets and deficits in learning processes. While the test yields a composite psycholinguistic age, its principal diagnostic value lies in the information provided by a child's pattern of behavior on the various subtests.

Certain tests assess a child's proficiency in performing specific language or auditory tasks. The Peabody Picture Vocabulary Test (Dunn, 1965) and the Full Range Picture Vocabulary Test (Ammons and Ammons, 1958) are measures of auditory comprehension of single words. The receptive portion of the Northwestern Syntax Screening Test (Lee, 1969) and the Test of Auditory Comprehension of Language (Carrow, 1973) are designed to evaluate children's comprehension of certain grammatical structures. The expressive subtest of the Northwestern Syntax Screening Test (Lee, 1969) and the Carrow Elicited Language Inventory (Carrow, 1974) assess a child's productive control of grammatical forms through a sentence-imitation task. The Wepman Auditory Discrimination Test (Wepman, 1958) and the Goldman-Fristoe-Woodcock Test of Discrimination (Goldman et al., 1970) are designed to measure children's ability to differentiate among speech sounds. Commonly used tests of children's ability to articulate sounds include the Goldman-Fristoe Test of Articulation

(Goldman and Fristoe, 1969) and the Templin-Darley Test of Articulation (Templin and Darley, 1960). Each of these measures provides important information about specific aspects of a child's auditory and language functioning, but none is inclusive enough to permit accurate generalization to other behaviors on the basis of the score or performance on a single text.

Frequently used tests of visual–motor functioning include the Visual Motor Inventory (Beery, 1967), the Developmental Test of Visual Perception (Frostig, 1964), and the Bender Visual Motor Gestalt (Bender, 1949). Each of these provides information about visual perception, eye-hand coordination, and fine motor skills. The Southern California Test of Sensory Integration (Ayres, 1975) is designed to obtain information about tactile and kinesthetic functioning, visual abilities, eye-hand coordination, and general motor coordination.

Some inventories used with auditorially disordered children consider the child's level of independence in daily living and his achievement of developmental skills. Instruments used with infants include the California First-Year Mental Scale (Bayley, 1933), the Cattell Infant Intelligence Scale (Cattell, 1947), and the Denver Developmental Screening Test (Frankenburg and Dodds, 1970). The Vineland Social Maturity Scale (Doll, 1947) provides a means of comparing a child with his peers in skills necessary for social adjustment and independence.

Numerous achievement tests are used to determine levels of performance in various academic skills. Most of these yield grade-equivalent or percentile scores, indicating the grade level on which the child is functioning or comparing the child's performance with norms for his grade placement. Diagnosticians can obtain pertinent information by noting whether a child is functioning at an appropriate level for his grade and his level of intelligence and whether he shows significant discrepancies among various academic skills. While all areas of academic functioning may be affected adversely by auditory disorders, spelling and reading are most frequently disrupted by these types of disabilities.

The diagnostician must be cognizant of inconsistencies in test results or test behaviors in interpreting previous test data. Diagnostically significant inconsistencies include discrepancies between verbal and nonverbal scores, fluctuation in performance on the same measure from one testing situation to another, differences between achievement and potential, and contradictions between test results and parent or teacher reports.

STRUCTURING THE EVALUATION SESSION

Diagnosticians must organize their contact time with a child so that they have opportunity for observation of receptive and expressive language and of nonverbal behavior. With young children or those with limited verbal abilities, toys and pictures appropriate for the child's age level should be available. The diagnostician and the child's parent can question and instruct the child during play activities. They are thereby able to observe the child's receptive language and evaluate his expressive abilities through his comments and responses during play activities. With older children, toys may not be necessary, although pictures and books can help stimulate conversation. Receptive and expressive language can be observed through questions, instructions, and general conversation. Social skills can be observed as the child manipulates toys, engages in symbolic play, and interacts with or reacts to persons and events. Motor proficiency can be observed by watching the child move to and from the examining room and noting coordination as the child manipulates objects, pictures, or a pencil.

In evaluating auditory functioning, diagnosticians should watch the child's reactions to sounds in the environment. Does Tim disregard sudden bursts of sound that would startle most listeners? Does he appear to be overly responsive or sensitive to ordinary but nonpertinent environmental sounds (for example, persons walking in the hall or talking in the background, typewriters, doors closing)? Diagnosticians should note how parents communicate with the child. Do they rely on verbalizations, gestures, or a combination of these to transmit information to the child? Does the parent simplify, rephrase, or repeat what the diagnostician says to Jerry? Does the parent address him in simplified language patterns? Does the parent attempt to converse casually with him? Quite often parents unknowingly have learned to phrase verbalizations so that the child will understand. Their verbal interactions may be limited to short, direct questions or instructions; they may make little or no effort to engage the child in conversation.

In addition to observing parent-child interaction, diagnosticians should provide time for direct verbal interchanges with the child. They should note whether the child responds appropriately both to structured questions and instructions and to social conversational speech. Do Betty's answers indicate that she understood the questions she was asked? Does she follow verbal instructions appropriately or does she require simplification or demonstration before she understands? Does she know factual information appropriate for her age level (for example, her age, names of her pets, parents, siblings, and teachers, her address)? Can she comprehend social conversation? Does she make overly literal interpretations of what is said?

Diagnosticians should listen to the child talk, noting any deviations in the child's expressive language. Does Sara label objects and actions appropriately? Is her sentence structure grammatically adequate for her age and linguistic background? Is the content of her speech appropriate and easy to follow? Does she ramble from topic to topic? Can her speech be understood easily? Is her voice normal in quality, pitch, and loudness?

Social and emotional behaviors should be evaluated in light of the child's age. Does Jack behave appropriately in the waiting room? Is his behavior disruptive? Is he unusually passive? Does he touch everything? Does he relate to objects appropriately? Is his behavior purposeful? Do his parents appear to trust his judgment or to be unusually directive with him? Is his affective behavior appropriate?

Diagnosticians should note a child's motor behavior. Is Sherry awkward or clumsy? Does she have an unusual gait or posture? Does she trip, drop things, or have difficulty manipulating objects? Does she fall or lose her balance easily? Is she overly active? Does she have an unusual grip when using a pencil or crayon?

Abnormalities or unusual patterns of behavior, such as those described in the previous section, should be considered symptomatic of deficits in language and learning. Observed behavior patterns, either normal or abnormal, should be corroborated by information obtained from parents or other persons with whom the child has frequent contact.

ACQUISITION AND INTERPRETATION OF CASE HISTORY INFORMATION

An important component in differential diagnosis is the compilation and interpretation of information about a child's history and present behaviors in his daily environment. Medical, developmental, environmental, emotional, intellectual, and educational background should be explored (Mecham, 1966a). Bangs (1969) and Berry (1969) suggest formats for obtaining and recording pertinent historical data. Diagnosticians should note conditions or experiences that may have disrupted normal development.

Family History

Children whose family members either have experienced difficulties in school achievement or have a history of developmental, medical, or emotional disorders are high-risk subjects for abnormalities in their own maturational patterns. Age of the mother during pregnancy and any previous miscarriages can increase the probability of abnormal prenatal conditions.

Prenatal Conditions

A mother's illness, injury, drug use, emotional stress, or diet during pregnancy affects the developing fetus (Bricker and Bricker, 1974). Any abnormal events or conditions affecting the mother during pregnancy increase the probability that a child will have some handicapping condition.

Birth History

Prematurity or injury occurring during birth increases the likelihood of abnormalities in the child (Bricker and Bricker, 1974). Prolonged or precipitous labor, breech presentation, or any condition producing anoxia can adversely affect the infant. A description of the condition of the child immediately after birth can provide clues to possible prenatal or birth traumas. Jaundice, delay in starting to breathe, or cyanosis may indicate abnormalities in the newborn child.

Medical History

The probability of disorders in development or learning is higher for children who have had convulsions, prolonged high fever, injuries to the head, viral infections affecting the central nervous system, severe or prolonged diarrhea at an early age, unusual emotional trauma, or nutritional deprivation. Children with physical anomalies, chromosome disorders, metabolic disturbances, or sensory deficits should be considered high risk for disabilities in a number of areas of functioning (Bricker and Bricker, 1974).

Developmental Patterns

The age and pattern of development of linguistic and nonlinguistic skills may reveal significant diagnostic information. Comparing the age at which a child achieves developmental milestones with normative data will indicate whether he has progressed at an appropriate sequential rate in some or all areas of development. Gesell (1940), Bangs (1969), and Uzgiris and Hunt (1975) have compiled information about normal stages of development. Comparison of a child's progress in different aspects of development can help the diagnostician identify significant patterns of development or specific areas of strengths and weaknesses. For children suspected of having auditory disorders, details of hearing deficits and language development should be emphasized.

Social-Emotional Development

How children interact with other people during the developmental process can give valuable clues to auditory, linguistic, and emotional development. If social or emotional problems are reported, detailed information should be obtained in an effort to uncover related problems or traumas to which they can be attributed.

Academic Progress

As was described previously in this chapter, poor academic progress can be the result of auditory disorders. Parents or teachers should be questioned about the adequacy of academic performance and the details of learning deficiencies.

Sources of Case History Information

Parents generally are the most valuable source of information about their children, although teachers, physicians, and other professionals should be consulted if they have had sufficient contact with the children.

Interviewing Parents. Through skillful questioning and listening, diagnosticians can obtain valuable information from parents early in the evaluation process. Sensitivity to parents' reports of background and behavioral information can help professionals identify a problem and ultimately make an accurate diagnosis. Rarely do parents express unjustified reservations about their child's development or functioning. The diagnostician should explore reasons for such concerns rather than dismissing the complaints as insignificant. All too often parents report that they had sought help for their child on previous occasions but had been told, "Give him some time and don't worry so much about him," or "You're an over-anxious parent. Your child probably will outgrow the problem, but if not, you can get help for her when she starts school." This advice can be frustrating and confusing to parents and detrimental to the child. If children are not developing or learning as parents feel they should, vague reassurance without careful investigation will not alleviate parental anxiety. Parents may follow the advice but continue to worry. For children with significant learning or developmental deficits, early intervention is crucial to later success (Johnson and Myklebust, 1967; Evans and Bangs, 1972). Delay in diagnosis and remediation compounds the problem. Diagnosticians should take parental concerns seriously and explore them in detail.

As an initial step in the diagnostic process, parents should be encouraged to voice their concerns and to state the questions they want answered. Most professionals have done unnecessary testing and have been in the embarrassing position of telling parents what they already know without either addressing the primary issue or diagnosing the problem.

Diagnostician: Mrs. Jones, I tested Sally's hearing and it is normal.

Mrs. Jones: I know her hearing is fine; she passed the hearing screening test at school last week. I wanted to know why she never remembers what I tell her to do.

The labels or terms parents use to state their concerns may be misleading. They should be asked to cite examples of specific behaviors that worry them.

Diagnostician: Tell me what concerns you about Paul.

Mother: I think he has a hearing loss.

Diagnostician: What does he do that makes you question his hearing?

291

Mother: He covers his ears and screams when I run the vacuum cleaner or the dishwasher or when there is a loud noise outside.

The questions found on case-history forms often require parents to report specific ages at which developmental milestones were reached. This information is important because it permits comparison with developmental norms and provides an opportunity to focus on abnormal variations among different areas of development. Parents also should be encouraged to give their subjective impressions about the adequacy of their child's development. Sometimes these recollections provide diagnostic clues.

Diagnostician: Tell me about Tommy's learning to sit up, crawl, and walk.

Mother: He did those things at a normal age, but he never was well coordinated. He fell often and was much more awkward than my other children.

Other Sources of Information

Other professionals who have been involved with the care or education of a child may have information valuable to the diagnostic process. They should be consulted only with the parents' written permission and should be told that information is being sought at the parents' request. The nature of the professional's dealings with the child will determine the type of information available from him. For example, an otolaryngologist who saw a child once for an ear infection probably will not have information about general development or other health problems. The same open-ended interviewing procedures used with parents may be successful with a teacher who has had extended daily contact with the child. Specific questions can be asked if pertinent information is not covered in the general discussion. If other professionals, such as speech pathologists or psychologists, have evaluated the child, the contact with them should include requests for reports of their testing or therapy as well as general impressions about the child.

ETIOLOGY

An etiological diagnosis should specify conditions that have a functional relationship to observed deficits (Perkins and Curlee, 1969). Identification of etiology is useful to persons immediately responsible for a child if it suggests beneficial treatment procedures, provides prognostic data, or improves understanding and acceptance by parents anxious to know the cause of a disorder. Common etiological categories used in an effort to explain the causes of behavioral and learning differences in children with nonsensory auditory disorders include mental retardation, brain damage or neurological dysfunction, and emotional disturbance.

Brain damage or neurological dysfunction, terms used interchangeably in this chapter, can cause disorders in audition. Some children with nonsensory auditory deficits have verified histories of brain damage or positive signs on an EEG or on classical neurological examinations. In some auditorially defective children, neurological dysfunction is inferred even when observed behavioral abnormalities cannot be correlated with specific brain damage (deHirsch, 1967). When brain damage is inferred but not verified, the diagnostician should acknowledge that the statement of etiology is speculative. Attributing auditory disorders to neurological dysfunction denotes the physical basis for the deficits but does not describe the disruptions in functioning and frequently does not indicate appropriate treatment or prognosis for change (Bangs, 1969).

Nonsensory auditory deficiencies may be attributed to mental retardation or emotional disturbance. A diagnosis of mental retardation implies an overall below-normal capacity to learn and to adapt behaviorally (Lillywhite and Bradley, 1969). The term *emotional disturbance* connotes severe and continued disruptions in interpersonal relationships. Specification of mental retardation or of emotional disturbance as causes for specific abnormal behaviors implies that the deficits under consideration are a part of a general pattern of dysfunction (Myklebust, 1954). Unlike a diagnosis of brain damage, these diagnostic categories do not specify the physical cause of the disorder.

Accurately identifying the cause of a disorder often is a complex process. Erroneous judgments can result if etiology is inferred on the basis of limited observations and reports of linguistic and nonlinguistic behaviors considered characteristic of certain abnormalities. In discussing the diagnosis of autism, which is a specific type of emotional disorder, Ornitz and Ritvo (1976) suggest that the probability of making an accurate diagnosis is increased if children are seen for at least three separate diagnostic examinations at weekly intervals. In describing assessment procedures for language-disordered children, Berry (1969) recommends diagnostic teaching over an extended time period to permit observations, testing, taking of case histories, and assessments of progress rather than assigning diagnostic labels and planning remediation procedures on the basis of limited observations or testing. Weiner (1968) describes severely handicapped preschool children whose auditory processing disorders were diagnosed accurately only after several months of contact and interaction with the children.

The similarities in developmental and behavioral patterns among children from different etiology groups complicate the process of differential diagnosis. Baltaxe and Simmons (1975), Ornitz and Ritvo (1976), and Ratusnik and Ratusnik (1976) identified echolalia, impaired receptive and expressive skills, auditory inattention, concrete thought processes, and unusual modulation of voice and rhythm as common linguistic behaviors in psychotic and autistic children, who could be placed in the general etiological category of emotional disturbance. These authors stated that problems in speech and language development frequently are the earliest recognized symptoms of emotional abnormalities, although defective motor and social development are common also. Children diagnosed as having auditory disorders resulting from neurological dysfunction or of undetermined etiology may display similar characteristics in language development and functioning (Myklebust, 1954; de Hirsch, 1967). Commonalities in abnormal nonlinguistic behaviors also are reported for emotionally disturbed children and those with auditory and language problems. Impaired ego functioning, limited or abnormal interpersonal or social interactions, acting-out behavior, preoccupation with sameness, perseveration, hyperactivity, and limited self-help skills occur frequently in emotionally disturbed children (Baltaxe and Simmon, 1975; Ratusnik and Ratusnik, 1976) and in those with auditory disorders (deHirsch, 1967; M. Berko, 1966; de Ajuriaguerra et al., 1976).

Certain behavioral commonalities can make differentiation among mentally retarded, emotionally disturbed, and brain-damaged children difficult. Developmental and behavioral characteristics observed in mentally retarded children include echolalia, delayed development of receptive and expressive speech and language skills, immature social behavior and emotional reactions, and inadequate gross and fine motor functioning (Smith, 1968; Lillywhite and Bradley, 1969). As indicated previously, these behaviors also may appear in emotionally disturbed and auditorially handicapped children; therefore, they cannot serve as the only source of information for identifying etiology.

The documented evidence of the range in type and severity of disorders within a given etiological category shows the futility of trying to make decisions about treatment or prognosis on the basis of general classifications. The scope and severity of problems manifested by mentally retarded children vary greatly (Lillywhite and Bradley, 1969). Some have limited meaningful responses to language; others understand most simple verbal stimuli. Some have intelligible speech patterns that permit effective communication in most situations; others use no intelligible speech. Motor abilities among retardates range from immobility to mild deficits in gross and fine motor skills. Bangs (1969) and Cromer (1974) emphasized that all children diagnosed as mentally retarded do not present the same strengths and deficits in language and learning. A given child may function in one or more areas at a level significantly below that expected for his mental age. Unless the differential diagnostic process identifies the child's assets and deficits, the information essential for guiding clinicians, teachers, and parents in their interactions with the child is omitted.

Behavioral and learning deficits in children with emotional disturbances vary (Myklebust, 1954). Rubin, Bar, and Dwyer (1967) noted that psychotic children differ in vocabulary, grammatical proficiency, articulation patterns, and willingness to use language. Ornitz and Ritvo (1976) described abnormal responses to sound ranging from hypersensitivity to hyposensitivity, and differences in degree of disturbances in relating to people varying from subtle and intermittent to consistent, overt inabilities. The variations in behaviors of disturbed children, and even within more specific categories such as psychotic or autistic, demonstrate that the specific label used to describe the child is not sufficient to denote the unique characteristics of his problem.

Neurologically based auditory disorders result in a wide range of behavior patterns (Myklebust, 1954; deHirsch, 1967; Eisenson, 1968). The variety of behavioral manifestations described in the previous section of this chapter demonstrates the diverse linguistic and nonlinguistic characteristics associated with auditory disorders resulting from neurological deficiencies or from other causes. Specification of brain damage as the etiology does not reveal the nature or severity of the deficit in functioning.

A major problem in identifying etiology of abnormalities in behavior and learning is the frequency with which multiple handicaps occur. Brain damage, mental retardation, and emotional disturbance are not mutually exclusive conditions. Children with auditory and language disorders resulting from brain damage frequently develop emotional problems because of their inability to communicate with others (deHirsch, 1967; Wyatt, 1969; Ornitz and Ritvo, 1976). Perceptual problems can result in misinterpretations of environmental occurrences, thus making a child fearful or distrusting of certain persons or situations. Overly aggressive behavior or withdrawal may occur when a child is unable to function successfully. Because children's emotional reactions to perceptual and linguistic deficits resulting from neurological dysfunction may be the most disturbing and obvious to those around them, they may be mislabeled as emotionally disturbed when the basis for their disruptive behavior is an inability to perceive, interpret, or express information.

The unusually high incidence of hearing loss in mentally retarded children (Lillywhite and Bradley, 1969) and among those with language deficits attributed to brain dysfunction (Mecham, 1966b; Eisenson, 1968) exemplifies how multiple handicaps can affect learning and behavior. Ornitz and Ritvo (1976) called attention to the coexistence of mental retardation and autism and observed that autism probably results from central nervous system pathology of a specific type. Baltaxe and Simmons (1975) suggested that the differences between children with severe language disorders and psychotic children may be in degree and not in type of impairment. They postulated that the extent of impairment of auditory perception, assumed to be related to neurological integrity, may determine whether a child is psychotic or is diagnosed as having a language disorder. Lillywhite and Bradley (1969) described mental retardation resulting from neurological dysfunction or damage to the brain.

The differential diagnostician should not feel compelled to specify the cause of a disorder unless there is strong evidence to support his judgment. It may be appropriate to identify multiple causes or to indicate primary and secondary etiological factors. For some children, etiology cannot be determined even after thorough testing and observations have been completed by a multidisciplinary team and detailed background information has been obtained.

Speculative judgments of cause made on the basis of incomplete information are likely to be erroneous and can result in mishandling of a child.

Susie at age 3 was diagnosed by one professional as deaf because she did not respond to speech. A member of another profession stated that Susie was mentally retarded, basing this judgment on the child's failure to comprehend or use speech for communication. A third person diagnosed her as autistic because she echoed speech and lacked appropriate social interaction skills. After a period of diagnostic therapy at age 4, it was determined that Susie's lack of oral communication skills resulted from a severe deficit in the ability to attach meaning to verbal symbols. Her hearing sensitivity was within normal range, and on nonverbal intelligence tests she scored in the superior range. As her comprehension of language improved during the course of therapy, she used speech as a tool for interaction with people and her social skills improved. The diagnoses of deafness, mental retardation, and autism had all been erroneous. Her family had been through unnecessary distress in trying to adjust to each of these labels, and appropriate help for Susie had been delayed by more than a year as the family groped for assistance.

INTERPRETATION OF DIAGNOSTIC INFORMATION

After the screening or evaluation data have been compiled and the diagnostician has made decisions about the nature of the problems and appropriate follow-up assessment or treatment, the results and recommendations must be explained to parents and others responsible for the child. Children's ability to cope with their deficits depends on how the people important to them respond to the problems (deHirsch, 1967; Hirsh, 1967). If parents are to react constructively, the diagnostic information presented must be meaningful and not in conflict with observations they have made about the child. The diagnostician who sees the child early and identifies problem areas has an opportunity to serve as facilitator and guide in locating appropriate services for the child. The report to parents should contain descriptions of their child's behavior, not labels that could frighten or confuse them and thereby interfere with their seeking proper help for the child. Unless a complete assessment has been made, the diagnostician should state clearly the tentative nature of the conclusions and the need for extended evaluation.

As the culmination of their testing and observations, some diagnosticians categorize or label abnormal patterns of development, behavior, and achievement. Familiarity with the meaning of common classifications may be important to persons responsible for reporting and interpreting diagnostic information. Some descriptive categories are intended to convey information about patterns of behavior and to specify etiology. The term *aphasia* refers to deficiencies in the use of verbal symbols as a result of brain damage (Eisenson, 1968). *Auditory agnosia* is an inability to interpret auditory stimuli. *Dysarthria* refers to a partial lack of motor control in the speech mechanism. Both auditory agnosia and dysarthria result from injury to the brain (Myklebust, 1954). *Psychoneurological learning disabilities* are disruptions in learning processes resulting from neurological dysfunction (Johnson and Myklebust, 1967). Other descriptive labels are used to indicate the presence of deficits in audition and language, but do not imply cause. *Aphasoid* (deHirsch, 1967), *language-disordered* (Bangs 1969; Menyuk and Looney, 1976), *auditory vocal channel disabilities* (Kirk and Kirk, 1971), and *specific learning disabilities* (Peterson, 1967) are terms used to describe children with language-learning deficits. If diagnostic categories are used when reporting information, operational definitions must be given to insure that the interpretation is meaningful and explicit.

Talking With Parents

If a child has nonsensory auditory deficits, the interpretation of diagnostic information to parents should explain the difference between hearing sound and using or interpreting sound. Parents should understand that although a child can hear, he may not respond appropriately to sound or learn from what he hears. An example related to their child's suspected deficit can help clarify the problem for some parents. For example, if a child appears to have limited understanding of speech, the diagnostician might explain that the combinations of sounds that we call words carry meaning only if one can associate that grouping of sounds with the object, action, or idea it represents. Comparing our inability to understand an unfamiliar foreign language with the child's comprehension deficits may aid the parents in understanding the necessity of associating a word with its referent in order to comprehend speech. If the child's deficits are in areas other than comprehension of speech, concrete examples of those deficits are needed.

The diagnostician should explain to parents that children can have deficiencies in some aspects of behavior and function substantially better in others. A deficit in auditory functioning does not necessarily signal a generalized incapacity to learn. When possible, the diagnostician should point out how the child seems to learn best and on what types of tasks the child has difficulty. For example, the child may learn adequately if he sees an activity or experiences a series of movements, yet he may fail to learn from what he hears people say. Everyone has strengths and weaknesses in learning, and the parents must recognize that the diagnostician is not attempting to exaggerate normal individual differences but rather is identifying significant deficits that may require special help and that the child probably will not outgrow.

Parents may find the results of the evaluation or screening more meaningful if they are given an opportunity to verify the examiner's conclusions with their own observations of the child. The diagnostician should attempt to use parent-reported behaviors as examples of the child's specific deficits.

Parent's Report

Ben does not mind me. I tell him to pick up his toys and get his coat, and he never gets past the stairs.

Diagnostician's Explanation of Observations

We noticed that Ben does not always follow directions or answer simple questions. He may not understand everything you say to him. We found that he had a difficult time learning how to take the hearing test. We had to remind him each time to raise his hand when he heard a pure-tone. Once we demonstrated what we wanted him to do, he seemed to understand and he responded consistently without further instructions. What you describe and what we saw seem to indicate that he has some problems in understanding speech.

Parent's Report

Patty ignores me when the TV is on. Sometimes she acts like she is deaf, or maybe she is just stubborn. I think she hears what she wants to hear.

Diagnostician's Explanation of Observations

We found that Patty does not sort out sounds when she hears several types of noise at the same time. She may have trouble paying attention to more than one thing at a time. That could account for her not responding if you talk to her while the TV is on.

Parent's Report

Robin never seems to hear her homework assignments. I think she is trying to get out of something by playing dumb.

Diagnostician's Explanation of Observations

Robin may have trouble remembering what she hears. We noticed that she followed directions quite well if we told her only one thing at a time. If we told her two or

three things at the same time, she
usually remembered only one of
them. Possibly she hears her homework assignments but cannot
remember them. Some children
have unusual problems in this type
of memory. Your reports and our
observations suggest that this may
be a problem for Robin.

In some instances, diagnosticians will not uncover evidence of a problem. On
the basis of their observations, the parent's reports, and the case history information, they will conclude that the child is functioning adequately in all areas. In
these cases, the diagnostician should ask the parents to verify this conclusion
with their impressions of the child. If the diagnostician has reasonable doubt
that the child is developing normally, but has no clear justification to support
this doubt, the parents should be given this opinion. If the parents agree that a
problem seems to exist, additional assessment should be recommended to confirm or deny the presence of a significant problem.

When a deficit is suspected and additional evaluation is recommended,
parents should understand that further assessment can lead to remediation. The
diagnostician should make it clear that the evaluation process is an integral part
of any remediation program, and the objective of testing is to designate appropriate remedial procedures. Some parents will want immediate and specific
assistance in finding appropriate sources of help for the child. Audiologists
should help the parent by recommending or contacting an appropriate center
and should offer to forward their evaluation data. Parents will want to know
what services are available and to which questions answers are being sought. The
diagnostician should follow up the referral with a call to the parents or the
center to which the child was referred to determine that appropriate services are
being pursued.

Referring to Other Professionals

When contacting other professionals and agencies to make a referral, information should be provided concerning specific observed behaviors and possible
auditory deficits. Parental permission should be obtained to send confidential
information, such as case history records and test results, to these agencies.
Interdisciplinary teamwork, often required for diagnosis of auditory disorders,
requires shared information, discussion and interaction, not just serial testing of
the child by various specialists operating independently. It may be necessary to
share the information, conclusions, and recommendations concerning the child
with several specialists working cooperatively for the child's best interests. With-

out this interaction, the differential diagnosis process may be incomplete and erroneous judgments and recommendations may be given.

SUMMARY

Children with intact auditory processing systems use their hearing to interpret and relate to their environment. Some children have nonsensory auditory disorders that interfere with their perception and interpretation of sounds. This chapter discusses certain diagnostic procedures for identifying and describing children who fail to use what they hear for communication and learning.

The purpose of differential diagnosis is to identify the nature and scope of a disorder and to describe the parameters of the problem in terms of normal and deficient learning processes. Contributions from an interdisciplinary team of professionals may be necessary for accurate diagnosis of auditory disorders in children. As members of the diagnostic team, audiologists are responsible both for defining losses in hearing sensitivity and for identifying symptoms of nonsensory auditory deficits. If audiologists recognize behavior patterns suggestive of abnormal utilization of sound and understand the significance of observed or reported auditory deficits, they can make appropriate referrals to other professionals and effectively explain to parents the need for additional assistance.

Children with nonsensory auditory disorders present certain patterns of behavior that reflect their strengths and weaknesses in auditory functioning. Auditory reception, verbal expression, social-emotional, and academic behaviors and patterns of functioning on formal tests often indicate the presence and nature of auditory deficits. A list of behaviors that often are diagnostically significant is given in the appendix to this chapter.

Certain deficits in nonverbal abilities frequently occur in association with auditory disorders or may reflect deviations in other aspects of learning. The diagnostician should recognize and report indications of problems in visual, motor, or tactile functioning. Diagnostically significant behaviors in these areas may include gross motor incoordination, problems in eye-hand coordination, lack of hand dominance, visual perception deficits, unusual reactions to touch, and spatial disorientation.

If deficits in auditory functioning are recognized, the diagnostician is responsible for interpreting information so that parents will understand the nature of the suspected disorder and the sources of appropriate assistance. It is important that parents recognize the relationship between the observations reported by the diagnostician and the behaviors that caused them to bring the child for evaluation. Parents should be given descriptions of the specific behaviors considered to be deviant and explanations of process breakdowns that may be causing the difficulties. Labeling the behavior according to etiology or using general categorical terms probably will not be meaningful or helpful to parents.

The diagnostician should consider all observed and reported behaviors and work interactively with the parents and other professionals to provide complete differential diagnostic services. Speculative judgments and overgeneralizations are likely to result in erroneous diagnosis and mishandling of the child.

RESEARCH NEEDS

The similarities in linguistic and nonlinguistic behaviors of children with varying types of auditory disorders illustrate the need for research directed toward objective means of differentiating between nonsensory and sensory impairments and among different types of auditory dysfunction. Additional objective assessment procedures are needed for screening purposes as well as for indepth evaluations. The identification of symbolic and conceptual deficits in children with peripheral hearing loss is vital in the differential diagnostic process but is often not pursued because of the absence of quantifiable information describing the differing and overlapping symptoms. Information regarding the variety of verbal and nonverbal behaviors in multihandicapped children would assist in accurate identification and more efficient management of these children.

REFERENCES

Ammons, R., and H. Ammons, *Full Range Picture Vocabulary Test.* Missoula, Mont.: Psychological Test Specialists, 1958.

Aram, D., and J. Nation, "Patterns of Language Behavior in Children with Developmental Language Disorders," *Journal of Speech and Hearing Research,* 18 (1975), 229–243.

Arthur, G., *The Arthur Adaptation of the Leiter International Performance Scale.* Washington: Psychological Service Center Press, 1952.

Ayres, J., *Sensory Integration and Learning Disorders.* Los Angeles: Western Psychological Services, 1972.

Ayres, J., *Southern California Sensory Integration Test.* Los Angeles: Western Psychological Services, 1975.

Baltaxe, C., and J. Simmons, "Language in Childhood Psychosis: A Review," *Journal of Speech and Hearing Disorders,* 40 (1975), 439–458.

Bangs, T., *Language and Learning Disorders of the Pre-academic Child.* New York: Appleton-Century-Crofts, 1969.

Bayley, N., *The California First-Year Mental Scale.* Berkeley: University of California Syllabus Series, No. 243, 1933.

Beery, K., *Developmental Test of Visual Motor Integration.* Chicago: Follett Educational Corporation, 1967.

Bender, L., *Bender Visual Motor Gestalt.* Los Angeles: Western Psychological Services, 1949.

Berko, F., "Special Education for the Cerebral Palsied: A Group Language Learning Experience," in *Communication Training in Childhood Brain Damage,* edited by M. Mecham, M. Berko, F. Berko, and M. Palmer. Springfield, Ill.: Charles C. Thomas, 1966, pp. 261–376.

Berko, M., "Psychological and Linguistic Implications of Brain Damage in Children," in *Communication Training in Childhood Brain Damage,* edited by M. Mecham, M. Berko, F. Berko, and M. Palmer. Springfield, Ill.: Charles C. Thomas, 1966, pp. 144–260.

Berry, M., *Language Disorders of Children: The Bases and Diagnoses.* New York: Appleton-Century-Crofts, 1969.

Black, F., "Use of the Leiter International Performance Scale with Aphasic Children," *Journal of Speech and Hearing Research,* 16 (1973), 530–532.

Bloom, L., "Talking, Understanding, and Thinking," in *Language Perspectives—Acquisition, Retardation, and Intervention,* edited by R. Schiefelbusch and L. Lloyd. Baltimore: University Park Press, 1974, pp. 285–312.

Bowerman, M., "Discussion Summary—Development of Concepts Underlying Language," in *Language Perspectives—Acquisition, Retardation, and Intervention,* edited by R. Schiefelbusch and L. Lloyd. Baltimore: University Park Press, 1974, pp. 191–209.

Bricker, W., and D. Bricker, "An Early Language Training Strategy," in *Language Perspectives—Acquisition, Retardation, and Intervention,* edited by R. Schiefelbusch and L. Lloyd. Baltimore: University Park Press, 1974, pp. 431–468.

Bruner, J., J. Goodnow, and G. Austin, *A Study of Thinking.* New York: Wiley and Sons, 1967.

Carrow, E., *Carrow Elicited Language Inventory.* Austin, Texas: Learning Concepts, 1974.

Carrow, E., *Test for Auditory Comprehension of Language: English/Spanish.* Austin, Texas: Learning Concepts, 1973.

Cattell, P., *The Measurement of Intelligence of Infants and Young Children.* New York: The Psychological Corporation, 1947.

Columbia Mental Maturity Scale. New York: Harcourt, Brace and World, 1959.

Cromer, R., "Receptive Language in the Mentally Retarded: Processes and Diagnostic Distinctions," in *Language Perspectives—Acquisition, Retardation, and Intervention,* edited by R. Schiefelbusch and L. Lloyd. Baltimore: University Park Press, 1974, pp. 237–267.

deAjuriaguerra, J., A. Jaeggi, F. Guignard, F. Kocher, M. Maquard, S. Roth, and E. Schmid, "The Development and Prognosis of Dysphasia in Children," in *Normal and Deficient Child Language,* edited by Donald Morehead and Ann Morehead. Baltimore: University Park Press, 1976, pp. 345–385.

deHirsch, K., "Differential Diagnosis Between Aphasic and Schizophrenic Language in Children," *Journal of Speech and Hearing Disorders,* 32 (1967), 3–10.

Denhoff, E., and J. Novack, "Syndromes of Cerebral Dysfunction: Medical Aspects that Contribute to Special Education Methods," in *Methods in Special Education*, edited by N. Haring and R. Schiefelbusch. New York: McGraw-Hill, 1967, 351–383.

Doll, E., *Vineland Social Maturity Scale*. Minneapolis: American Guidance Service, 1947.

Dunn, L., *Peabody Picture Vocabulary Test*. Los Angeles: Western Psychological Services, 1965.

Eisenson, J., "Developmental Aphasia: A Speculative View with Therapeutic Implications," *Journal of Speech and Hearing Disorders*, 33 (1968), 3–13.

Evans, J., and T. Bangs, "Effects of Preschool Language Training on Later Academic Achievement of Children with Language and Learning Disabilities," *Journal of Learning Disabilities*, 5 (1972), 5–12.

Fay, W., and B. Bulter, "Echolalia, IQ, and the Developmental Dichotomy of Speech and Language Systems," *Journal of Speech and Hearing Research*, 11 (1968), 365–371.

Frankenburg, W., and J. Dodds, *Denver Development Screening Test*, rev. Denver: University of Colorado Medical Center, 1970.

Frostig, M., *Developmental Test of Visual Perception*. Chicago: Consulting Psychologist Press, 1964.

Gesell, A., *The First Five Years of Life: A Guide to the Study of the Preschool Child*. New York: Harper and Brothers, 1940.

Goldman, R., and M. Fristoe, *Goldman-Fristoe Test of Articulation*. Circle Pines, Minn.: American Guidance Service, 1969.

Goldman, R., M. Fristoe, and R. Woodcock, *Goldman-Fristoe-Woodcock Test of Discrimination*. Circle Pines, Minn.: American Guidance Service, 1970.

Hegrenes, J., N. Marshall, and J. Armas, "Treatment As An Extension of Diagnostic Function: A Case Study," *Journal of Speech and Hearing Disorders*, 35 (1970), 182–187.

Hirsh, I., "Information Processing in Input Channels for Speech and Language: The Significance of Serial Order of Stimuli," in *Brain Mechanisms Underlying Speech and Language*, edited by C. Millikan and F. Darley. New York: Grune and Stratton, 1967, pp. 21–27.

Johnson, D., and H. Myklebust, *Learning Disabilities: Educational Principles and Practices*. New York: Grune and Stratton, 1967.

Kirk, S., and W. Kirk, *Psycholinguistic Learning Disabilities: Diagnosis and Remediation*. Urbana, Ill.: University of Illinois Press, 1971.

Kirk, S., J. McCarthy, and W. Kirk, *Illinois Test of Psycholinguistic Abilities*, rev. ed. Urbana, Ill.: University of Illinois Press, 1969.

Lee, L., *The Northwestern Syntax Screening Test*. Evanston, Ill.: Northwestern University Press, 1969.

Lillywhite, H., and D. Bradley, *Communication Problems in Mental Retardation: Diagnosis and Management*. New York: Harper & Row, 1969.

Mecham, M., "Appraisal of Speech and Hearing Problems," in *Communication*

Training in Childhood Brain Damage, edited by M. Mecham, M. Berko, F. Berko, and M. Palmer. Springfield, Ill.: Charles C. Thomas, 1966a, pp. 49-69.

Mecham, M., "Disorders of Speech and Hearing," in *Communication Training in Childhood Brain Damage,* edited by M. Mecham, M. Berko, F. Berko, and M. Palmer. Springfield, Ill.: Charles C. Thomas, 1966b, pp. 21-48.

Menyuk, P., "Early Development of Receptive Language: From Babbling to Words," in *Language Perspectives—Acquisition, Retardation, and Intervention,* edited by R. Schiefelbusch and L. Lloyd. Baltimore: University Park Press, 1974 pp. 213-235.

Menyuk, P. and P. Looney, "A Problem of Language Disorder—Length Versus Structure," in *Normal and Deficient Child Language,* edited by D. Morehead and A. Morehead. Baltimore: University Park Press, 1976, pp. 259-279.

Myklebust, H., *Auditory Disorders in Children.* New York: Grune and Stratton, 1954.

Nelson, K., "Structure and Strategy in Learning to Talk," *Monograph for the Society for Research in Child Development,* 149 (1973).

Ornitz, E., and E. Ritvo, "The Syndrome of Autism: A Critical Review," *The American Journal of Psychiatry,* 133:6 (1976), 609-621.

Panagos, J., "Persistence of the Open Syllable Reinterpreted as a Symptom of Language Disorders," *Journal of Speech and Hearing Disorders,* 39 (1974), 23-31.

Perkins, W., and R. Curlee, "Causality in Speech Pathology," *Journal of Speech and Hearing Disorders,* 34 (1969), 231-238.

Peterson, W., "Children with Specific Learning Disabilities," in *Methods in Special Education,* edited by N. Haring and R. Schiefelbusch. New York: McGraw-Hill, 1967, pp. 159-167.

Ratusnik, C., and D. Ratusnik, "A Therapeutic Milieu for Establishing and Expanding Communicative Behaviors in Psychotic Children," *Journal of Speech and Hearing Disorders,* 41 (1976), 70-92.

Rubin, H., A. Bar, and J. Dwyer, "An Experimental Speech and Language Program for Psychotic Children," *Journal of Speech and Hearing Disorders,* 33 (1967) 242-248.

Smith, R., *Clinical Teaching: Methods of Instruction for the Mentally Retarded.* New York: McGraw-Hill, 1968.

Spellacy, F., and F. Black, "Intelligence Assessment of Language-Impaired Children by Means of Two Nonverbal Tests," *Journal of Clinical Psychology,* 28 (1972), 357-358.

Stutsman, R., *Guide for Administering The Merrill Palmer Scale of Mental Tests.* New York: Harcourt, Brace and World, 1948.

Templin, M., and F. Darley, *The Templin-Darley Test of Articulation.* Iowa City: Bureau of Educational Research and Service, Division of Extension and University Services, 1966.

Terman, L., and M. Merrill, *Stanford-Binet Intelligence Scale (Form L-M).* Boston: Houghton Mifflin Company, 1960.

Uzgiris, I., and J. Hunt, *Assessment in Infancy: Ordinal Scales of Psychological Development.* Urbana, Ill.: University of Illinois Press, 1975.

Vogel, S., *Syntactic Abilities in Normal and Dyslexic Children.* London: University Park Press, 1975.

Wechsler, D., *The Measurement and Appraisal of Adult Intelligence,* 4th ed. Baltimore: Williams and Wilkins Co., 1964.

Wechsler, D., *Wechsler Intelligence Scale for Children—Revised.* New York: The Psychological Corporation, 1974.

Wechsler, D., *Wechsler Pre-school and Primary Scale of Intelligence.* New York: The Psychological Corporation, 1967.

Weiner, P., "Auditory Discrimination and Articulation," *Journal of Speech and Hearing Disorders,* 32 (1967), 19–28.

Weiner, P., "The Emotionally Disturbed Child in the Speech Clinic: Some Considerations," *Journal of Speech and Hearing Disorders,* 33 (1968), 158–166.

Weiner, P., "Stability and Validity of Two Measures of Intelligence Used with Children Whose Language Development Is Delayed," *Journal of Speech and Hearing Research,* 14 (1971), 254–261.

Wepman, J., "Approaches to the Analysis of Aphasia," *Human Communication and Its Disorders—An Overview.* Bethesda, Md.: National Institutes of Health 1969, pp. 127–141.

Wepman, J., *Auditory Discrimination Test.* Chicago: University of Chicago, 1958.

Winitz, H., *Articulatory Acquisition and Behavior.* New York: Appleton-Century-Crofts, 1969.

Wyatt, G., *Language Learning and Communication Disorders in Children.* New York: Free Press, 1969.

Appendix

DIAGNOSTICALLY SIGNIFICANT BEHAVIORS OF CHILDREN WITH NONSENSORY AUDITORY DISORDERS

I. Auditory Reception

    A. Disregard of speech or all sounds

    B. Better responses in quiet than in noise

    C. Hypersensitivity to sound

    D. Echolalia

    E. Difficulty following verbal instructions unless accompanied by visual demonstrations

    F. Difficulty learning in group situations

    G. Failure to remember what people say

    H. Failure to generalize information from one experience to another

II. Verbal Expression

    A. Reduced quantity of verbalization

    B. Inadequate vocabulary

    C. Defective sentence structure

    D. Inability to verbalize experiences using a series of utterances

    E. Incorrect pronunciation (articulation) of words

    F. Disorganized content within or among utterances

    G. Dependence on gestures to express information

    H. Unusually literal content in ideas expressed

III. Social–Emotional Behaviors

    A. Problems in attention to pertinent tasks

    B. Inability to inhibit behavior

    C. Inability to cope with change

    D. Disorientation in space and time

    E. Immature self-help skills

    F. Perseveration

    G. Hyperactivity

    H. Inappropriate emotional reactions

    I. Social isolation

    J. Extreme aggression

    K. Limited interpersonal relationships

IV. Academic Behaviors
   A. Difficulty following verbal instructions or learning from verbal explanations in the classroom
   B. Difficulty learning phonics
   C. Inadequate reading or spelling
   D. Poor comprehension of what is read
   E. Disorganization in content of written material
   F. Poor sentence construction in written work
   G. Discrepancy between achievement level and potential for learning

V. Test Behaviors
   A. Significant discrepancy between verbal and nonverbal scores
   B. Low scores on verbal tests
   C. Discrepancy between test-retest scores on same measure or on tests designed to measure similar abilities
   D. Low achievement test scores

Management

 Knowledge of the etiologic factors and sequellae of hearing loss, as well as appropriate diagnostic procedures, are useless without correct amelioration when indicated. Too often correct history and diagnostic data are filed away on a child who never realizes the benefits to be derived from this information. The task of the habilitative or rehabilitative audiologist is usually to work around those auditory disorders that are nonreversible. While these efforts involve the handicapped child directly, to a great extent they also include his parents and family.

Too often the abilities of audiologists as counselors have been largely determined by their natural talents at communicating with people. In Chapter 9, on counseling parents, the Streams show that before the audiologist can become an effective conveyor of information, he must be a careful receiver—a good listener. Through a knowledge of the meanings behind the words and facial expressions of the family the audiologist-counselor selects what he will say and the manner in which it will be said. Dr. Simmons-Martin also deals with the child through his parents in Chapter 10, but she discusses direct habilitative and rehabilitative methods as well.

CHAPTER NINE

Counseling the Parents
of the Hearing-Impaired Child

RICHARD W. STREAM, KATHRYN S. STREAM

INTRODUCTION

Clinical experiences of the last decade have yielded substantial information about identifying and quantifying hearing loss in children. Though the methods for obtaining information on the status of the auditory system have become more sophisticated, the skills necessary for meaningfully translating our findings to parents have received little emphasis. The disparity between our knowledge of appraisal techniques and our knowledge of counseling techniques is cause for concern, since inadequate presentation can cause parents to ignore or reject the most appropriate recommendations for management of their hearing-impaired children, even though they have obtained accurate diagnostic information.

During the course of services to the hearing-impaired child and his family, the audiologist must consider amplification, language enrichment, auditory training, speech training, special education, and parent counseling. Although numerous publications provide information on the first six areas, audiologists have given only cursory attention to parent counseling. In the past, the term "parent counseling" for audiologists has connoted (1) explaining audiologic findings to parents and (2) explaining to parents the steps needed for habilitating their child. Some of our colleagues (Weiss and Duffy, 1974; and Rosen, 1967) as well as parents (Martin, 1975) have reported that this concept of counseling falls short of the real meaning of the parent counseling process.

This chapter highlights the counseling processes and emphasizes the practical aspects of counseling parents of children with hearing impairment. It is designed to encourage the audiologist to explore methods of creating a communicative environment in which parents may become active participants in making the decisions regarding the management of their children. Parental involvement in this decision-making process reduces their anxiety, allowing them to use their energy to understand and help their child.

CHAPTER OBJECTIVES

This chapter reviews some of the major theories currently used in parent counseling. This background information will allow the clinician to choose an approach for more intensive study. Also discussed are the personal qualities that we find helpful when counseling parents. Guidelines and principles of counseling that the clinician may employ to gain additional insight and become more sensitive in his role as a facilitator of communication are given. These guidelines are applied in specific case studies of various types of auditory disorders.

BACKGROUND TO COUNSELING PERSPECTIVES

We believe that a well-founded background of knowledge in the developmental milestones for speech, hearing, and language is essential when counseling parents of children with hearing impairment. With this prerequisite in mind, our counseling goals are to (1) present information on the current hearing status of the child as it relates to factors that affect the child's potential, (2) develop realistic, supportive educational plans for school or home training programs, (3) support parents in dealing with their feelings regarding the many ramifications of the handicap, and (4) allow parents to enhance their understanding and acceptance of the disorder as it relates to the impact on the child's development, adjustment, and ultimate self-actualization.

Through academic training and experience, audiologists are usually well prepared to achieve the first and second of these goals. The third and fourth goals deal with the emotional and behavioral adjustments of parents. In some clinical settings allied professional workers are available to assume major responsibility for counseling in these latter two areas. However, few of our colleagues in these allied disciplines are familiar with the unique problems confronting the family of the hearing-impaired child. Also, in many clinical programs budgetary restrictions limit the number of trained personnel from other professions who are available to work with these parents. For these reasons the audiologist, although he is often untrained in counseling skills, must attempt to bridge the gap between explaining the factual interpretation of the disorder to the parents and understanding the emotions of these parents as they receive the information.

Our experience suggests that audiologists often avoid or fail to recognize the need to deal with the emotions and feelings of parents. When the audiologist does not recognize or confront these issues, the parents may be unable to cope with the information presented. Therefore, the audiologist must be willing to become involved in emotionally charged situations. The extent to which he is willing to risk this kind of involvement seems to be related to his knowledge of himself and his reactions to others. If he understands some of the basic theories of human development and personality growth, the clinician increases his ability to comprehend the nature of the counseling process (Solnit and Stark, 1961).

Many different approaches are employed in the counseling process. Although some approaches were developed for use with people having severe emotional disorders, other approaches are more adaptable to the clinical situations most frequently encountered by audiologists. The audiologist's primary concern is with individuals who have no severe emotional deficiency or handicap, but who are experiencing difficulty adjusting to a specific situation. *Therefore, the task of counseling parents of hearing-impaired children requires that the counselor guide the parents as they identify alternatives and make decisions.*

Hearing loss introduces a new dimension to which parents react, and their personality factors will determine their perception of the problem. The reality of substance for parents is not the fact of hearing loss, but rather how they perceive the fact. Moreover, perceptual differences are related to personality constructs.

It follows, therefore, that theories of counseling interface with theories of personality development. Since personality is a conglomerate of personal traits, properties, and attributes that influence behavior, many factors determine its dynamic structure. As Kroth (1973) points out,

> Personality is involved in how well we deal with stress, how we react to anxiety, what cognitive styles we develop to solve problems, what motives push us into activity, how well we maintain control, integration and organization in our lives as well as how we express ourselves and live a rich, affective and enjoyable life. (p. 24)

Human Development Theories

Given the influence personality will have on parental reaction, an awareness of some theories of personality should help the audiologist understand how parents may cope with the problem of hearing loss in their child. Since it is impossible to review all of these theories, we have chosen an organization of major theories similar to that outlined by Kroth (1973) and Luterman (1976). This overview of some approaches to understanding behavior, included in the Appendix to this chapter, may serve as a reference for further study in this area.

The application of these approaches provides direction in working with parents and in understanding some aspects of human behavior that the clinician will encounter in parent counseling. In the counseling setting, the personal growth of the clinician becomes as important as his professional growth and development.

Attributes of a Counselor

Essential to a satisfactory encounter with parents is the clinician's ability to maximize the interaction between himself and the parents. How well he and the parents exchange and integrate information reflects the clinician's effectiveness. Certain personal qualities, present in varying degrees in all clinicians, will enhance a clinician's ability to communicate. Through greater awareness of these qualities, the potential for utilizing them can be realized. We believe that the following five factors characterize the most desirable qualities of a counselor.

Warmth and Nurturing. Perhaps one of the more important, yet least acknowledged, attributes of a counselor is the ability to nurture. Recognizing that our society often confuses tenderness with weakness and concern for overprotection, we define nurturing as the verbal and nonverbal communication transmitted from one person to another to support, reassure, and warmly, genuinely express one's caring for another. Nurturing establishes a favorable climate for personal growth. To go one step further, a nurturing environment is shaped by what we say and how we say it. The most meaningful information, when given in a matter-of-fact manner, is of questionable worth. Beck (1959) has pointed out that parents tend to reject unpleasant or distressing information when it comes to them through a seemingly disinterested or unfeeling source. By nurturing we do not mean creating a smothering, over-protective atmosphere in which one is not responsible for his actions. Rather, a warm and nurturing person permits the parent to feel that someone cares and that that person can see both parent and child as real people with whom he would like to relate.

Honesty. The ability to be honest with oneself is another attribute required of the counselor. Hamilton (1951) states that this characteristic differentiates a professional relationship from a social conversation. Honesty, in this instance, refers to the degree to which a professional can be sensitively aware of and accept his own feelings. Since each of us has our particular biases that enter into our interpersonal relationships, the adage to "know thyself" is particularly apropos.

Recognizing that *all* behavior is motivated, we believe that an awareness of one's own motivations and defense mechanisms helps prepare an individual to be more effective in his interpersonal relationships. For example, the audiologist who feels uncomfortable as a counselor will present only the facts of the hearing loss, rationalizing that "other" professionals will talk with the parents about their feelings and reactions. The difficulty arises when the "other" professionals possess the same anxieties and defense mechanisms: The physician talks about the medical aspects; the audiologist discusses the hearing tests; the teacher concentrates on the educational aspects of the hearing problem. Each has conven-

315

iently avoided confronting the problems of the family by focusing on the problems of the child. The parents have met with the required specialists who deal with children who have a hearing loss, but no one has discussed the parents' feelings.

In a mistaken attempt to exclude personal feelings from the professional relationship, some clinicians may withdraw behind an aloof facade of professionalism, an attitude of "I'm the expert," which prevents anything but the most sterile and impersonal contact. By acknowledging his own personal biases and determining their basis, the audiologist can choose to use this self-information to enhance his relationships with parents.

Objectivity. When listening to parents tell how they perceive the problem, the audiologist may be drawn into making value judgments about what has been said. This attitude of judging is neither appropriate nor conducive to good counseling techniques. The clinician who interjects his values or judgments into the counseling process diminishes the willingness of the parents to share their feelings. For example, a parent may say, "I became so frustrated with Jeremy not being able to understand, I wanted to shake him as hard as I could." Communicating your agreement or rejection of this comment, either verbally or nonverbally, would not be helpful. When the clinician judges, the parents will not reveal thoughts or actions that they think will be unacceptable. An appropriate response in the foregoing situation might be, "It's easy to become frustrated when you have to repeat so many times," thus acknowledging the feeling, but not condoning the resulting behavior.

Active Listening. Good communication requires active listening. Schulman (1974) points out that active listening is the bridge between hearing and understanding. Gordon (1970) describes active listening as a technique for insuring the correct interpretation of statements made by others. This technique emphasizes the listener's conscious attempts to understand clearly what the speaker means by what he has said. A listener may decode the message correctly or incorrectly. Only if he checks back with the sender, can the listener guarantee that what he has understood is what was meant. That is, the listener will translate the message into his own words and verify it by transmitting it back to the sender. The listener only says what he interpreted the sender to mean. In active listening, one does not send a message containing advice, opinions, analysis, evaluations, or questions. In the dialogue of active listening below, a statement is incorrectly decoded:

Parent: People cannot understand Johnny when he talks.

Audiologist: You are concerned about the way Johnny talks.

Parent: Not really, I'm concerned because people laugh at him.

Many different thoughts may be the basis for a single statement. For example, the statement "I'm not sure I want Johnny to have a hearing aid now," may reflect any of the following thoughts:

that it would make him appear "different";

that he will lose it;

that it will not be comfortable;

that it's too expensive;

that it won't help him;

that he won't wear it;

that he won't be accepted.

Active listening permits: (1) the parents to feel that they have been heard and (2) the audiologist to understand the feelings underlying the parents' concerns. Thus, by focusing on the thoughts of the parents and avoiding preoccupation with his own opinions, the clinician will establish a clearer picture of the problem as the parent sees it.

Awareness of Ambivalence. The audiologist in the counseling role must understand the concept of ambivalence. Ambivalence means that both positive and negative feelings regarding a single idea exist at the same time. We are aware of this feeling when we say "I want to, but on the other hand I don't want to."

The presence of such opposing thoughts may be noted when we ask for help, but don't want it; when we ask for advice, but don't use it; when we agree to plans, but don't carry them out; when we say one thing while our behavior indicates an opposing viewpoint (Garrett, 1942). Many audiologists tell parents the best course of action for them to take with their child and expect those plans to be followed implicitly. In actuality, we believe that the plans that are carried out are the ones that the parents view as reasonable for them. Although the audiologist presents the various alternatives, the parents make the choice. Awareness of this precept of ambivalence permits the audiologist to allow the parents to help themselves. We are reminded of the anonymous quotation used by the staff at the John Tracy Clinic in Los Angeles:

Anxiety cries for answer.

The answer-giver ties the asker.

He who makes the asker answer,

Makes the asker answer master.[1]

Although no textbook can supply human qualities, we believe that we can be better counselors when we develop characteristics of warmth and nurturing, honesty, objectivity, active listening, and when we are aware of ambivalence.

[1]Personal communication from Dr. A. J. Smith, John Tracy Clinic, Los Angeles, Cal., 1976.

THE COUNSELING PROCESS

The counseling process begins with the initial introduction of clinician and parents. Its termination depends on the nature of the disorder and the needs of the parents to receive additional support and to review options. The amount of interaction between the clinician and the parents varies, depending on the severity and permanence of the disorder. Consequently, the duration of counseling experiences may be as brief as a few hours, or may extend to months or years. Regardless of the number of visits, there is a logical sequence in which information is obtained and integrated and during which decisions are made. A first step is to establish an atmosphere in which the information one wishes to impart can be not only heard, but also understood.

The Audiologist as a Consultant or Manager

Whether the audiologist is a consultant or a primary manager for a child with a hearing loss depends upon the particular clinical setting, the team with which he functions, and the specific auditory problem. For example, middle-ear problems requiring surgical intervention and medical treatment are obviously the primary responsibility of the physician. On the other hand, the management of children who possess sensorineural hearing losses should be referred to the audiologist so that he may make recommendations and coordinate these recommendations with those of educational and medical specialists.

The audiologist must define his role and establish a clear understanding of his responsibilities and those of the referral source. As consultant, the audiologist must evaluate hearing and forward the results and recommendations to the referral source; the referral source coordinates, considering the audiological findings and recommendations, then decides what courses of action to pursue. Even in the consulting role, the audiologist has a responsibility to explain the results of his testing. He also has an obligation to make clear to the parents that he will be sending his results to the referral source, who will give the parents additional explanation and interpretation.

As a manager, on the other hand, the audiologist discusses results, makes recommendations, and works closely with the parents in following through on these recommendations. In this role, the audiologist is obligated to keep the referral source apprised of what steps are being taken.

Initial Interview

The interview, which is probably the first encounter the parent and the clinician have after the initial introduction, is integral to the counseling process. We believe its basic purpose is to obtain an understanding of the problem as the parents see it. The events leading to a decision to make an appointment for a hearing evaluation usually cause some degree of disruption in family relationships. Since both the parents and their child are already experiencing some anxiety, the young child should not be separated from the parents initially.

In the interview, the clinician allows the child to play with appropriate toys. Toys that produce excessive noise can disrupt the interview and should not be selected. Since children naturally possess short attention spans, the clinician should have several toys available to give to the child, one at a time as he needs additional amusement. This also gives the clinician the opportunity to establish rapport and to evaluate informally the self-directed play behavior of the child.

In this initial phase of the interview, besides attending to the child, the clinician is also relating to the parents. When the parents see the child becoming more at ease, they begin to relax. We would hope that they decide that the clinician is a person who relates well to children. Also, having both the parents and their child at the interview lets the clinician observe the relationship between them. At one extreme we find parents who constantly interrupt and correct the child's play, not letting him play by himself. At the other extreme are parents who provide no boundaries for the child's behavior, not only allowing complete freedom but also permitting destructive behavior. When either of these relationships is noted, it is important that later in the counseling process the parents be encouraged to discuss their ideas about how they relate to the child.

In addition to observing the parent-child relationship, the clinician must obtain background information about the current problems. Two methods are commonly employed: One involves having parents complete a questionnaire form prior to the appointment; the second is simply for the clinician to ask the parents direct questions as they occur on the questionnaire form. The first method is more desirable and efficient because it permits the clinician to seek additional specific information in pertinent areas. It also allows the clinician to familiarize himself with responses prior to the interview, then supplement this information with additional questions.

When eliciting information, the clinician should avoid phrasing questions so that parents can respond with a "yes" or "no" answer. In other words, questions should be designed to allow the parents to expand. For example, "Did you have any trouble when Johnny was born?" will most often receive either a "yes" or "no" answer, thus forcing the clinician to ask more specific questions. A more appropriate way to obtain this information is to say, "Tell me about Johnny's birth." Beginning a question with "How," "Where," "When" or "What," is more productive than beginning with "Did" or "Why" (Edinburg, Zinburg, and Kelman, 1975). McDonald (1962) also emphasizes the need for phrasing questions carefully to permit parents maximum opportunity to express their feelings. An example of this type of question is, "What are your concerns about Johnny?" Questions should not be phrased in a manner that causes parents to feel defensive about their child. Simmons (1974) suggests that parents' defensiveness is heightened if they are asked to tell what is "wrong" or what they think is wrong with their child. Questions permitting parents to describe or tell about their child are usually not threatening and provide an opportunity for parents to express their concerns in the manner most acceptable to them.

Parents can give information about their child at at least three levels of consciousness. At the most obvious level is knowledge that they will readily share, such as factual information and opinions. The child's birth date and age of walking or their opinion as to why he was a finicky eater would fall into this category. At a second level of consciousness is information they do not mention because of embarrassment, distrust, shame, or fear of rejection—for example, such circumstances as illegitimacy or the parent's hospitalization for nervous disorders. The third level of awareness, and the one least likely to emerge in the interview, represents information that is "repressed or forgotten because of its emotional charge" (Simmons, 1974, p. 118). Some feelings may be so stressful—for example, a death wish for a defective child—that parents will not discuss them because they cannot bear the pain of confronting them at this point.

Important as it is to give your undivided attention to what is being said, most authorities agree that some notes must be made. But bear in mind that extensive note-taking detracts from the interview and will impede the transfer of information. A thorough knowledge of and familiarity with the content of the interview form will permit the audiologist maximum flexibility in formulating questions and directing the discussion.

Some writers question the wisdom of a case-history interview, believing that the information obtained may bias the clinician (Northern and Downs, 1974). Proponents of this philosophy assume that the audiologist functions as an integral member of a team of specialists. In instances where team efforts consistently focus on children with hearing impairments, we would agree wholeheartedly with this philosophy. Unfortunately, most audiologists are not part of a cohesive, on-going, multidisciplinary team. Notwithstanding the obvious counseling advantages available in a team approach, obtaining the information and recording it is usually the task of the clinician.

Regardless of whether the method used to obtain initial information is based on a written questionnaire, a multidisciplinary approach, or a clinician-directed interview, we believe the clinician should ask the parents four crucial questions before terminating the interview:

1. "Where has your child been evaluated previously?"
2. "What were you told?"
3. "What did you think about what you were told?"
4. "What information do you want from me?"

The responses to these questions provide knowledge of the parents' awareness and understanding of the present situation and allow the clinician to gain insight into some of the parents' specific needs.

Testing

In the testing phase we invite one of the parents to stay in the test room if the child is 4 years old or younger. Having a parent present who appears relaxed is a cue to the child to react the same way. Requesting that a parent remain in the test environment is a critical part of the counseling procedure because it: (1) constitutes continuation of the rapport already established with the parent in the interview; (2) allows the parent to observe the child in the test situation; (3) aids in the explanation of the results. Furthermore, the presence of the parent alleviates the "hocus-pocus" aura of a clinician who suddenly announces to a parent who has been in the waiting room during testing, " Your child has normal hearing," or "Your child has a profound hearing loss." Attempts to explain, after the fact, the process involved in the test situation—for example, earphone versus sound-field testing—are never as effective as having a parent see it for himself. Detailed protocols for testing children are discussed in other chapters of this book.

Interpretive Interview

After acquiring data on a child's auditory performance levels, the audiologist must relay this information to the parents. Whenever possible, both parents should attend the interpretive interview without the child (Levine, 1960). Presenting the facts about a child's disorder is not enough, even if those facts are presented simply and honestly. The audiologist must present this information in a way that will be understood by the parents. Audiologists often forget that our terminology of dB, SRT, sound-field, and so forth have little meaning to parents. Parents will need help in organizing what has been said and assessing what that information means to them. As a general rule, the more severe and permanent the hearing loss of the child, the more support the parent will need. The interpretations of findings alone may require additional visits; some parents need to hear the findings and recommendations several times before they can fully comprehend them.

To assist the clinician in maximizing the exchange of information, the concepts of *stop, look,* and *listen* are helpful.

Stop. Counseling sessions where audiological findings are to be presented require careful preparation. The audiologist must stop and examine the specific information, assess what statements can be made on the basis of these data, and anticipate the ability of the parents to understand and accept the information. In most cases, the parents are anxious and are waiting for their suspicions to be confirmed. The audiologist must plan specifically what information he wishes to communicate. It is irresponsible for the clinician to go into this meeting with the parents without a complete grasp of the facts. The better the factual material is mastered, the easier it will be to handle the session without being pressed to minimize the situation or to hold out false promises. It is also important to thoroughly formulate the plans for follow-up and the recommendations that are to be presented.

Information should be presented to the parents unhurriedly, with assurance, and in a manner most easily understood by these particular parents. Ross (1964) notes that "shopping around" by parents usually indicates that they have not received the help they need in a way that they can use it. Therefore, during the stop phase we formulate the approaches and techniques that will clarify the information we are about to present. After compiling the available data and carefully formulating the recommendations, we feel better prepared when we stop to consider how to approach this particular family.

Look. While presenting the information, we look for nonverbal clues that reveal how the parents are handling the information. Do the things they say and the way they look go together? Nonverbal communication, including body language, is very powerful, and audiologists who observe this aspect of communication closely can tell how parents are accepting what they are hearing. Developing the habit of observing the nonverbal behavior of the parents during the interpretive interview is important.

Listen. After the initial explanation of findings, we anticipate questions from the parents. Garrett (1942) observes that the first question is often a "trial balloon," used to test the situation while the parents gather courage to ask what they really want to know. Listening attentively to these questions is one of the most crucial factors in the counseling process.

Three distinguishable types of questions are usually asked by parents: (1) content questions; (2) confirmation questions; (3) affect questions (Luterman, 1976). The first category, content questions, implies that the asker wants specific information from the audiologist. An example of this type of question is "Does Johnny hear the same in both ears?" These information-seeking questions are the easiest for the audiologist to answer and usually enable him to feel comfortable in his role as an information-giver.

The second type of question is used to confirm their own ideas. Parents may have a specific position on an issue; yet, instead of stating their position, they ask a question phrased in such a way that the answer will support their opinion. "Will a school that has an oral approach be best for my child?" may be a confirmation question. A monologue at this point regarding the clinician's opinions of oralism is a response indicating that this question has been interpreted as a content question. A more appropriate response would be to determine the type of question involved by asking the parents for their ideas on the subject. For example, "You must have done some thinking in that area," or "You must have some good ideas about that," will allow the parents to express their opinion.

Some questions may be either content questions, confirmation questions, or affect questions. For example, our original question, "Does Johnny hear the same in both ears?" may be either a content question or a confirmation question. To distinguish between the two, the audiologist must check with the parent. "What have you noticed in Johnny's reaction to sounds?" The parent may say, "I haven't noticed anything, I was just wondering," or "They tried to tell me before that his hearing was the same in both ears, but he keeps turning his right ear toward me all the time." In this example, the first parental response indicates that he is seeking information and his question was one of content. The second response in this example indicates that the parent had some preconceived notion about the answer. Therefore, his question was one of confirmation. After hearing the parent's response, the audiologist can determine the implication of the question. Some clinicians respond to all questions as if they were content, not confirmation, questions. However, the astute clinician realizes that if the parents are continuing to ask the same questions, specific information is not what they are seeking.

The third type of question, an affect question, involves some feeling of the parents that they are too insecure to mention or that they are not even aware of. For example, "Can an airplane flight in the later months of pregnancy cause deafness in a child?" reflects the possibility that the parents may feel guilty and be searching for the cause of their child's deafness. One response to this as an affect question could be, "It is natural to feel responsible and to search for reasons why your child has a hearing loss." A response to an affect question causes the parent to look within himself for a new awareness. This question could be responded to as a content question, a confirmation question, or an affect question. Luterman (1976) states that none of the responses is right or wrong; each is appropriate at some point. However, the counseling audiologist should be able to recognize content questions, confirmation questions, and affect questions when they are asked. If an audiologist feels that no parents are asking questions other than ones of content, he should remember the guideword for this section: listen.

Explanation of the Audiogram

At some stage in the interpretive interview, the audiologist must explain his objective findings. When the child is old enough to take a pure-tone air-conduction and bone-conduction test, we explain the findings to the parents by using the audiogram. We discuss the coordinates of the audiogram, indicating that pitch is represented from low to high across the top of the graph, while loudness is plotted along the side of the chart. The parent is told that red denotes the right ear and blue the left ear responses. The concept of threshold is defined as the softest sound that can be heard at each frequency. Further description is provided by discussing the relative position of the thresholds on the loudness scale of the audiogram and comparing these levels to known environmental sound levels.

The terms *mild, moderate, severe,* and *profound,* which indicate degrees of hearing loss, are unfamiliar to parents. The concept that one either hears or that he is hard-of-hearing is a prevalent one; for this reason, through demonstration and examples, we explain what the child can or cannot be expected to hear. The frequencies involved in hearing speech and the level of normal conversational speech should be indicated on the audiogram. These explanations might include statements such as, "He may be able to hear that you have called his name, but not hear well enough to be certain of exactly what has been said," or "If you speak to him when he is standing about three feet away, he will be able to hear, but if you are farther away, your voice will be too soft," or "When you get his attention, he must be able to watch you closely as well as listen to you if he is to understand what you are saying." Anatomical charts, diagrams of the ear, and a chalkboard can help supplement these explanations.

When children cannot respond appropriately to a pure-tone test under earphones, the results of alternate procedures and their significance must be explained. In this situation, it is equally important to explain what is not known. For example, "We do not know which ear is responding to the sounds," or "We cannot be certain how he responds to high-frequency sounds." When further information is needed, we set up additional appointments on specific dates and at specific times for continued evaluations. "We need to see him again in three weeks" does not leave the parents with the same assurance as "We will see you again on July 10 at 9 a.m."

Before the interpretive interview is terminated, determine if the parents comprehend what has been said. Asking the question, "What is your understanding about what has been said?" provides an opportunity to clear up any misconceptions the parents may have. Simply asking, "Do you have any questions?" will provide no clues to what the parent has understood and whether or not he has understood correctly. Many times it is not that the parents have no questions, but rather that they do not know what to ask or how to ask it.

Recommendations and Follow-Up

By the time the audiologist makes his recommendations, he should have established: (1) rapport with the parents; (2) insight into how the parents have handled the information he has presented; (3) an understanding of some of their concerns; (4) an idea of how the parents will accept his recommendations and incorporate them into a plan of their own. Recommendations related to specific hearing problems will be discussed later in this chapter.

In some cases, the follow-up visits will be scheduled for retest to check the child's hearing levels after medical management or surgery. In most cases, additional visits should be scheduled so that the information already presented can be reorganized and new information can be added. Follow-up counseling sessions have three purposes. According to Webster (1971), these sessions provide an opportunity to: (1) present additional information, (2) develop alternate methods for promoting better communication; (3) provide an atmosphere in which parents can verbalize freely and frankly about their needs, fears, and goals.

To summarize briefly, the counseling process includes the initial interview, testing, the interpretative interview, and discussion of appropriate follow-up procedures. It has a threefold purpose for parents in allowing them the opportunity to: (1) understand the hearing status of the child, (2) discuss their feelings regarding the implications of the loss, (3) make appropriate decisions in the best interests of the child.

CASE HISTORIES

Recognizing that every child and his parents present a new situation, we have selected the following representative case histories to illustrate some of the practical applications of the counseling process. The recommendations and follow-up procedures will vary with the degree and type of hearing loss, but the elements of the counseling process remain the same.

Mild Conductive Hearing Loss

The conductive hearing loss differs from other types of hearing impairment in that it offers the opportunity to be optimistic regarding the return of hearing to normal levels.

In one such case, Robert, age 6, was referred for a hearing evaluation by his physician who reported that he had bilateral perforations of the tympanic membranes. Our results revealed bone-conduction thresholds at 0dB HL and air-conduction thresholds at 35dB HL. On the basis of these data, we concluded that Robert had a mild bilateral, symmetrical, conductive hearing loss. In our experience, most parents have heard that nerve losses are permanent, but they have little or no concept of what mild, bilateral, symmetrical, and conductive mean. Consequently, we focused our explanation on each of these terms. In this case, we told the parents that the results indicate the possibility of a medically treatable problem and that they should return to their physician. An audiologist must not be drawn into a conversation about whether or not surgery is indicated or might be helpful. His opinion, although well-intentioned, can cause problems.

After the interpretive interview, our next task was to communicate to Robert's physician our findings and our recommendation that the child's hearing be monitored during the period of medical treatment. Routinely in cases of conductive hearing losses, we strongly urge that the child receive audiologic follow-up after medical treatment. Shortly after Robert's next medical appointment, his physician telephoned to state that while medical treatment was in progress, he felt that it was advisable to delay surgical intervention for four to six months. He requested that we follow Robert audiologically and educationally during this time.

The educational dilemmas created by a mild conductive hearing loss should not be minimized. During our next appointment with Robert, we discussed with the parents the necessity for having him preferentially seated in the classroom. His parents were informed of the recommendations that would be made to his teachers. These recommendations included seating Robert close to the teacher when she addressed the class and where the chalkboard was easily visible. Our recommendations would also include the necessity of seating Robert away from noise sources such as hallways, air conditioners, and playground windows, where competing noises could interfere with his instruction. Children in elementary schools often change classes during the day or have different teachers come to them for instruction. Therefore, we impress upon the parents the necessity of checking with each teacher to insure that our recommendations have been followed during this transition period.

One final point that should be made to parents of children with losses in this category is that hearing often fluctuates. Hearing may be better one day than the next; therefore, parents are cautioned not to make the assumption that their child hears equally well at all times.

Unilateral Hearing Loss

If a child has a unilateral hearing loss from birth, the child as well as his parents may remain unaware of the problem for a long time. Since speech, language, and vocabulary develop normally in these children, they are most often identified when they fail a school hearing screening test or develop otitis media in the good ear. The diagnostic information, "Your child has a profound hearing loss in one ear," given to the parents usually produces responses such as "What does that mean?" and "How could it have been present all this time without our realizing it?" Parents should be reassured that language, vocabulary, and learning will continue to progress because the child has one normally hearing ear. Unfavorable listening conditions arise when: (1) noise is on the side of the good ear; (2) he is unable to localize the source of sound. Inability to localize makes it difficult for him to position himself in listening situations so that the noise source is nearer the poor ear.

Gregory, age 4, was referred to us by a physician for audiological testing after the child's mother reported her concern about Gregory's inconsistent responses to sounds in the past few weeks. When asked what information she wanted from the evaluation, she replied that she wanted to know whether her son was ignoring her or if he really had a hearing problem. Our evaluation of Gregory indicated a profound sensorineural hearing loss in one ear and a mild conductive loss in the other ear. Our first task was to recommend that Gregory return to the physician for medical treatment of the pathology causing the conductive problem. We discussed with his mother the possibility of evaluating Gregory with a CROS hearing aid after the conductive problem had been corrected. In this discussion we pointed out that a CROS hearing aid could offer appreciable help in localizing the source of sounds.

Specific suggestions were made to the mother regarding ways to minimize listening difficulties in the classroom. We scheduled a conference with Gregory's mother and preschool teachers to discuss the need for preferential seating and to emphasize the importance of assuring that Gregory understands instructions clearly. His mother was given the responsibility for checking on the seating arrangement with the teachers in each class, especially as he progressed to higher grades. If Gregory changes schools, his mother has been instructed to notify us so that additional letters can be written to appropriate school personnel.

Parental anxiety concerning a unilateral hearing loss in a child usually centers on the question, "Will something happen to the good ear?" Even if genetic factors do not explain the hearing loss, we cannot guarantee that the other ear will remain normal. Therefore, we counsel in terms of our experience: that is, we see no reason to expect an additional hearing loss in the good ear any more than we expect a severe loss of hearing in the ear of any other child. We mention the illnesses and medicines that are known to be causal factors in hearing losses. We also discuss the necessity of protecting the good ear against noise exposure, being alert to symptoms of early otitis media, and seeking immediate medical attention for any suspected ear problems. Since speech and language are not appreciably affected by a unilateral hearing loss, strong parental feelings are rarely prolonged. Furthermore, the prognosis for educational and vocational growth is good, and these positive aspects should be emphasized. Nevertheless, the audiologist must be looking and listening for parental reactions that indicate lack of understanding or distress.

Nonorganic Hearing Loss

Children who have normal hearing and choose to pretend a hearing loss do so for a variety of reasons. In some cases, it is an attention-getting device. In others, it is an attempt to focus parental concern on hearing and away from real problems, such as poor grades or reported behavior problems in school. In a few cases, pretended hearing loss is an indication of serious emotional problems, which require referral for psychological or psychiatric counseling. Most audiologists have evaluated perplexing young children who have chosen not to attend to any stimulus, visually or auditorily. Obviously, these children and their parents will need long-term, specialized care. This discussion is focused on the child who consciously chooses to "acquire" a hearing loss, not on the truly autistic child. The audiologist has the responsibility to consider carefully the appropriateness of referring any child with a nonorganic hearing loss for psychological or psychiatric evaluation.

The majority of children we see who exhibit nonorganic hearing losses are between the ages of 7 and 14. In the interview, they usually will answer questions and exhibit no apparent difficulty in hearing. Although some of these children have a history of previous ear infections, most of them have no history that would indicate hearing problems.

An example is Susan, age 12, whose mother bought her to us for evaluation. While talking with her mother, we learned that Susan was doing poorly in math and was sent to the school nurse to have her hearing screened. She failed the screening test. A few days later follow-up testing by the school nurse also indicated a hearing loss. Susan was referred to a physician who checked her ears. A hearing test in his office showed her voluntary air-conduction thresholds were 45dB HL bilaterally. Susan was then referred to a hearing-aid dealer who tested her and recommended an ear level aid for one ear. Her mother made a down payment on the hearing aid, and they were to pick it up a few days later. A relative of Susan who works at our center insisted that she be tested in our facility before purchasing the hearing aid.

By the time we evaluated Susan, she had been through several tests and was very good at choosing consistent voluntary "thresholds" of about 45dB HL by air and bone conduction. However, she was not as sophisticated with speech tests, and she began repeating spondaic words within the range of normal hearing. At this point, her mother was brought into the control room to observe Susan's ability to respond to faint levels of speech. Although permitting parents in the control room is not the usual procedure, when parents have become convinced that their normally hearing child has a hearing loss, first-hand evidence is most useful in enabling them to accept the diagnostic findings. To reiterate, if in the interpretive interview parents hear information that they are totally unprepared for, they usually suspect that the findings are invalid and will seek another evaluation elsewhere.

When a child commits himself to pretending a hearing loss, he has a substantial investment regardless of the reason behind his choice. He is unsure of the repercussions if his pretense is discovered, and the fear of embarrassment and/or punishment causes him to be anxious and feel threatened. Particularly in the case of nonorganic problems, the concerns of both parents and child must be considered fully.

When Susan's mother realized that her child's hearing was normal, she asked "What should I do to her now? I've been worried and spent so much time and money for nothing. Why would she rather wear a hearing aid she doesn't need than tell us the truth?" Our reply to that confirmation question is to indicate our concern by saying, "That's a good question," then add, "You probably have some good ideas about the answer." After thinking for a few minutes, the parents usually develop some ideas and decide that punishment would not help, that they would like to be supportive of the child. We did not press Susan to reveal true air-conduction thresholds on her initial visit. Instead, we told her that we had been able to determine the level of her hearing and that we would like for her to come back in a month for another test.

Susan's mother was seen twice during the next few weeks and reported that both she and her husband had been supportive of Susan. As Susan walked down the hall to the test room for her re-evaluation she said, "My hearing is better now. I don't think I'll have that problem again." Her air-conduction thresholds during this evaluation were well within the range of normal hearing, and we told her that her hearing was normal. We encouraged her to return to us for a re-evaluation in the future if she felt she had a hearing problem.

Children sometimes get themselves into corners and cannot find a way out by themselves. Audiologists who are concerned about the effect of such a situation can provide options that will allow both parents and children to be truthful without fear. Parental support is a key deterrent to the establishment of defense mechanisms by children. As Ginott (1968) points out, once the child no longer needs defenses, the behavioral manifestation disappears.

Bilateral High-Frequency Sensorineural Hearing Loss

Children whose hearing is within normal limits for low frequencies but show a sharply sloping loss through the high frequencies are familiar to the clinical audiologist. These are the children who turn when someone calls their name and who develop speech and language, although they may have articulation problems.

These children frequently misunderstand instructions, use self-taught speech-reading cues, and are often accused of being inattentive. As a matter of fact these children are labeled with as many different tags as there are misinterpretations of their behavior. The child is called lazy, stupid, uncaring, and shy; he is viewed as a behavior problem while all the time he is just himself, a hard-of-hearing child (Levine, 1960).

The hearing loss of these children is often undetected until they fail a school hearing screening test or are referred to the school speech pathologist because of their poor articulation. Some children with this problem are not identified until the third or fourth grade, and an unfortunate few are not identified until much later.

A typical case is that of Carl, age 7, who was referred to our center because of an articulation problem. As a routine part of the diagnostic battery, the speech pathologist requested a hearing evaluation. During the initial interview phase of the audiologic evaluation, Carl's parents expressed concern over the child's poor grades, his speech production, and his teacher's comments that he did not pay attention. They also wanted to know if their child might be simply ignoring them. They stated that their family physician had seen the child and could find no obvious pathology in the ear to account for a hearing problem. The physician had recommended a hearing test, but since their child had suffered no discomfort with his ears, they had not followed through on the recommendation. Our audiologic evaluation indicated that Carl had a mild hearing loss in both ears for frequencies 250 through 1000 Hz and then a drop to 45 to 55dB HL bilaterally for the frequencies 1500 through 8000 Hz.

In the interpretive interview, the explanation of the audiogram was supplemented by explaining the range of frequencies in conversational speech and pointing out the particular consonant sounds that Carl was missing. One helpful statement in this type of explanation is, "He will know that you are talking, but may not be able to distinguish whether you have said cat, bat, mat, pat, or that." We explain that the low-frequency components of background noise tend to interfere with the high-frequency consonant sounds that he needs to hear in order to differentiate among the various words. Carl's parents expressed relief following this explanation; at least now they had gained insight into some of the difficulties their child had experienced.

If the child is old enough to understand the implications of our discussion, and many school children are, he is included in the interpretive interview. Most often, he, too, is relieved that someone has determined the basis for his difficulty to hear clearly. Now is a good time to reassure the child that not only do we realize the stress he has experienced but also the additional energy he has expended in listening.

Two specific areas emphasized in counseling parents of a child with a high-frequency hearing loss are plans for education and amplification. The recommendations for these children need to be explained in an unhurried manner, giving the parents time to assimilate the information and to ask questions as they arise.

Educational Planning

We explained to Carl's parents that the principal, teacher, speech pathologist, and school nurse would be informed of the findings, and specific suggestions for working with Carl would be included in letters to them. Carl was in an open classroom where work was done in groups, circles, and such. Our experience suggests that the child with a hearing handicap is at a greater disadvantage in an open classroom.

Teachers, in particular, need specific suggestions regarding their role in helping this child. They should be encouraged to check each situation closely for the most advantageous seating for the child. They should be alert to different noise sources in the classroom and the learning difficulties that noise creates for this child. Along with the report to the school, sending a copy of a "Letter to the Teacher of a Hard-of-Hearing Child" (Pollock and Pollock, 1971) can provide many helpful suggestions for the teacher.

Amplification

In the past many clinicians have assumed that children with a precipitously sloping high-frequency hearing loss would not benefit from amplification. Current technology in hearing-aid design and the use of the open-mold fittings have enabled us to provide vital amplification for these children.

A hearing aid was recommended for Carl and, once it had been selected, counseling sessions were held with him and his parents to discuss his adjustment to the hearing aid and their acceptance of it. We recommended that we see Carl and his parents every four to five months for additional counseling sessions and to recheck his performance with the hearing aid.

Acceptance of the concept of amplification by both the parents and the child is the first prerequisite toward satisfactory adjustment. Parental acceptance is needed for support, but it is the child as he grows older who will use or reject the hearing aid. The child should be encouraged to verbalize his feelings about wearing a hearing aid, and we often observe that many of his questions are the same as those of his parents: "What will it look like?" "When would I have to wear it?" "Can it be seen?" "What difference will it make?" "What will my friends think?" Dale (1976) states that the fear of being rejected is one of the most powerful feelings in individuals. That fear is accentuated in an adolescent or school-age child who is hard-of-hearing and wears a hearing aid. Years of failing, being ridiculed, meeting new people, being slighted, being singled out, and being in new situations are all fears of the hard-of-hearing child (Levine, 1960).

Counseling sessions with the child allow him an opportunity to examine his feelings about wearing a hearing aid and to develop positive attitudes toward it. Without follow-up counseling the child's acceptance of amplification is often questionable. This statement is substantiated by the following case.

Terry, a 13-year-old girl, was first seen by us three years after a recommended hearing aid had been purchased for her; she had not had subsequent counseling. We found that she had a mild bilateral hearing loss for 250 through 1000 Hz. The audiometric configuration showed a precipitous slope to 85 to 90dB HL bilaterally in the frequency range from 2000 through 8000 Hz. Unaided speech discrimination performance was poor in her left ear and only fair in the right ear. With her ear-level hearing aid on the right ear, she received substantial benefit. Although she readily admitted that amplification helped her, Terry did not wear her aid all the time, made every effort to hide her aid, never put it on in the presence of anyone, and never told any of her friends that she had a hearing aid. In our discussions with Terry about her experiences with her hearing aid she asked, "What do you tell someone who asks, "Are you deaf?" A content question? Hardly! An affect reply could be, "It can be embarrassing when you are not able to hear." This reply would allow her the opportunity to discuss the embarrassment she feels about wearing a hearing aid. We need to provide counseling for children experiencing these adjustment problems.

Moderate-to-Severe Sensorineural Hearing Losses

Marked language deficiencies and articulation problems are the two concerns most frequently mentioned by parents who bring a child with moderate-to-severe sensorineural hearing loss for audiologic evaluation. We find that these parents have usually discussed their questions about the child's hearing with family members, friends, and/or physician. Since these children often make some progress in speech and language, well-meaning suggestions to wait awhile before pursuing evaluation of hearing may have sounded reasonable to these parents.

This circumstance is illustrated by the case of Harold, age 7, who had minimal speech when his mother brought him in for an evaluation. He used his voice to attract attention and turned to the talker when his name was called. He had been in kindergarten for two years and was now in a first-grade classroom. His mother reported that both she and the teachers felt that he could hear because, when they called him, he would scan his environment. Harold had a 70 to 85dB HL sloping loss in the left ear with no measurable hearing beyond 4000 Hz. The right ear had a hearing loss that sloped sharply from 35dB HL at 250 Hz to 110dB HL at 1500 Hz. He had no measurable hearing above 1500 Hz in the right ear. In the interpretive interview, we explained that sensitivity in the right ear would allow him to be aware of loud conversational speech, but that his residual hearing was not sufficient to permit him to understand normal conversational speech. Harold's mother admitted that she had been using gestures along with her speech for quite some time in order to communicate with Harold. Following our explanation of the audiogram, we used additional techniques to demonstrate what Harold might be expected to hear when speech is presented at normal conversational levels.

Currently available are recordings which simulate how one hears normal conversational speech with various degrees and types of hearing loss. Two such recordings are "How They Hear" (RCA Victor, 1964) and "Getting Through" (Zenith Radio Corporation, 1971) (see Appendix). Having parents listen to these records helps explain the magnitude of their child's problem. In addition, we often present very soft speech to parents through the earphones as a method of demonstrating the difficulties their child encounters when constantly straining to understand what is being said.

Using the foregoing devices often raises questions by the parents. In Harold's case we used the questions his mother asked as a guide to explain that many steps could be taken to reduce the effects of his problem. We focused on the two areas that needed our immediate attention. First, we discussed the benefits of amplification and the procedures to be followed in choosing an appropriate hearing aid for Harold. Second, we suggested: (1) getting the child's attention before speaking to him; (2) talking to him at close range and at eye level; (3) using visual clues to supplement his hearing.

Because a critical aspect of counseling in the early stages is to avoid presenting too much information too quickly, we did not dwell on the limitations of hearing-aid use at this time. Nor did we discuss the mechanics of checking and maintaining the hearing aid. On the other hand, we believe parents feel better if they are given some structured activities to perform following this session. Going away from the evaluation empty-handed perpetuates their feeling of helplessness. Therefore, Harold's mother was given some simple homework assignments. For example, she was asked to make a list of objects in their home which combines both auditory and visual cues such as the electric can opener, vacuum cleaner, and running bath water. Before the visit was terminated, we checked about what she understood us to have said. She had some misconceptions, which were rediscussed at that time. We ended this session by saying, "Between now and the next time I see you, you will probably have some thoughts or several questions. Write them down as you think of them and we will discuss them when we see you next Wednesday."

In the second session, we began by saying, "You have had several days to think over what we said when you were here before. How are you feeling about it now?" She expressed a broad range of feelings from relief at knowing what the problem was to anxiety and guilt. Her questions varied from "What do I do next?" to "Why did this happen to me?" Once again, the audiologist must listen closely to the question and evaluate whether it is one of content, confirmation, or affect. At the appropriate point in the conversation, we again discussed the audiogram. Parents seldom understand the audiogram the first time it is presented.

During this second session Harold was evaluated for a hearing aid, and additional information about hearing aids was presented to his mother. This time we became more specific regarding the benefits and limitations of amplification. This discussion enabled Harold's mother to be realistic in her expectations from amplification. If parents are left with the idea that a hearing aid will solve the problem, not only will they place unrealistic demands on the child, but also they will be less prepared to accept further suggestions regarding auditory training, speechreading, language enrichment, or special educational placement. In particular, they must understand the child's needs for visual communication, a comprehensive term for utilizing all aspects of the visual channel (Sanders, 1971). One week later, after Harold and his mother had purchased the recommended hearing aid, she was again counseled about the aid.

Keith (1974) and Sanders (1975) suggest some specific areas of information about hearing aids that should be mentioned to parents. These suggestions include the component parts of the aid, how it works, how to clean the earmold, effects of moisture on aids, removal of batteries when the aid is not in use, effects of ambient noise, accidental loss insurance policies, and daily checks for malfunction. Hanners and Sitton (1974) present a checklist and designate the equipment needed for daily use in troubleshooting the child's hearing aid: we strongly encourage using their approach. McConnell and Horton (1970) also make some practical suggestions for hearing-aid management procedures with young children who use body aids. Helpful suggestions to make the parent's life easier include securing the hearing-aid harness in a comfortable position, wrapping receiver cords around the harness if they are too long, and using receiver-savers. We also emphasize that we would have to make new earmolds periodically as the child grows. The concept of acoustic feedback in relation to the fit of the earmold is also explained.

The following series of questions were posed by his mother and are typical of those often asked by parents: "Will the hearing get better if he wears the aid?" "If he wears his aid, will other people think he's different?" "When can he stop wearing the hearing aid?" "How long do these aids usually last?" Following our discussion of hearing aids, we directed his mother's thoughts to Harold's needs in speech and language development.

In general it is imperative that the audiologist be familiar with all programs for hearing-impaired children in the geographical area. Each available program must be explained, along with the approaches and methods used in that particular program. For the preschool child, we mention that in addition to special education placement, the parents may want to send him to a regular nursery school. Parents are given the names and telephone numbers of people at various programs who can provide them with additional information. We cannot make these decisions for the parents, but we do help them to formulate their thoughts in this important area.

If the age of the child or other factors preclude making a specific recommendation for a hearing aid, we evaluate his performance with various hearing aids by trying them on a loan basis. The parents are required to help with this evaluation by reporting their impressions of the child's listening behavior at home. Parents are asked to maintain a record that designates the aid in use, the ear in which it is worn, and the child's responses to a variety of sounds in the home.

If the child is school age, as Harold was, information and recommendations for him are sent to his school's principal and to the director of special education in the school system. Harold's mother was encouraged to meet with these professionals to gain a specific understanding of what is being done in that school's program for children like her son who have moderate to severe hearing losses. We recommended that she meet with these school administrators because she needed to know how decisions were made regarding placement in a regular classroom and the frequency of meetings with the staff members and parents. Harold was moved from a regular classroom to a special classroom for hearing impaired children. Once he had been placed and his mother knew who the teacher would be, we made her aware that frequent meetings between parents and the child's teachers are mandatory. We gave Harold's mother the responsibility for making certain that these meetings are held.

Once decisions had been made regarding educational placement for Harold we continued to evaluate his hearing periodically and to assess his adjustment to his hearing aid. We continued to work with him and his mother and maintained contact with his teachers. When his teacher changes, we have the responsibility of familiarizing the new teacher with the hearing problems of this child.

Each new situation presents new factors to which children with moderate-to-severe sensorineural hearing losses must adjust. One overriding factor with children who have these losses is that some psychological problems can arise from even a mild hearing loss. However, emotional problems seem to increase with the severity of the hearing loss (Goetzinger, 1972). A good parent-child relationship can help to minimize the psychological effects associated with a hearing loss. Therefore, in our discussions with parents we counsel them about the importance and pleasures of seeking a rewarding parent-child relationship, rather than becoming absorbed in the mechanics of planning for the child.

Profound Sensorineural Hearing Loss

From birth to 3 years of age, each child differs in his pattern of development (Gesell et al., 1940). In attempting to allow for these individual differences, parents of a profoundly hearing-impaired child may, during the early stages of their child's development, alternately ponder the question of the child's hearing and then dismiss it. At some point, however, parents decide to seek professional opinions regarding the child's hearing. In some cases the decision is made on the urging of relatives and friends who have also observed the child's behavior. Regardless of events leading to the evaluation, no parent is ever prepared for the confirmation that his child is handicapped. Whenever the suspicion of a severe hearing impairment is confirmed, the identification of their role as the mother and father of a handicapped child is always painful (Barsch, 1968).

When the factual information is presented in the interpretive interview, the parents' fears are now being discussed as a reality. Their child is not normal; all the plans, hopes, and dreams they had for their normal child are lost. Suddenly, they must cope with both the reality of a child with a defect and the emotional turmoil of feeling the loss of a normal child (Solnit and Stark, 1961). The realization of this loss dominates the parents, who experience a period of bereavement and grief (Wright, 1960). This period of grief has been termed a period of mourning (Wright, 1960; Solnit and Stark, 1961; Ross, 1964; Kübler-Ross, 1969; McCollum and Schwartz, 1972; Moses, 1974). The theories on this mourning period designate specific stages through which an individual must pass before he can reach a psychologically healthy level of acceptance. These stages are denial, anger, guilt, anxiety, and acceptance. Parents whose child has a hearing loss of a lesser degree than profound often pass through these same emotional states. On the other hand, parents whose child has a profound hearing loss are most likely to manifest these stages and discuss their feelings with the clinician. Moreover, the parents of a profoundly hearing-impaired child tend to remain in these stages longer and experience them with greater intensity because of the pervasive magnitude of the problem. For these reasons it is particularly appropriate to discuss stages as they relate to profound sensorineural hearing loss.

When parents evidence grief, their ability to recognize, evaluate, and adapt to reality is often significantly impeded. During this period counseling is a continuing process used to help parents establish a sense of confidence and an understanding of the child's defect. Parents need an opportunity to discuss their inner reactions of disappointment, resentment, humiliation, and loneliness. The period of mourning facilitates the transition from disbelief to reality through a gradual, repetitive re-experiencing of the memories and expectations of the parents (Solnit and Stark, 1961). This mourning period may be summarized as a process of moving through the states of denial, anger, guilt, and anxiety toward acceptance of the profoundly hearing-impaired child.

Denial. When the parents are confronted with test results, their initial reaction, whether verbalized or not, is denial. The phrase, "Oh no! This can't be true. It can't be happening to me!" passes through the mind of every parent who is told that his child has very limited hearing. Parents use denial as a defense mechanism to cope with their anxieties as they are told that their child possesses a profound hearing impairment. The magnitude of this reaction may vary, depending upon preceding events. For example, if a loss has been suspected for an extended period of time, parents will be less likely to reject these findings. Parents who have been elsewhere, who have "shopped around" for evaluations, are also aware that a problem may be present. Nevertheless, in attempting to obtain support for their disbelief, they will seek confirmation from professionals that the condition is transient, reversible, or curable. However, it is a disservice to the family to respond to the defense mechanism of denial by minimizing the seriousness of the loss or by holding out false hopes. It is important to be honest.

During the denial stage, it is difficult for parents to assimilate information. The audiologist who attempts to "unload" management information on the parents at this juncture will create confusion and will be ineffective. Parents are ready to receive information only when they ask for it. When parents begin asking for information, it may be a sign that they are emerging from the denial stage. Questions regarding the etiology and complexity of the problem are usually the first asked by the parents. We provide pamphlets or brochures on hearing loss designed specifically for parents so that they may educate themselves at their own leisure and in a more neutral environment. (Some sources for obtaining excellent materials that can be adapted for use in this area are cited in the appendix at the end of the chapter.) Sheimo (1951) suggests that centering attention on the impaired child rather than on the parental feelings focuses on the least relevant factor of the denial stage.

Anger. The second stage of mourning begins when the parents seek a focal point to which they can displace their rising anger as they work toward acceptance of the problem. Thus, feelings of anger, rage, envy, and resentment gradually replace feelings of denial (McCollum and Schwartz, 1972, Kübler-Ross, 1969). Anger may be transferred to others: loved ones, marital partner, God, physician, or audiologist; anyone and anything is vulnerable. To attack others because of their child's deafness is only natural as the parents try to protect their own personalities (McDonald, 1962). When we can tolerate the anger and resentment, we are allowing parents to move toward acceptance without guilt. If we respond by becoming angry ourselves or blaming them for their feelings, we ultimately prolong the personal grief, thus impeding acceptance. The audiologist's ability to be objective at this point enables parents to acknowledge anger, recognize its displacement, and discharge it through nondestructive channels.

Guilt. A third stage in the mourning period is guilt. Since guilt is a pervasive emotion in the general population, it is not surprising to find these feelings in parents of defective children. The simple fact that the child is theirs makes them particularly vulnerable to this emotion (Schmideberg, 1956). Guilt-laden feelings associated with the concept of punishment are often deep-seated.

Some parents search for causal factors in an attempt to place the blame on something or someone. Occasionally, parents go through a period of blaming each other; if these feelings are not resolved, they may disrupt an otherwise satisfactory marriage. In talking with divorced parents, we learned that marital dissension became more pronounced when the hearing loss was first discovered in the child. Elements that might otherwise remain dormant in a marriage are brought to the surface and seem to be aggravated by this stress (Stream and Stream, 1972). However, divorce does not seem to be more prevalent among parents of hearing-impaired children. A recent study on the psychosocial problems of deaf children and their families has indicated that in a large population sample, the divorce and separation rate was not higher for parents with hearing-impaired children than for those in the population as a whole (Malkin, Freeman, and Hasting, 1976a, b).

Parents who never get over feeling guilty may react by (1) overprotecting the child to the exclusion of other members in the family or (2) manifesting strong feelings of intolerance coupled with an irresistible impulse to deny their relationship to the child (Solnit and Stark, 1961). Since neither of these reactions is in the best interest of the child, we encourage parents to acknowledge and accept these negative feelings of guilt as an understandable response to the circumstances. At the same time, we ask them to emphasize the positive components in their feelings toward care of the child. In fact, the discussion of both their positive and negative feelings often enables the parents to minimize the need to place the blame on themselves. When parents no longer need to blame themselves, their guilt feelings are reduced.

Anxiety. When parents have too many questions to answer or too many decisions to make at one time, they may become confused. Unrecognized and unmanaged feelings of confusion can lead to deeper feelings of anxiety. McDonald (1962) defines anxiety as an uneasiness of mind accompanied by restlessness or nervousness. Anxiety interferes with parental effectiveness. A basic premise of counseling the parents of the handicapped child is that too much information given too soon can be as confusing as having too little information or getting the information too late. Anxiety can occur because of concern over any number of things: marital relations, sibling rivalry, acceptance of the child by the neighborhood, choice of schooling, discipline problems, possible vocations, toilet training, or communication methods. Often parents need to be reminded to deal with one thing at a time. At this stage, the audiologist should be attuned to anxiety as it arises. By watching and listening for signs of confusion, the audiologist can help parents to focus on issues that they can productively work with at that time.

According to the principle of satiation, individuals can maintain an emotional state for only a limited period of time. The length of time that parents are in one of the foregoing stages will depend on their past experiences and personal influences. It is clinically unwise to attempt to rush parents through any of these stages, but, as Wright (1960) points out, suddenly the person will be tired of mourning and will be ready for new and different approaches to the problem.

Acceptance. When parents are satiated with mourning, they enter a new phase called *acceptance*. In this stage, they are ready to confront a new reality. Furthermore, they can approach the goals and demands required of them without being overwhelmed by irrelevant concerns over which they have no control. As parents learn to cope with their problems in the best way they know how, their anxiety levels are proportionately diminished. The vast majority of these parents, with guidance and nurturing, can gradually pass through these stages of denial, anger, guilt, and anxiety to face reality and restructure their lives in a positive manner. The clinician's first responsibility is to address the parents' feelings and attitudes; and later he can concentrate on appropriate language and auditory stimulation for the child (Northcott, 1972). Complete acceptance may take years, even all of a parent's life. The growth of feelings of acceptance of the problem cannot be hurried and will develop gradually if the parents' capacities to think, feel, and talk about their disappointment, sense of failure, and feelings of helplessness are not hampered by the attitudes of the clinician.

Central Auditory Processing Problems

Children who come to us for evaluation of auditory processing problems usually have had many different kinds of psychometrics. Typically, their sensory and cognitive performance has been evaluated through the usual battery of tests administered by the diagnostic clinicians in the school system. Parents have been told that previous testing did not indicate any problems, yet the parents feel that something is awry. The child's teacher continues to indicate that the child does not follow directions well and is inattentive in class. As this child progresses in school, reports to parents may contain the terms "disruptive" and "a behavior problem."

By the time we evaluate the child, it is not uncommon to observe that both the child and the parents are confused. The child is aware that he is not doing as well in school as his peers. Yet, he feels he is probably just as smart as they are. He can cope with neither the demands of the teacher nor the demands made of him at home. Increasingly, people in authority are displeased with him, and he is beginning to conclude that he must be a "bad" child. Parents are confused, alternating between believing that their child simply does not listen and attempting to discover a logical reason to explain his behavior.

Robb, age 6, was referred to us for a hearing evaluation which was part of a comprehensive battery of diagnostic tests. In fact, his parents had specifically requested a hearing test. During the interview Robb's parents stated that he had had a hearing evaluation elsewhere and that the audiologist had reported that he heard normally. Questioning the accuracy of the previous test, the parents remarked that they would like a second opinion. When the audiogram reflecting Robb's normal hearing was interpreted to the parents, they both sat stone-faced. The father then slapped his knee and said, "Well, that's that." Observation of the parents' nonverbal cues by the audiologist indicated that the parents did not yet have the answer they sought. Therefore, we pursued the matter further by asking if they had additional concerns or questions about Robb that they had not mentioned in the initial interview. Immediately the mother asked, "If he can hear, why can't he listen?" Without waiting for an answer, she related that they were confused about his being a behavior problem at school, that he could not seem to remember things that he had been told repeatedly, and that he often did just the opposite of what he had been told. Based on the secondary information plus our own observation, we suggested further assessment for a central auditory processing problem. On the central auditory perception test battery Robb performed very poorly on two of the four tests. His performance indicated that he did have substantial difficulty in the area of auditory perception (Willeford, 1976).

The term "auditory perception problem" had little meaning for Robb's parents. However, this concept became clearer when we explained that Robb did not process auditory information as well as other children his age, particularly in noisy situations. Although he could hear well, he was at a disadvantage in situations where he had to separate the message he wished to hear from irrelevant background sounds. His parents were relieved to find that someone had identified a plausible explanation for his behavior, and they were eager for suggestions. We counseled them about controlling the home environment, with specific emphasis on the need for quiet. We called attention to various noise sources in the home such as the dishwasher, washing machine, television, radio, record player, and vacuum cleaner. The noise of these appliances as well as talking or laughing will distract this child when he is trying to attend to conversation. Willeford (1976) advises using simple language, learning to avoid important conversations in noisy places, moving to a quieter environment, and finding quiet conversational periods on a regular basis during the course of each day.

Children with special problems such as Robb's are at a decided disadvantage in an open classroom or when seated by doorways, windows facing playgrounds, air conditioners, or pencil sharpeners. Specific, written suggestions to Robb's teachers are needed if he is to thrive in the auditory jungle of the modern classroom. Earmuffs are one therapeutic recommendation for school and work periods at home (Willeford, 1976). Robb's parents will be unable to communicate effectively with him from room to room or "on the run." Since maturation may influence the child's ability to separate background from foreground auditory stimuli, we emphasized the need for annual rechecking.

In counseling Robb's parents we recommended that they praise him for his achievements. For example, we suggested that they: (1) look for things he does right and mention them first; (2) recognize the extra effort that goes into his work; (3) check themselves to see if they are critical of most things he does. Positive reinforcement of achievements will encourage him and do much to improve his self-image. No genes carry self-worth; it is learned (Satir, 1972) and the majority of the learning takes place in the family. After all, the nuclear family provides our primary training in who we are and how we behave. We figure out ways to survive in our family unit and use what we have learned in our approach to other people (Purcell, 1976). We are particularly concerned that parents of children with central auditory processing problems realize how important it is to be positive and nurturing with their child. How the child thinks of himself will largely determine how he handles the criticism and labeling he may encounter from those outside the family.

Hereditary Hearing Loss

The question of genetically transmitted deafness invariably arises when counseling parents of a congenitally hearing-impaired child, especially when no other apparent etiology explains the hearing loss. While some parents may be looking for the cause of the deafness, others may be seeking answers regarding the question of having additional children.

Genetic counseling, a service conducted by genetic specialists, determines the risk of occurrence or statistical chance that an abnormal trait can occur or recur in a family. Risk factors can be determined only after obtaining a thorough and extensive family history and developing a family pedigree. Despite technological advances, the family pedigree is still the single most powerful tool of the genetic counselor.

Current statistics reveal that more than 50% of congenital deafness is hereditary (Fraser, 1964; Brown, 1967; Nance and Sweeney, 1975). Although the basic patterns of inheritance are well known, it is often difficult to compile the information necessary to make an intelligent prediction on the probabilities of having a deaf child. It becomes a relatively easier task if the family has exhibited the characteristic syndromes associated with one of the dominant patterns of inheritance. The three patterns of inheritance are dominant, recessive, and sex-linked. However, as Proctor and Proctor (1967) point out, most genetically related deafness (40%) is of the recessive type. Recessive deafness is the most difficult to identify and predict because the trait only appears when both genes on an autosome are abnormal. Case-history information from both sides of a family is usually sketchy at best, thus making it difficult to create a case for recessive transmission (Wedenberg, 1972).

The parental concern about information on hereditary deafness seems to be related to the order of birth of a hearing-impaired child in a family (Meadow and Meadow, 1971; Roberts, 1962). When the impaired child is the first-born, there may be more need for genetic counseling as contrasted to families where normal children have preceded the handicapped child. Misconceptions about genetic transmission may affect several aspects of the marital relationship and subsequent decisions about having more children. Recently Stream and Stream (1973) reported results from interviews of eight couples, each of whom had a deaf child. Whether for conscious or unconscious reasons, all of them had decided not to have additional children following the identification of deafness in the child.

It is the role of the genetic counselor to provide a couple with enough information to allow them to make a rational decision concerning their plans for a family. The choice is theirs; they are given no instructions or advice as to what they should do. In this situation, the genetic counselor's task is to explain the genetic and environmental factors involved, expecting the couple to make an appropriate decision. Data indicate a high correlation between the number of couples who seek this information and those who plan their families accordingly (Northern and Downs, 1974).

Currently, geneticists are able to predict the possibility of having a defective child. Northern and Downs (1974) emphasize that the prediction must be made correctly since this information will be used in a decision-making process. For this reason audiologists should not undertake genetic counseling but should refer concerned parents to genetic counseling centers. (A source for a listing of locations of these centers as well as supplemental materials relevant to hereditary deafness can be found in the appendix at the end of this chapter.) Many materials are available and can be purchased at a nominal charge. These materials are routinely distributed to parents in our program who make an inquiry about genetic problems.

Hereditary deafness was a concern of Peter's parents when they brought him to be evaluated at 6 months of age. His father was deaf from birth, and his mother had normal hearing. Both parents were alerted early to the need for hearing surveillance because of the father's deafness. A series of tests established that Peter possessed a profound bilateral hearing loss. In the interview the mother discussed the history of hearing loss in Peter's father's family. Peter's paternal great-grandfather was deaf and his father's two brothers had unilateral hearing losses. Peter's parents wanted to investigate the possibility of genetic counseling before making a decision to have another child. This family was referred to a genetic counseling center in our area for a genetic study.

Since the results of a genetic study are so important to a family, we do not discuss genetic probabilities with parents. Of related interest is Reed's (1957) comment that parents would rather be told that their child had a rare disease or had undergone a severe trauma than be told that a genetic cause was probably the basis of the problem. A genetic counselor can reduce feelings of shame or guilt and restore parents' self-esteem by assuring them that we all, without exception, carry at least one abnormal gene which, if duplicated by our partner, can cause serious defects in or the death of our offspring (Roberts, 1962; Nance and Sweeney, 1975).

SUMMARY

In this chapter we emphasized the need for the audiologist in a counseling situation to increase his awareness of the parents' feelings and to allow parents to become a vital part of the decision-making process regarding the audiologic management of their child. Parents will follow through only on recommendations they have decided are reasonable for them. In contrast to diagnostic information-giving, counseling is not a quick and easy solution for problems. Rather, it provides an avenue for allowing parents to express their thoughts and feelings in an accepting environment.

The audiologist can establish a favorable counseling environment. Warmth and nurturing, honesty, objectivity, active listening, and understanding ambivalence are essential elements of the counseling process. Application of these qualities combined with specific suggestions is presented in relation to the various types and degrees of hearing impairment in children.

Many audiologists have mistakenly considered the audiometer to be the primary tool of their profession. The essence of clinical audiology is not the manipulation of instruments; the clinician is the key. We strongly agree with McDonald (1962), who states that unless the feelings of parents are properly understood and guided, handicapped families can develop around handicapped children.

RESEARCH NEEDS

Currently, the data available on parent-child relationships and deafness are of a sociodemographic nature. These descriptive data are of limited use in understanding parental attitudes and feelings related to a hearing impairment in their child. We note an absence of valid and reliable data on changes in parental attitudes. Two reasons why this kind of data has been difficult to acquire are (1) the large number of variables to control, such as socioeconomic and ethnic backgrounds, parental expectations, and population mobility, and (2) the problem of quantifying subtle psychological states in a longitudinal manner.

Several indices and inventories are available which might be adapted for use with parents of hearing-impaired children. Inventories such as the Family

Relations Test and Personal Observations Inventory may provide an initial framework for evaluating self-actualization, self-acceptance, and culture-locked attitudes towards a handicap. A particularly fruitful area of investigation is the psychosocial problems encountered by the families of hearing-impaired children. Relevant to this topic is the need to extend our knowledge of how family members cope with crises and stresses while living in a complex society.

Another research need involves the accumulation of pertinent data correlating the attitude of the audiologist with his approach to counseling. In particular, it would be beneficial to know which of the audiologist's qualities help create a positive feeling on the part of the parents.

REFERENCES

Barsch, R.H., *The Parent of the Handicapped Child: The Study of Child-rearing Practices.* Springfield, Ill: Charles C. Thomas, 1968.

Beck, H.L., "Counseling Parents of Retarded Children," *Children,* 6 (1959), 225-230.

Berne, E., *Principles of Group Treatment.* New York: Oxford University Press, 1966.

Brown, K.S., "The Genetics of Childhood Deafness," in *Deafness in Childhood,* edited by F. McConnell and P.H. Ward. Nashville: Vanderbilt University Press, 1967, pp. 177-202.

Dale, S., "Fear: The Dirtiest Four-Letter Word." Paper presented at the Conference on Counseling in the Rehabilitation Process, Pomona, Cal: January, 1976.

Edinburg, G.M., N.E. Zinberg, and W. Kelman, *Clinical Interviewing and Counseling: Principles and Techniques.* New York: Appleton-Century-Crofts, 1975.

Ellis, A., and R.A. Harper, *A Guide to Rational Living.* Hollywood, Cal: Wilshire, 1974.

Frazer, G.R., "Profound Childhood Deafness," *Journal of Medical Genetics,* 1 (1964), 118-151.

Garrett, A., *Interviewing: Its Principles and Methods.* New York: Family Service Association of America, 1942.

Gesell, A., H.M. Halverson, H. Thompson, F.L. Ilg, B.M. Castner, L.B. Ames and C.S. Amatruda, *The First Five Years of Life: A Guide to the Study of the Preschool Child.* New York: Harper & Row, 1940.

Ginott, H.G., "Interpretations and Child Therapy," in *Use of Interpretation in Treatment: Technique and Art,* edited by E.F. Hammer. New York: Grune and Stratton, 1968, pp. 291-299.

Goetzinger, C.P., "The Psychology of Hearing Impairment," in *Handbook of Clinical Audiology,* edited by J. Katz. Baltimore: Williams and Wilkins, 1972, pp. 666-701.

Gordon, T., *P.E.T. Parent Effectiveness Training.* New York: Peter H. Wyden, 1970.

Haley, J., "A Review of the Family Therapy Field," in *Changing Families: A Family Therapy Reader,* edited by J. Haley. New York: Grune and Stratton, 1971, pp. 1–12.

Hamilton, G., *The Theory and Practice of Social Case Work,* 2nd ed. New York: Columbia University Press, 1951.

Hammer, E.F., "Interpretation as Interpersonal Structuring," in *Use of Interpretation in Treatment: Technique and Art,* edited by E.F. Hammer. New York: Grune and Stratton, 1968, pp. 62–70.

Hanners, B.A., and A.B. Sitton, "Ears to Hear: A Daily Hearing Aid Monitor Program," *Volta Review,* 76 (1974) 530–536.

James, M., and D. Jongeward, *Born To Win: Transactional Analysis with Gestalt Experiments.* Reading, Mass: Addison-Wesley, 1971.

Keith, R.W., "Evaluation Procedures for Children," in *Interpreting Hearing Aid Technology,* edited by K. Donnelly. Springfield, Ill: Charles C. Thomas, 1974, pp. 159–180.

Kroth, J.A., *Counseling Psychology and Guidance: An Overview in Outline.* Springfield, Ill: Charles C. Thomas, 1973.

Kübler-Ross, E., *On Death and Dying.* New York: Macmillan Co., 1969.

Levine, E.S., *The Psychology of Deafness: Techniques of Appraisal for Rehabilitation.* New York: Columbia University Press, 1960.

Luterman, D., "The Counseling Experience," *Journal of the Academy of Rehabilitative Audiology,* 9 (1976), 62–66.

McCollum, A.T., and A.H. Schwartz, "Social Work and the Mourning Parent," *Social Work,* 17 (1972), 25–36.

McConnell, F., and K.B. Horton, *A Home Teaching Program for Parents of Very Young Deaf Children.* Final report, project no. 6-1187, grant no. O.E.G. 32-52-0450-6007. Nashville, Tenn: U.S. Dept. of Health, Education, and Welfare, Office of Education, Bureau of Research, 1970.

McDonald, E.T., *Understanding Those Feelings.* Pittsburgh: Stanwix House, 1962.

Malkin, S.F., R.D. Freeman, and J.O. Hasting, "Psychosocial Problems of Deaf Children and Their Families: A Comparative Study," *Audiology and Hearing Education,* 2 (1976a), 21–29.

Malkin, S.F., R.D. Freeman, and J.O. Hasting, "Psychosocial Problems of Deaf Children and Their Families: A Comparative Study," *Audiology and Hearing Education,* 2 (1976b), 31–38.

Martin, V.S., "What It Means to Be the Parent of a Deaf Child," *Otolaryngologic Clinics of North America,* 8 (1975), 59–67.

Meadow, K.P., and L. Meadow, "Changing Role Perceptions for Parents of Handicapped Children," *Exceptional Children,* 38 (1971), 21–27.

Moses, K.R., "Issues of Parent Counseling: An Introduction to Mourning Theory." Presented as a Mini-Seminar at the Annual Convention of the American Speech and Hearing Association, Las Vegas: November, 1974.

Nance, W.E., and A. Sweeney, "Genetic Factors in Deafness of Early Life," *Otolaryngologic Clinics of North America,* 8 (1975), 19–48.

Northcott, W.H., *Curriculum Guide: Hearing-Impaired Children—Birth to Three Years—and Their Parents.* Washington, D.C.: Alexander Graham Bell Association for the Deaf, 1972.

Northern, J.L., and M.P. Downs, *Hearing in Children.* Baltimore: Williams and Wilkins, 1974.

Pollock, M.B., and K.C. Pollock, "Letter to the Teacher of a Hard-of-Hearing Child," *Childhood Education,* 47 (1971), 206–209.

Proctor, C.A., and B. Proctor, "Understanding Hereditary Nerve Deafness," *Archives of Otolaryngology,* 85 (1967), 23–40.

Purcell, J., "Survival Roles and Family Rules for Survival." Paper presented at the Conference on Counseling in the Rehabilitation Process, Pomona, Cal.: January, 1976.

Reed, S.C., "Counseling in Medical Genetics," *Acta Genetica Statistica Medica,* 7 (1957), 473–480.

Roberts, J.A.F., "Genetic Prognosis," *British Medical Journal,* 1 (1962), 587–592.

Rogers, C.R., *Counseling and Psychotherapy: Newer Concepts in Practice.* Boston: Houghton Mifflin, 1961a.

Rogers, C.R., *On Becoming a Person: A Therapist's View of Psychotherapy.* Boston: Houghton Mifflin, 1961b.

Rosen, J., "Distortions in the Training of Audiologists," *Journal of the American Speech and Hearing Association,* 9 (1967), 171–174.

Ross, A.O., *The Exceptional Child in the Family: Helping Parents of Exceptional Children.* New York: Grune and Stratton, 1964.

Sanders, D.A., *Aural Rehabilitation.* Englewood Cliffs, N.J.: Prentice-Hall, 1971.

Sanders, D.A., "Hearing Aid Orientation and Counseling," in *Amplification for the Hearing-Impaired,* edited by M.C. Pollack. New York: Grune & Stratton, 1975, pp. 323–372.

Satir, V., "The Family as a Treatment Unit," in *Changing Families: A Family Therapy Reader,* edited by J. Hayley. New York: Grune & Stratton, 1971, pp. 127–132.

Satir, V., *Conjoint Family Therapy.* Palo Alto, Cal.: Science and Behavior Books, 1964.

Satir, V., *Peoplemaking.* Palo Alto, Cal.: Science and Behavior Books, 1972.

Schmideberg, M., "Multiple Origins and Functions of Guilt," *Psychiatric Quarterly,* 30 (1956), 471–477.

Schulman, E.D., *Intervention in Human Services.* Saint Louis, Mo: C.V. Mosby, 1974.

Sheimo, S.L., "Problems in Helping Parents of Mentally Defective and Handicapped Children," *American Journal of Mental Deficiency,* 56 (1951), 42–47.

Simmons, J.E., *Psychiatric Examination of Children,* 2nd ed. Philadelphia: Lea and Febiger, 1974.

Solnit, A.J., and M.H. Stark, "Mourning and the Birth of a Defective Child," *Psychoanalytic Study of the Child,* 16 (1961), 523–537.

Steiner, C.M., *Scripts People Live: Transactional Analysis of Life Scripts.* New York: Grove Press, 1974.

Stream, R.W., and K.S. Stream, "Problems in Counseling." Paper presented at the Symposium on Educational Audiology, Galveston, Tex.: February, 1973.

Stream, R.W., and K.S. Stream, "Profound Deafness: Its Effect Upon the Family." Paper presented at the Southwest Regional Meeting of the American Orthopsychiatric Association, Galveston, Tex.: November, 1972.

Webster, E.J., "Parent Counseling by Speech Pathologists and Audiologists," in *Counseling Parents of the Ill and the Handicapped,* edited by R.L. Noland. Springfield, Ill: Charles C. Thomas, 1971, pp. 285–298.

Wedenberg, E., "Endogenous Hearing Impairments," in *International Symposium on Speech Communication Ability and Profound Deafness,* edited by G. Fant. Washington, D.C.: Alexander Graham Bell Association for the Deaf, 1972, pp. 3–17.

Weiss, M.A., and M.R. Duffy, "Counseling in Speech and Language Disorders," *Pediatric Psychology,* 2 (1974), 2–5.

Willeford, J.A., "Central Auditory Function," *Communicative Disorders: Learning Disabilities,* edited by K. Donnelly. Boston: Little, Brown, 1976.

Wright, B.A., *Physical Disability—A Psychological Approach.* New York: Harper & Row, 1960.

SUGGESTED READINGS

Alpiner, J.G., "Hearing Aid Selection For Adults," in *Amplification for the Hearing Impaired,* edited by M.C. Pollack. New York: Grune and Stratton, 1975, pp. 145–205.

Bone, H., "Two Proposed Alternatives to Psychoanalytic Interpreting," in *Use of Interpretation in Treatment: Technique and Art,* edited by E.F. Hammer. New York: Grune and Stratton, 1968, pp. 169–196.

Cutter, A.V., and E.A. Miller, "The Interpretive and Summing-up Process with Parents During and After Diagnostic Studies of Children," in *Counseling Parents of the Ill and the Handicapped,* edited by R.L. Noland. Springfield, Ill: Charles C. Thomas, 1971, pp. 62–77.

Downs, M.P., "Overview of the Management of the Congenitally Deaf Child," *Otolaryngologic Clinics of North America,* 4 (1971), 223–226.

Ellis, A., "A Rational Approach to Interpretation," in *Use of Interpretation in Treatment: Technique and Art,* edited by E.F. Hammer. New York: Grune and Stratton, 1968, pp. 232–239.

Fenlason, A.F., *Essentials in Interviewing: For the Interviewer Offering Professional Services.* New York: Harper and Brothers, 1952.

Fraser, G.R., "The Genetics of Congenital Deafness," *Otolaryngologic Clinics of North America*, 4 (1971), 227–247.

Frick, E., "Ensuring Successful Adjustment to Integration," in *The Hearing Impaired Child in a Regular Classroom: Preschool, Elementary, and Secondary Years*, edited by W.H. Northcott. Washington, D.C.: Alexander Graham Bell Association for the Deaf, 1973, pp. 177–187.

Frick, W.B., *Humanistic Psychology: Interviews with Maslow, Murphy and Rogers*. Columbus, Ohio: Charles E. Merrill, 1971.

Gray, B.B., and B.P. Ryan, *A Language Program For The Nonlanguage Child*. Champaign, Ill.: Research Press, 1973.

Haley, J., "Approaches to Family Therapy," in *Changing Families: A Family Therapy Reader*, edited by J. Haley. New York: Grune and Stratton, 1971, pp. 227–236.

Jackson, D.D., and J.H. Weakland, "Conjoint Family Therapy: Some Considerations on Theory Technique and Results," in *Changing Families: A Family Therapy Reader*, edited by J. Haley. New York: Grune and Stratton, 1971, pp. 13–35.

Johnson, E.W., "Let's Look at the Child, Not the Audiogram," in *The Hearing Impaired Child in a Regular Classroom: Preschool, Elementary, and Secondary Years*, edited by W.H. Northcott. Washington, D.C.: Alexander Graham Bell Association for the Deaf, 1973, pp. 18–23.

Kahn, R.L., and C.F. Cannell, *The Dynamics of Interviewing: Theory, Technique, and Cases*. New York: John Wiley and Sons, 1957.

Lassman, G.H., *Language For The Preschool Deaf Child*. New York: Grune and Stratton, 1950.

Liversidge, E.B., and G.M. Grana, "A Hearing Impaired Child in the Family: The Parent's Perspective," *Volta Review*, 75 (1973), 174–180.

McConnell, F., "A New Approach to the Management of Childhood Deafness," *Pediatric Clinics of North America*, 17 (1970), 347–362.

McConnell, F., "The Psychology of Communication," in *Speech for the Deaf Child: Knowledge and Use*, edited by L.E. Connor. Washington, D.C.: Alexander Graham Bell Association for the Deaf, 1971, pp. 170–182.

Meadow, K.P., "Parental Response to the Medical Ambiguities of Congenital Deafness," *Journal of Health and Social Behavior*, 9 (1968), 299–309.

Meadow, K.P., "Self-Image, Family Climate, and Deafness," *Social Forces*, 47 (1969), 428–438.

Minuchin, S., *Families and Family Therapy*. Cambridge, Mass.: Harvard University Press, 1974.

Myklebust, H.R., *Your Deaf Child: A Guide for Parents*. Springfield, Ill.: Charles C. Thomas, 1950.

Noble, W.G., and G.R.C. Atherly, "The Hearing Measure Scale: A Questionnaire for the Assessment of Auditory Disability," *Journal of Auditory Research*, 10 (1970), 229–250.

Patterson, G.R., *Families: Applications of Social Learning to Family Life*. Champaign, Ill.: Research Press Company, 1971.

Patterson, G.R. and M.E. Gullion, *Living With Children, New Methods for Parents and Teachers.* Champaign, Ill.: Research Press, 1968.

Perls, F.S., *Gestalt Therapy Verbatim.* New York: Bantam Books, 1971.

Public Service Programs, *What Every Person Should Know About Heredity and Deafness.* Washington, D.C.: Gallaudet College, 1975.

Reid, E.S., "Helping Parents of Handicapped Children," in *Counseling Parents of the Ill and the Handicapped,* edited by R.L. Noland. Springfield, Ill.: Charles C. Thomas, 1971, pp. 52–61.

Rogers, C.R., *Carl Rogers on Encounter Groups.* New York: Harper & Row, 1970.

Shontz, F.C., "Reactions to Crisis," *Volta Review,* 67 (1965), 364–370.

Silverman, S.R., and H. Davis, "Hard-of-Hearing Children," in *Hearing and Deafness,* 3rd ed., edited by H. Davis and S.R. Silverman. New York: Holt, Rinehart and Winston, 1970, pp. 426–434.

Stassen, R.A., "I Have One in My Class Who's Wearing Hearing Aids!" in *The Hearing Impaired Child in a Regular Classroom: Preschool, Elementary and Secondary Years,* edited by W.H. Northcott. Washington, D.C., Alexander Graham Bell Association for the Deaf, 1973, pp. 24–31.

Stern, V., *Never Too Young.* New York: Lexington School for the Deaf, 1975.

Stewart, L.G., *Selecting a School for Your Deaf Child.* Tuscon, Ariz.: Center on Deafness, 1974.

Tracy, L.S., "What Can A Mother Do For Her Deaf Child?" in *If You Have a Deaf Child.* Urbana, Ill.: University of Illinois Press, 1953, pp. 7–18.

Tyler, L.E., *The Work of the Counselor.* New York: Appleton-Century-Crofts, 1953.

Wedenberg, E., and J. Lindsten, "Endogenous Hearing Impairments," in *International Symposium on Speech Communication Ability and Profound Deafness,* edited by G. Fant. Washington, D.C.: Alexander Graham Bell Association for the Deaf, 1972, pp. 3–17.

Appendix A

SUMMARY OF HUMAN DEVELOPMENT THEORIES

The Traditional Psychoanalytic Approach. Generally, this approach stresses the importance of early childhood experiences to explain, interpret, and provide insight into current behavior. The underlying tenet of the traditional psychoanalytic approach, as developed by Freud, is that early experiences influence behavior and that the organism seeks to maintain balance. According to Freud, all behavior is motivated by drives or instincts that are biological in origin and release mental energy. Freud correlates personality traits with various stages of psychosexual development. Important constructs of this theory are the Oedipus complex and the id, ego, and superego. The subconscious mind plays an important role, influencing the various defense mechanisms the individual uses to meet tension and stress (Kroth, 1973; Hammer, 1968). Variations on this theory have been proposed by Jung and Adler.

Rational Therapy. The rational approach focuses on the intellect; it views the person as he is at the present time, regardless of his past experiences. This approach stresses the importance of replacing irrational thinking and ideas with rational thoughts. Albert Ellis, a developer of this approach, points out that man can live a most self-fulfilling, creative, and emotionally satisfying life by intelligently organizing and disciplining his thinking. A recurring theme in rational therapy is that "you feel as you think." Thus, if a person feels that he must have the approval of others or that it is bad when his desires are not fulfilled, he can change these feelings by questioning them. In other words, a person can restructure his inappropriate feelings and thinking into rational thinking and behavior if he so chooses (Hammer, 1968; Ellis and Harper, 1974).

Behavior and Learning Theory. Proponents of a third approach to counseling, Salter, Wolpe, and Lazarus, contend that all changes in behavior and growth are the direct result of learning (Kroth, 1973). Some of the basic concepts of behavior therapy are counterconditioning, positive reconditioning, and experimental extinction. One of the most prominent techniques employed in behavior therapy is systematic desensitization. The underlying tenet of this approach is learning through selective reinforcement.

The Human Potential Movement. Many approaches to counseling are based on the following two concepts: (1) individuals possess the capacity to develop a high level of self-concept, but their efforts are often thwarted by their environment, and (2) an atmosphere consistent with nurturing and trust can create a psychological climate favorable to growth. We have chosen to present three approaches—the client-centered approach, family therapy approach, and transactional analysis—as examples of this philosophy.

Carl Rogers, the father of the *client-centered* approach, sees the individual as existing in a field of experiences through which he develops, from infancy, an awareness of himself. In interaction with parents and others, the child develops a need for self-esteem. He learns to feel more or less worthy of the positive regard of others as he grows. Self-regard and self-worth are important concepts of this model. This approach emphasizes the individual's capacity for self-direction. Rogers (1961a) states that it is the client who knows what hurts, what directions to go, what problems are crucial, and what experiences have been deeply buried.

The client-centered approach is concerned with failure of communication—first, with oneself and, second, with others. The major barrier to mutual interpersonal communication, according to Rogers (1961b), is a tendency on the part of the listener to judge. Communication occurs when the listener avoids this tendency and listens with understanding. The technique of "ownership restatement" is used as a primary method in establishing good communication with oneself. For example, a parent may state, "My mother-in-law makes me feel guilty when she refers to my deaf relatives." An ownership restatement of this feeling would be, "I allow myself to feel guilty when my mother-in-law refers to my deaf relatives."

A second approach, *family therapy*, which involves working with the whole family, arose toward the end of the 1950s, when treatment began to emphasize the need for changes in the structure of a family rather than changing the individual's perception of his behavior (Haley, 1971). Assuming that early experiences and the feedback received from them have the greatest impact on how we see ourselves, then it is the nuclear family that provides the most training in who we are and how we should act. In a family setting, the effects of the behavior of one individual are not isolated. For instance, Satir (1964) states that when one person in a family exhibits symptoms of a problem, all family members' feelings are affected in some way.

Family therapy focuses on the repetitive communications that occur among family members—for example, "You're not able to follow through on anything" or "You can't get anything right" are messages that can recur consistently. Satir (1972) believes that by observing and learning to understand the transactions that occur among family members, it is possible to uncover the rules governing each person's behavior. Though the family is often unaware of these rules on a conscious level, they do influence behavior of family members relative to survival, growth, identity, productivity, and closeness. In family therapy it is absolutely necessary to deal with the feelings of all members of the family as a group. Exclusion of any one member from the group can impede appropriate changes.

A third approach, *transactional analysis,* was originated by Eric Berne, who states that this approach to understanding behavior encompasses many of the major tenets of personality theory (Berne, 1966). Three concepts associated with transactional analysis are that: (1) people are born O.K.—that is, people by their basic nature are inclined to live and are capable of living in harmony with themselves, each other, and nature; (2) people are capable of understanding their problems and the processes which liberate them from their difficulties; (3) emotional difficulties are curable, given adequate knowledge and the proper approach (Steiner, 1974).

Transactional analysis is concerned with four kinds of analysis. First, structural analysis examines the individual personality and looks at the questions "Who am I?" and "How did I get this way?" The basic method involved in this type of analysis concerns an awareness of three ego states—parent, adult, and child. Second, actions between people involve a transaction between the ego states of each person. Transactional analysis looks at the interaction of people, what they do, and what they say to one another. Third, game analysis looks at the ulterior motives involved in an interaction between people. Fourth, script analysis involves becoming aware of the decisions which dictate the way one has chosen to follow his plan for living. James and Jongeward (1971) point out that when people come to a time in their lives when they are provoked to define themselves, transactional analysis provides a method that can be understood and that individuals can put to use in their own lives. This method focuses on intellectual insight into one's needs, feelings, basic motivations, and interactions with others.

Appendix B

SOURCES FOR PARENT TRAINING INFORMATION AND MATERIALS:

Bureau of Education for the Handicapped
Office of Education
Department of Health, Education and Welfare
Washington, D.C.

A.G. Bell Association for the Deaf
3417 Volta Pl., N.W.
Washington, D.C. 20007

John Tracy Clinic
806 W. Adams Blvd.
Los Angeles, Cal. 90007

American Speech and Hearing Association
10801 Rockville Pike
Rockville, Md. 20852

Bill Wilkerson Hearing and Speech Center
Division of Language Development Programs
1114 19th Ave. South
Nashville, Tenn. 27212

The Center on Deafness
1034 East Adams
Tucson, Ariz. 85719

National Association of the Deaf
814 Thayer Avenue
Silver Spring, Md. 20910

SOURCES OF INFORMATION ON GENETIC COUNSELING:

Public Service Programs
Gallaudet College
Washington, D.C. 20002

National Foundation March of Dimes
Box 2000
White Plains, N.Y. 10602

354

SOURCES OF INFORMATION FOR PURCHASE OF RECORDED MATERIALS

"How They Hear"
Gordon N. Stowe and Associates
Northbrook, Ill.

"Getting Through"
Zenith Radio Corporation
6501 W. Grand Ave.
Chicago, Ill. 60635

CHAPTER TEN

Early Management Procedures
for the Hearing-Impaired Child

AUDREY SIMMENS-MARTIN

INTRODUCTION

One of the purposes of this textbook is to increase the cooperation between clinical and educational audiology in early management programs for the hearing-impaired child. On one hand, we find clinical audiologists who traditionally define the sensory capacity of the auditory system as accurately as possible, recommend a hearing aid, then dismiss the child and his family. On the other hand, there are teachers or educational audiologists who may pick up and independently manage the intervention. Far more beneficial is a team approach where all members of the team, including parents, contribute valuable information for the overall benefit of the hearing-impaired child.

Regrettably, we still find clinical audiologists who, on the basis of a single hearing evaluation, make conclusive statements about a child's potential for language learning (Hanners, 1976) and give parents bewildering advice about their child's ability to communicate (Sander, 1976). We observe teachers attenuating down to the young child procedures traditionally used with older children. We see programs where adult grammar is taught in a formal way to young children. It is time that we consider not only the hearing or its deficit but the child and his family as individuals in successful habilitation.

Audiological testing must be incorporated into the management of the child; *hearing aids must be selected,* monitored, and maintained. But all this should be accomplished within the framework of a total development program in which language acquisition is paramount. Knowledge about language development, strategies children employ in its acquisition, the role of the family, the relation of perception and thinking to language, and the effects of the child's experiences is an important component of the early management of the hearing-impaired child. Only with team commitment and cooperation, with both audiologic treatment and educational procedures, can a strong early-intervention program succeed.

CHAPTER OBJECTIVES

This chapter will discuss the cooperative effort of clinical and educational audiologists in managing young hearing-impaired children. Diagnosis and measurement of auditory capacity will be treated elsewhere in this book; we will be concerned with helping parents capture the smallest residue of hearing, train it, and utilize it effectively in developing their hearing-impaired child's linguistic and cognitive behavior.

ROLE OF THE PARENTS

Language acquisition and thinking ability are the primary goals of any habilitative program with children. The appropriate model is the natural one of the child's home environment, where parents universally have had critical roles in developing language and activating intelligence. Procedures that allow parents to become participants, rather than either spectators or, at the other extreme, therapists, are our concern. We want to develop parents' natural ability in stimulating, responding, and interacting with their child.

Such activities are not learned through didactic formal sessions but instead through "reality-based" experiences that guide parents in utilizing hearing for speech, stimulating thought within the child, and matching it with language. Parents are in the ideal position for constant interacting and for utilizing verbal concepts that interest their child. According to theorists, this give and take appears to be the important factor in all children's development (Hess and Shipman, 1965). Parents of handicapped children have no less responsibility. The rationale for *parent* education, rather than *child* education, comes from several disciplines, which we present in this chapter.

Language Development

When parental interaction is lacking, all children demonstrate a decline in mental ability and school achievement as they mature (Schaefer, 1972). Obscuring the meaning of verbal cues, restricting verbal input, and dealing with events as unrelated incidents causes a child to be an ineffective language user (Bernstein, 1971). Because parents are important in language development, we must educate them to function as good delivery agents. To do so, we must know how parents perform this role with hearing children, and then predict how this relates to parents of deaf children.

The various aspects of mother-to-child language have been the focus of a significant amount of recent research. Brown and Bellugi (1964), among the first to study such language, found a mother's speech to be simple but always grammatical. Furthermore, they observed mothers employing a strategy of imitating the child's utterance and expanding it to include function words—words that carry meaning only in context, such as: "the," "if," "but," and "as." The strategy is interesting because the researchers hypothesized that function words, having only secondary stress, were low in acoustic power. The technique that mothers employed to expand the hearing children's telegraphic utterances is applicable for children who probably will not hear those function words.

Not only is it important that parents talk to their children, but equally important are the manner and style in which they do so. Observations of effective mothers have provided information about "motherese" that needs to be incorporated into an understanding of language development. Mothers, for instance, interact to a high degree with first-borns (Rubenstein, 1967). If the first-born is deaf and does not reciprocate, the probability of the interaction continuing without outside guidance is questionable. Part of the educational audiologist's task is to foster parental responsibility and supply the reinforcement necessary for continued activity.

Babies use facial expressions and body movements as well as vocalizations to communicate (Ambrose, 1961). If parents are expecting the first utterances to be words, counseling must be given for them to understand the early forms of communication their deaf baby uses before meaningful vocalizations start.

Mothers of normal children use eye contact along with such other modes of communication as body posture, demonstrations, and vocalizations (Ling and Ling, 1974). Certainly eye contact between parent and child is the beginning of lipreading. "Eyeing" the speaker gives the hearing-impaired child a model for speech production and assists in developing the child's competence in language. Competence depends not only on understanding the language code but also on using it. Production information is not available auditorily to many deaf children. For them, the speech signal, even with amplification, will always be at a very low acoustic level. Through listening alone, all they may ever achieve are gross temporal patterns and minimal discrimination cues. They will always need to search the visual field for consonant information. Lipreading and listening have to be synchronized. Since this appears to be normal behavior for a hearing child, it follows that the multisensory approach is a comfortable route for the hearing-impaired child.

Mothers of hearing children talk more to young children than to their older siblings; they use simpler syntax and a more concrete vocabulary of "here and now" (Phillips, 1973). The implications for parents of deaf children are obvious. Many of them need help in knowing what to talk about, how to talk, and when to talk.

With hearing toddlers, mothers employ a slower rate and fewer disfluencies, repeat their utterances more frequently and single out parts of phrases for emphasis more often than they do with older children (Snow, 1972). These procedures are the ones that educational audiologists should emulate.

Fathers certainly should be part of the habilitative program, although the literature has given little attention to their role in their hearing child's language development. In one report, a father was observed using simple sentences when talking to his infant daughter, but he rarely repeated his utterances (Giattino and Hogan, 1975). He seemed to give more attention to the content of the interaction, using descriptions, explanations, and questions about ongoing events and activities, than to teaching the form of the language.

All young children are motivated to communicate by an instinctive *need* to communicate, whether they are hearing or deaf. The form and content of language that has special significance in the development of the young normal child should be presented with particular salience to the young hearing-impaired child. The mother-child interactions with normal-hearing children provide the model. It is the task of the educational audiologist to learn the nature of such interactions and set the models for parents of young hearing-impaired children.

Some years ago, McNeill (1966) noted with bewilderment that adult grammar was used in teaching deaf children and, in turn, was expected of them. Since normal hearing children do not learn a few words, then start stringing them together as adult utterances, he questioned why it was expected of deaf children. That it requires a great deal of motivation to learn a language in a formal manner was similarly expressed by Furth (1974). He considered the case of the deaf child not receiving therapy until he arrived at school at the age of 4. By then language had no place in his development; therefore, it was difficult to motivate him to learn it.

Our thrust must be toward the first months and years. Along with Menyuk (1974), we emphasize the importance of considering how mothers talk to their hearing infants and toddlers. The language-meaning and language-form features need to be analyzed for sensory input and carried into training for effective spoken communication between mother and child. This *is* the primary role for the educational audiologist—teaching mothers to interact verbally and meaningfully with their child.

Learning verbal communication is an active, evolving procedure between parent and child. For the deaf child and his family, it is important to get the process into motion as soon as possible. Reciprocal interaction between parent and child involves linguistic, cognitive, and emotional components that reinforce each other.

Cognitive Development

Language does not develop in a vacuum. Infants who are reared in institutions staffed by few and inconsistent caretakers demonstrate not only severe language deficits but also marked retardation on all indices of physical and psychological maturation. If nutrition and cleanliness are maintained at a high level but specific enrichment of adult-infant social interaction is not provided, the lag in adaptive behavior continues and results in developmental quotients in the defective range (Dennis and Najarian, 1957). If these conditions are allowed to persist throughout childhood, the youngsters exhibit mental deficiency and become adults who function as poorly as those with intrinsic brain pathology. It is not known with certainty how long severe psychosocial deprivation can be tolerated before the functional retardation becomes irreversible. Rapid recovery is possible with adoption into family life before the end of the first year, while the central nervous system is still developing.

Case studies show that children so deprived are retarded in symbol learning, which is in fact language—that is, symbols manipulated by rules of the code. Language is the code system in which symbols strung together represent the thought of the speaker. The listener needs the same code to unlock that thought. In other words, the listener and the speaker must be capable not only of comprehending and producing the same code, but they can exchange ideas, thoughts, percepts, and concepts only by using the code.

Cognition then is the base of communication and, addressing this thesis, Slobin (1973) proposed:

> The pacesetter in linguistic growth is the child's cognitive growth, as opposed to an autonomous linguistic development which can then reflect back on cognition (p. 184).

MacNamara (1972) goes so far as to say:

> Infants learn their language by first determining, independent of language, the meaning which a speaker intends to convey to them, and by then working out the relationship between the meaning and the language. To put it another way, the infant uses meaning as a clue to language, rather than language as a clue to meaning (p. 1).

As Clark (1974) views it, much of the cognitive basis for early language consists of the perceptual information that the child has interpreted and organized by the time he starts to work directly on language. This is particularly observable in the child's acquisition of word meanings. Piagetian-oriented theorists would differ from Clark in emphasizing not perception but rather actions as the sources for acquiring meaning. They view the ability to represent a thing with a word as the more fundamental cognitive prerequisite for language development (Sinclair-de-Zwart, 1969).

Perceptions are acquired through the child's action upon objects. Such perceptions are not passive observations of pictures, for example. Experience mediated with language is the medium through which children develop. In talking about early education of young children, Read (1960) stated:

> If young children are to learn, they must have first-hand experience. They profit very little from experiences which are second-hand out of books or through being told about a thing. They must first form concepts from actual first-hand experiences of their own if their thinking is to be sound. Later, on the basis of what they know from experience, they can understand reports by others of related experiences or grasp generalizations (p. 52).

The parental role consists of a rich fabric of interrelated cognitive processes. Programs need to shape these processes by assisting parents to interact, stimulate their children, and provide meaningful experiences. Hess (1968) has found that, when the parents' role in a functional-cognitive system is learned, it relates significantly to the child's intellectual development. When parents demand high achievement, maximize verbal interaction, give attention to the child, use parental teaching strategies, and diffuse intellectual stimulation, the children achieve (Brofenbrenner, 1974). It is no different for children with hearing impairment.

Parent Education

Parent education is not new. Within the last decade educational programs for young children and their parents have become a societal goal of major importance. Many of these programs have shown that educational experiences in the first three years of a child's life can enhance intellectual development. Moreover, conclusive evidence shows the *long-term* effect resulting when *parents* are trained to be the delivery agents. When children are involved in an intensive program of parent intervention during and, more important, prior to their enrollment in preschool or school, they achieve greater and more enduring gains than those children only in child-oriented group programs (Gilmer, Miller, and Gray, 1970; Gordon, 1973; and Radin, 1972).

The evidence points so decidedly to parents as educators in the broad sense that Schaefer (1972) concluded his review of research on the outcome of parent-training programs by stating that this type of program provided an *alternative* for preschool education rather than just an effective supplement.

Bronfenbrenner's (1974) conclusions to his extensive longitudinal evaluations of early intervention are worth noting in some detail.

> The strengths of the parent-child approach are clearly impressive both in terms of productiveness, permanence and practicality. This form of family centered intervention, when applied in the first three years of life, produces initial gains which are as great as or greater than those obtained either through group programs in preschool settings or tutoring conducted in the home.
>
> More significantly, even when parent intervention is introduced after three years of age, the gains are substantially more resistant to erosion after formal intervention is discontinued. This indicates that some of the forces enhancing and sustaining the child's development have been incorporated into his enduring environment in the home (p. 35).

The common generalizations underlying parent-education programs are described by Altschuler (1972):

1. The preschool years from birth to 5 are critical for cognitive and language development.
2. Parent behavior during this period significantly influences the child's cognitive and language development.
3. The parents *are* the primary agents for change in the life of the preschool child.

4. Parents are capable of absorbing and implementing much of the accrued knowledge concerning early childhood development and learning.
5. Parents can learn specific methods, techniques, and skills to promote their child's cognitive and language development.

While White (1975) endorses the view of the family as the first and most fundamental delivery system, he further finds that most families get their children through the first 6 to 8 months of life reasonably well in terms of education and development. But he believes that perhaps no more than 10% manage to get their children through the 8- to 36-month age period as well educated and developed as they could and should be. Yet, his studies show that the period that starts at 8 months and ends at 3 years of age is of primary importance in child development. He feels that if you begin to look at a child's educational development when he is 2 years of age, you are already too late, particularly for affecting social skills and attitudes that are in the domain of language.

Given the importance of the parental role in early childhood development, it is ironic that so few parents are properly prepared for parenthood. White (1975) maintains further that our society does not educate its citizens to assume the parental role. He proposes that we teach each and every prospective parent all the known and accepted fundamentals about four areas of child development—language development, child curiosity, social development, and cognitive development. These topic areas he believes to be the foundations of every child's educational capacity.

Parents of Deaf Children

If the evidence indicates that the family is the most fruitful system for fostering and sustaining the development of the hearing child, the findings must certainly hold true for families of the hearing-impaired child. Like parents of normal children, parents of the handicapped child most often do not understand, or are poorly informed about, the importance of the child's early months. They, too, lack knowledge of growth and development and information about language acquisition. All of them need to learn about the role of auditory and visual processes and ways to maximize the sensory input.

Parents of hearing-impaired children, however, unlike parents of normal children, have great psychological adjustments to make. Parents of a handicapped child experience trauma upon receiving the diagnosis of substantial hearing loss, especially if the parents themselves have normal hearing and expected an unimpaired child.

Deaf parents have already adjusted to deafness through personal experience and are prepared for the possibility that their child may be born deaf. Hearing parents, however, lack both the experience and the preparation; their trauma has profound influence on their child's total development. It emotionally affects the parents so as to disrupt the normal interaction of parent and child, interaction that is a necessary prerequisite for language development.

The implication from a study by Greenstein et al. (1976) is that teachers or educational audiologists must give priority to helping the parents adjust to the child's handicap and must facilitate the flow of communication between the parents and the child that was interrupted by the trauma caused by the diagnosis.

The intense feelings of disappointment because their child is not the idealized child they expected prevent the development of parents' warm loving feelings toward their child. They cannot establish a stable interpersonal system capable of fostering and sustaining the child's development. Without understanding why, or perhaps without being aware of their feelings, disappointed parents may find it increasingly difficult to play with, talk to, or interact in any way with their handicapped child. It should be noted that parents often can mobilize themselves in the presence of professionals and this may prevent or delay the staff's recognizing that the parents have a problem.

There are several stages that all people who encounter shock experience. These have been discussed elsewhere (Simmons-Martin, 1976). At this time let us just discuss the implications for the educational audiologists working with parents who are in these stages.

In stage one of the initial shock period the parents are coping with trauma. While they seem alert and perceive sharply, they often use that as a facade. Do not be misled and expect them to retain anything that is not written. In fact, for topics of serious magnitude it would be wise to delay a final discussion and even then it would be well to follow up with the written report.

In stage two you frequently find parents shopping around from one specialist to another. This produces an uncoordinated and generally ineffective approach. The teacher or audiologist handling the case should also anticipate that the parents, who shopped, will have received conflicting advice. Such situations are bound to arise from the confusing and widespread opinions on every aspect of habilitation and child management in our field.

Consider the parent who, having just coped with the shock of the diagnosis, receives conflicting advice ranging from "Use only the child's hearing. The unisensory route is the only way" to "No, use manual sign language" to "Oh no, use fingerspelling" to "Oh, do everything—lipreading, sign, talk, and listen at the same time." Lucky the parent who can ventilate as this one did in The Deaf American (Rhodes, 1972):

> When will it ever end? Why can't professionals understand that parents of deaf children cannot be constantly in the middle of the "big experiment"?
> My heart aches for mothers and fathers of deaf children who are being caught up in yet another methods battle. I could cry—and I do (p. 3).

The next stage, the escape stage, also includes many seemingly disconnected events but all have an impact upon the case management. Hoffmeyer (1976) reports that over 35% of parents of deaf children in Connecticut are divorced, separated, or have other marital problems. He suggests a counselor for these parents to help them relate to their deaf children and develop a better understanding of deafness. It is essential that teachers or educational audiologists who provide services to hearing-impaired infants have some training in counseling.

By the fourth stage, films, slides, and written materials focusing on the parent's role with normal children prove helpful. Parenting discussions are appropriate, but help comes also from knowing about children who are similarly handicapped. Seeing the graduates of programs for the deaf and viewing the school's facilities help parents see their own problems in better perspective. Group discussions where parents can ventilate are a must. Only after the parents have faced the problem are they ready to plunge into the task of *parenting* their own handicapped child. Only then do they realize that there is no cure, no gimmick, no magic hearing aid. If the road to effective parenthood requires rather basic changes in attitude for the parents of normal children (White, 1975), even greater changes are called for from parents of the hearing-impaired child.

We should not leave the topic of the affective domain without mentioning that brothers and sisters of the deaf child, like their parents, are similarly caught in a conflict. They struggle with how to be thoughtful of and attentive to their deaf siblings, and at the same time how to live their own lives and fulfill their own aspirations. Some may only question, but others worry. Malkin, Freeman, and Hastings (1966) gave global ratings of the overall impact of deafness on the siblings, and showed that most experience concern. However, they did not mention number of siblings or their position in the family, both of which certainly also have some effect.

The obvious recommendation in habilitation is that siblings be included and as much as possible be an integral part of family "teaching." In fact, we find family outings, picnics, and trips to the zoo worthwhile experiences. They are language opportunities for the deaf child and fun for his hearing siblings. However, we would caution the educational audiologist to avoid unusual demands on mother's time and energy. Strive to keep her aware that she must conserve energy for the normal activities of the *total* family life. Most of what is recommended for parents is just part of the normal day-to-day experiences of family living in which mother interacts with all of her children, but especially her child with a hearing impairment.

EARLY MANAGEMENT PROGRAM OF THE CENTRAL INSTITUTE FOR THE DEAF

For all the reasons given above—language development, parent education, and parent counseling—we focus on the parent rather than the child in our habilitative program at the Central Institute for the Deaf. To insure that the parent sees the important functional aspect of the interaction, the program is housed in a Home Demonstration Center rather than a clinic or school.

Originally we functioned in a clinical setting, but as our emphasis shifted increasingly to home experiences it became more and more difficult to act out such events as bathing the child and feeding him, cooking, and dusting. Furthermore, because it was a combination medical and academic setting parents seemed to have punitive feelings about the clinic. When we moved into a home demonstration center the parents' relaxation was readily apparent.

If programs do not have a home setting, the next best avenue would be to go to the child's home. If that is not possible, we would then recommend that the staff annex at least a kitchen from the sponsoring agency. The goal is to train the parents to include the child in daily tasks. Parents, like teachers and audiologists, need many and varied practical experiences.

Our center is a modest but comfortable two-family apartment on the Central Institute campus. The obvious advantages are that the audiologic services are nearby and the clinical audiologist and educational audiologist can meet at least weekly. Because of the proximity they check with each other much more frequently about individual children, their tests, their hearing aids, and their problems. The other main advantage of the location is the proximity to the school where parents can see other deaf children at the elementary level and thereby get help in setting goals. There are other benefits to the setting: students in the Teacher Education Program can observe children first-hand; research personnel are free to use the facility. Above all, the dialogue among school staff, audiologists, and educational audiologists (whom we call teacher/counselors) is the critical team process.

The teacher/counselor is a teacher of the deaf with an audiologic background and with supplemental training in child development and counseling. The teacher/counselor in one-hour weekly sessions works to shape the parents' behavior so that parents use every opportunity for interaction with their child.

While there are several components to the Parent-Infant Program—weekly family sessions, daytime discussion groups, evening information series, parent participation, nursery classes, and periodic auditory evaluation—the major thrust is the family session. These sessions meet for an hour once a week to prevent the parents from indulging in their frequent wish to have teachers assume complete responsibility for the child's education. An hour once a week is sufficient time to model for the parent, but not long enough to carry the entire intervention load. A home demonstration program is effective in that the target of intervention is neither the child nor the parent, but the parent-child system.

The weekly sessions are directed to the entire family if possible—siblings, grandparents, aunts, and sitters; however, it is usually the mother who attends regularly. Parents differ widely in abilities, temperament, knowledge, cultural backgrounds, health, and economic security. Parents also are at different stages of trauma (discussed earlier), which is the overriding determiner of what parents should be given and in what manner; equally important, it also determines what they learn. While some parents may be ready to cope with the problem, particularly parents who are themselves deaf, others are still in shock.

Infants differ from each other. Some are multi-handicapped. Some are the first-born. All differ in degree of hearing loss. Age is probably the greatest difference. Although we are seeing children at an earlier age than a decade ago, they are still older than we would like. Youngsters with marked losses of 55dB to 70dB are, on the average, over 20 months of age before their parents question the hearing and are around 37 months of age before they enroll in the program. The parents of children with profound losses note it earlier and, on the average, enroll by the time the child is 18 months (Ruland, 1976). Regardless of the child's degree of hearing loss, it has been our experience that all parents need help—some for a longer period than others. The time usually relates to the amount of assistance a child receives from amplification.

Because parents differ from each other and because each child is unique, we feel that each family constellation should be handled individually in the parent-counseling sessions. The teacher/counselor paces the tasks, feeds in the proper amount of information, and reinforces according to each family's needs.

Much as we would like to start immediately on the child's habilitation, we have found that we increase the long-term benefit if we wait until the parents are ready. Until then we emphasize helping them perceive their deaf child as a *child*. As the parents observe the infant passing through normal development in gross motor skills and other dimensions, they begin to see a lovable infant. The ears, so to speak, diminish in size. As their own grief subsides, parents can love, respect, and respond to the hearing-impaired toddler. Then they are ready for the reciprocal interaction so necessary for continued development, and especially cognitive and linguistic growth.

Parent's Training

The text used in the parents' course is *Chats With Johnny's Parents* (Simmons-Martin, 1975b), but techniques for transferring that information into functional behavior vary, depending on the particular parent. With some parents, the teacher/counselor talks about a topic in the booklet, then gives the material to the parent to read at home. With others, the teacher may discuss a topic after reading the appropriate sections with the parent. For still other parents she may go over it sentence by sentence, possibly even including a "test" to check comprehension of the chapters. Although this is usually part of the individual sessions, discussions naturally carry over into group sessions.

During the individual sessions the parent is given an assignment to apply a principle or a rule to a common daily recurring situation that involves interaction between parent and child. The parent, as it were, demonstrates or "practice teaches" with his child under the watchful eye of the teacher/counselor and periodically the videotape camera.

Mother might prepare cookies, sort clothing, dust, make a bed, clean out a drawer, or run the vacuum sweeper. Father might help with the tasks or he might play with the toys, plant seeds, build something, or feed the infant. The features of the activities are highly perceptual and those perceptual features have verbal labels associated with them, which in turn assist in the storage of the language. Through those perceptions the child develops appropriate concepts and some language connected with the experiences that have features in common. Fortunately, there is a built-in redundancy factor because daily living activities provide daily repetitions. The task is to get the parent to utilize those experiences and feed the linguistic information to the child for his storage bank (Simmons, 1971).

The essential technique is that the parents "tune in" to the child and capitalize on what it is that he is thinking. There must be a language *match* between the words and what the child is perceiving and thinking; the words must not be seen as just "talk, talk, talk."

Most parents need the tasks modeled for them for some time. Some go through the actions but remain mute; for them we literally have to put the words in their mouth. Some parents continue to need advance planning for six months or longer. Some need a great deal of structure, a cookbook as it were. Others move along rapidly and apply strategies and principles as easily as White's "super mothers" (Simmons-Martin, 1975a).

The teacher/counselor prefaces most demonstrations with discussions, but parents' questions take priority. Just as the parent must eventually communicate with his child, so must the teacher/counselor communicate with the parent. The discussion usually relates to the activity the parent has planned to do. The points considered are:

Why was the particular task chosen?

What language was planned?

What is of interest to the child?

How will it be implemented at home?

While performing the activity the parents are checked for language content and form, the concreteness of the input, the match to child's perception, the level of the parent's voice, the proximity to the child, capturing of the child's eye for lipreading, and the use of intonation and stress patterns.

The teacher/counselor guides the parents, but nevertheless she recognizes that, initially, mother is getting little reciprocal feedback from the child. Therefore, the teacher/counselor tries to provide positive reinforcement, and no matter how abysmal the lesson, finds something that warrants some praise.

Discussion Group

During the year, about 20 daytime discussion sessions are held. Attendance by the whole family is encouraged, but usually it is only the mothers who participate. The group discussion session is an unstructured open meeting in which parents may ventilate and express anger, awe, or their own intimidations. Because we view ourselves as an educational agency, however, we try to avoid in-depth explorations of feelings and attitudes. When parents have serious problems we are fortunate in that we can get assistance from a nearby agency, The Family and Children's Services.

We try never to underestimate the impact of one parent on another in a group setting. Topics are discussed by the parents, and although they reflect teacher/counselor inputs, the exchange of information with the peer group seems to hasten learning. Occasionally, discussions are deliberately contrived, such as developmental traits, and baby-sitting principles.

Evening Information Series

Fundamental to the parent's understanding of the handicapping condition is his knowledge of the handicap. For this reason the evening series tend to be didactic, with topics such as language development, hearing aids, genetics, hearing, and implant research. The speakers have been deaf adults, parents of deaf adults, school personnel, child psychologists, and researchers.

Parents need and want current and accurate scientific information about their child's handicap and the way the handicap may affect him. They want practical information about what they can expect their child to achieve, and they need assistance in goal-setting. However, they will assimilate only as much of this information as they are able. All too frequently they will hear only what they want to hear. Hence, follow-up is needed in the individual sessions to clarify misinformation and expand partial information. Furthermore, printed pamphlets on the topic assist in understanding.

Parent-Participation Nursery Class

Of particular importance for sustaining the child's learning in school is the involvement of parents. By supporting at home the activities the children engage in at school, parents can continue to be effective. Even though the parents are no longer the child's only teachers, they must still continue to function as the primary figures. They are the ones who will provide continuity to the child's development through the years.

It has been demonstrated that programs that place the parent in a subordinate role dependent on the teacher/expert are not likely to be effective in the long run (Bronfenbrenner, 1974). Therefore, we attempt to help parents prepare for the advancing levels of the child while remaining their child's primary change agent. In the nursery classes connected to the Parent-Infant Program, parents serve as observers, as teacher aides, and even as participating teachers, *not* in an attempt to have parents become teachers but rather to help parents understand the class situation from their child's standpoint. By understanding the classroom tasks, parents can be more supportive, can retain their power to sustain, and can give momentum to whatever development the child achieves within or outside the family setting.

Periodic Auditory Evaluation

Evoked Response Audiometry (ERA) and/or play audiometry are used with the infant in the Hearing Clinics either immediately before or shortly after the family's enrollment in the Parent-Infant Program. The teacher/counselor usually participates as a team member at that time and in all subsequent evaluations. Audiologic re-evaluations continue at regular intervals of three to six months, or more often if needed.

Acoustic Amplification

Decisions about amount and kind of amplification are made only after much consultation between teacher/counselor and audiologist, the teacher/counselor reporting the child's behavior in a variety of home-like settings and the audiologist checking against information gathered by testing, including observations of the child's responses under earphones at various sound pressure levels. This coordination of behavioral observation and test findings should continue throughout the child's enrollment in a Parent-Infant Program.

Since it is not the intent of this chapter to go into procedures for examination of electroacoustic response characteristics of hearing aids and the rationale for the clinical audiologist's selection procedures, we will dismiss the topic and refer the reader to Gengel, Pascoe, and Shore (1971), Zink (1972), and Ross (1976a,b). It is sufficient to say that the clinical audiologist, knowing the characteristics of the individual hearing aids, selects the most appropriate one for the infant or toddler in the Parent-Infant Program.

The initial selection for the very young child is made primarily through inference from available audiologic data, with judicious care given to avoid excessive power. Speech-detection thresholds, pure-tone thresholds, noise-band threshold measures, impedance, and otoscopic examinations are likely to be the audiologic data available (Erber and Alencewicz, 1976). Signs of discomfort and responses at different levels are all indications that an audiologist uses in ascertaining correctness of fit. The clinical audiologist must use his experience in matching acoustic characteristics of amplifiers with audiologic data and subjective responses obtained from older children. However, we are especially concerned that the aid for the young child has some kind of peak limiting or automatic gain control circuitry. The earmold preparation must assure proper fit for the aid to function at its optimal gain setting.

Once the first hearing aid has been selected and fitted, the second stage of acoustic amplification is under way. Careful observation of the child's responses with the amplifier are crucial now. Special attention in everyday situations as well as in the test situation should be given to the child's tolerance for maximum power output of the instrument. A hearing aid owned by the clinic or Parent-Infant Program may be lent to the family in order to assure surveillance and control over its use. Several instruments may be tried during this period until the clinical and educational staff is satisfied with the safety of the selection.

As soon as periodic testing demonstrates reliable audiometric data, the parents are urged to purchase the child his own hearing aid because we want to provide a consistent auditory signal. With continued amplification, the child's responses will become even more reliable. Therefore, we tend to encourage the purchase of aids that are flexible in tone and power control (Ross, 1975; Grammatico, 1976). Because of the age of the child, ruggedness should also be considered. Erber has addressed himself to these topics in hearing aid selection in several publications (1971, 1973, 1974).

In a third stage of acoustic amplification, the clinical audiologist continues to pursue more refined test data, now with the child wearing the hearing aid. The educational audiologist observes the child's response to a variety of stimuli, including those of planned auditory training, which, as indicated later in this chapter, is natural language filled with proper intonation matched to the child's thought and perception. To be sure, the parent points out the environmental sounds as they occur, because it is in the home that the sounds assume meaning and are likely to recur and provide a source for emerging recognition. However, as we state later, we want the infant and toddler to learn the *sound of language* that is *meaningful to him.*

For the child with mild-to-moderate hearing loss, the selection of hearing aids takes into account the child's own reports of his experiences with different amplifiers under a variety of conditions. Noisy and reverberant situations, similar to those that might be found in school classrooms, should be used for testing (Watson, 1964). These children, of course, should continue to be monitored with some degree of regularity throughout their school years.

In recommending the first hearing aid, we usually suggest monaural amplification. If the hearing loss is bilaterally symmetrical, amplification is alternated between the ears; hence, we encourage the making of two earmolds. Binaural amplification is not used until valid and reliable thresholds can be established, but frequent evaluations continue. While the evidence fortunately is small (Rintelmann, 1976), we do not want any of our infants sustaining a threshold shift because of overamplification.

We would prefer ear level hearing aids, but our experience has led us to recommend body worn ones in the beginning for several reasons. The physical problem with ears of small children is probably the greatest concern. Manipulation by the child is more difficult if the aids are in a carrier or in a pocket of the dress or shirt. Even then, the aids are not sufficiently rugged to withstand the abuse of everyday use by the average child. Cereal, gelatin, milk, and soup are spilled and seep into the mechanism; cords break, earmolds get clogged with wax, and receivers crack.

Parents need to be trained to calibrate their ear to monitor the instrument, at least daily. The clinical audiologist and technicians on the team are on call when the aid cannot be restored with a new battery or cord or a clean earmold. Monitoring by parents and educational audiologists assures that the child wears the carefully selected aid constantly and that the aid operates as it was meant to operate, and that the downtime is minimal. When an aid does not work, we attempt to lend a similar aid during the repair time, and we stress the importance of similar characteristics, because we want the transmitted signal to be the same as the signal the child is regularly receiving. In order to insure that its characteristics have not been altered, the aid is checked after repair.

The dissimilar acoustic patterns generated by different amplifying systems influence our use of individual rather than group amplification in the nursery class. Since our program is one that trains the child to function not in a structured setting but in his own home, group amplification is not appropriate. The individual aid with which the child is learning to listen to speech is the same all day and wherever he goes. Most of these considerations are discussed in depth by Ross (1976a), Madell (1976), and Rubin (1976).

Auditory Training

Training a child to use residual hearing is far more complex than just placing a hearing aid on him. We have found that all hearing-impaired children have significant amounts of residual sensory capacity, which, if trained, will greatly facilitate the child's speech acquisition, but only to the degree that the youngster is taught to listen. Training to listen involves giving active and conscious attention to spoken language and thereby deriving meaning.

It has been demonstrated that listening is not intuitive, but rather is something that a child learns to do in the same way that he learns to perceive in the other sense modalities. Listening, unlike walking, does not develop naturally in the child. That children with normal hearing need training to listen has been reported by the teachers of language arts. It has been demonstrated that children with minor hearing losses need listening training if they are to acquire adequate verbal memory (Allen, 1969). Recently, Clark (1976) has pointed out that children with losses of only 15dB, experienced early and caused by serous otitis media, failed to develop normal language skills with a cumulative effect that later resulted in poor school achievement. Furthermore, a mild hearing loss creates poor speech and pitch discrimination when listening training is not provided (Sommers, Meyer, and Furlong, 1969).

Giving a hearing-impaired child a hearing aid without training him to listen is futile. However, his training to listen must pervade his entire day. Listening is not something a child does at a given time with a set procedure.

Because auditory processing is not thoroughly understood, it is very difficult to establish goals for children. Sensitivity is the most available index of auditory ability, yet it is not an adequate predictor of a child's speech recognition ability. Recent investigators have supported the importance of differentiating the hearing-impaired population by relating their speech production and discrimination abilities to threshold levels (Boothroyd and Cawkwell, 1970; Erber, 1974). Even when threshold audiograms are similar, important differences in auditory abilities may be revealed by auditory disrimination tests (Erber, 1972). Regrettably, infants' speech discrimination cannot be tested but must be observed.

The contribution of acoustic phonetics adds to our growing understanding of speech perception. The presence of important speech information in low frequencies is valuable in the teaching of speech. Time and intensity information can cue speech sound duration, presence or absence of voicing in continuant consonants, stress of syllables, and other prosodic features. Blessor (1972) and Erber (1974) have established that these features are available even to the subject with a profound hearing loss.

Time and intensity are the dimensions of speech by which we communicate feelings, specify meanings, and clarify attitudes. Important messages are embedded in the nuances and prosody of speech—in the rhythm, duration, stress, accent, and pitch. Interestingly, these features—our spoken tools for conveying meaning—are the very ones missing in the speech of many hearing-impaired children who have been denied amplification (Calvert, 1962).

Meaning plays a critical role in language acquisition. MacNamara (1972) thinks a child uses meaning as a clue to language rather than language as a clue to meaning. A child determines the meaning a speaker conveys, then works out the relationship between meaning and the language. The match, then, of the parents' language to the child's thought is an outcome of the essential auditory input.

Lewis (1963) believes that children learn the meaning of intonation before the meaning of words. Children with normal hearing respond to intonation before they respond to phonemes. Intonation patterns express affective states as well as serve as syntactic markers. The rhythmic structures of the code, the pulsings and the stresses, give information and meaning. Therefore, the acoustical features of speech that should be made available to a hearing-impaired child should be presented as fluent, meaningful speech, not single words or noise-makers.

Simply exposing the child to continuous and louder speech, however, is also inappropriate. Ervin-Tripp (1973) reports on such situations, in which hearing children of deaf parents have had continuous and loud exposure to speech via TV. She found that those children had learned neither to understand nor produce speech. The important dimension of interaction in which the parent tunes in to the child and provides the structure that clothes his thoughts has been aptly called the Ping-Pong approach by Gordon (1976).

This reciprocal action draws vocalizations from the parent and the child. The feedback system is not only interpersonal but intrapersonal as well. The child needs to hear his own voice as he imitates his parents. They in turn need to match his efforts and model new structures for him to store. In this way he receives repeated examples of connected speech that are stored for later induction of language code rules. Herein lies the primary strategy for training in listening.

The whole process of learning to listen is not a passive stage of growth, but rather an immensely dynamic and energetic enterprise that calls on the highest capabilities a hearing child can mobilize, according to Friedlander (1970). Because it is such a large task, children should not have to learn to listen through noises, but instead through spoken language. Training in discrimination should not be with bells, whistles, and drums, but with spoken language units. The training, in fact, is to listen, not discriminate—that is, listening to natural language, not to vowels, consonants, formants, or frequencies; listening to *meaningful* global speech organized around the child's thought, not to phonemes nor to other discrete units.

Speech Perception Through Lipreading

Although we have put emphasis on the acoustic information available to hearing-impaired children, we do not want to reduce attention to lipreading as an avenue for language input. Lipreading gives children place-of-articulation speech information. By watching the movement of the lips, tongue, and jaw, hearing-impaired children can attain high levels of communication, particularly if they are receiving complementary voicing, manner-of-articulation, and vowel formant appreciation through their residual hearing. By obtaining through one sensory system that which is not available through another, children with severe hearing losses usually comprehend quite well (Erber, 1974). Children with profound losses need to receive considerable lipreading information in order to comprehend speech. This does not say that the profoundly deaf do not benefit from the auditory perception, but rather that they understand spoken language better when they look as well as listen (Van Uden, 1970). The pattern information in the form of time and intensity cues supplements the place-of-articulation information and aids in language acquisition.

The task, then, is to insure the use of the residual hearing and allow the child to "eye" the speaker so that he perceives both auditory and visual information. Perception is not innate any more than language is. He must learn to look just as he must learn to listen.

OTHER PROCEDURES

If one sensory channel—for example, audition—is the *only* one available for learning oral communication, profoundly deaf children would be at a tremendous loss. Although there are reports of profoundly deaf children who make surprisingly good use of aural approaches, these tend to be exceptions. Upon closer examination, these children are often found to have a conductive component to their hearing losses.

Regrettably, in today's professional settings, enthusiastic advocacy of the unisensory approach precludes the opportunity for a deaf child to learn to look at the same time he is making maximum use of very small amounts of residual hearing, if any. As was so aptly stated by Calvert (1976):

> The single strand of acoustic pulses of compression and rarefication of air molecules is too thin a thread upon which to hang the future of oral communication for hearing impaired children (p. 79).

Another group of educators of the deaf offer the option of one or another form of manual communication. Within that group are opinions on the relative merit of each of eight distinct systems of hand gestures. Although the manual system is combined with lipreading and the use of a hearing aid and is called Total Communication, some feel it is only manual.

Lloyd (1973) addressed himself to this when he wrote:

> The so-called total communication approaches have included: . . . an overemphasis on the manual with a corresponding de-emphasis of the oral-aural aspects. In some cases, total communication has really been a euphemism for the manual method.
>
> Those using the manual method usually say they are using the simultaneous method. Unfortunately, the signs and fingerspelling many times communicate a different message than does the oral presentation, if any spoken words are present. In other words, simultaneous and total communication are often misnomers (p. 61).

Trevoort (1975) more recently stated:

> There is no such thing as coexistence between oralism and total communication. This was true a quarter of a century ago when I began my work with the deaf; it still is true now (p. 3).

In an issue of *Gallaudet Today,* one of the discussants wrote:

> Children and their parents who were taught "Total Communication" in the Chicago area have found it totally incomprehensible in California. . . . Language in Southern California bears only faint resemblance to that of Northern California (Schreiber, 1974–75, p. 6).

An examination of Bellugi's (1972) work points up differences between spoken and signed communication and signs that are distortions when one thinks of learning of the language code. Part of the learning is the processing of language information whereby the child can induce the principles of the language in order to comprehend and produce it. There is disparity between speech and a signed system in rate of transmission. While speech in conversation averages 140 words per minute, fingerspelling is at best 80 to 90 words.

In comparisons of sign and spoken interpretation, there is loss of information through vocabulary alone. Bellugi reported that the spoken paraphrase of a story required 405 words, but the signed version required 274 words. When the subjects were deprived but hearing children, such reduction of the language input was considered a serious impoverishment (Bernstein, 1971).

Not only is the input diminished but the message is distorted. The distortions can best be illustrated with examples of Bellugi (1972). The task she gave was to paraphrase this sentence:

He would give her the best fish and the villagers would buy the rest from him.

As you would suspect, the spoken version ran:

"He remembered that he would give the best fish to his daughter and sell the rest to the villagers."

However, the signed English version was:

He (h-e) think past he (h-e) would (w-d) keep best fish for girl his (h-s) daughter, and left he (h-e) village.

By American Sign Language, the paraphrase was:

Think. "Best fish take, save for my son." (his) son save. "Left fish left give-them to people in town, give fish. Sell fish, sell, but best keep my son."

In order to amass knowledge of the predictability of the language code, the child must encounter the code. He needs to produce the same code that he comprehends. In giving a rationale for intensive auditory input Fry (1963) stated:

> If a deaf child learns the system (Language Code) he will be able to guess just as efficiently as the hearing person only he needs more listening practice than the normal child. He must hear more speech, more continuous and louder speech so that he may learn the phonemic system and acquire the statistical knowledge that we all use when we take in speech (p. 184).

AUDITORY/GLOBAL APPROACH

Although the hearing-impaired child has restricted sensitivity, which reduces the redundancy and linguistic cues available to him, constant amplification of abundant meaningful auditory experiences compensates to a great degree. Lipreading compensates or supplements to an even greater degree. Through combined auditory/visual perception, there are sufficient phonologic, syntactic, and semantic code cues available to him to facilitate his induction of code rules (Calvert and Silverman, 1975).

The language input, then, most certainly should be the natural language of the child's environment, sometimes colloquial but always complete. Invariably, the input must observe the integrity of meaning and all syntactic rules. Because the input is an entire sentence or phrase, we sometimes label it "global" and the process for preschoolers frequently is referred to as "auditory-global." Perhaps natural language appropriate to the child's thought might be substituted for the word "global" because there are times that one word or even two are indeed global, for example, "Pull" or "Throw it."

In the Parent-Infant Program we believe that the parent-child interaction should be mediated with appropriate language. We guide parents in using it and in developing strategies for maximizing the input. Spoken language is the focal point of all interactions.

Contrary to most general practice, we believe that the natural setting of the home, while informal, is superior to structured programs. In the home listening becomes an integral part of all activities. The content can be infinite, but it is usually redundant. It centers on here and now, on the child's things, on what he is doing, wants, or needs. The form is usually short sentences or phrases, but may be meaningful single words. Most important, it is simple language that gets repeated from day to day in the average home and is tangibly associated with meaning.

We want parents to label all the objects their child uses and sees every day. For example, when dressing they can say:

Let's put on your shoe.
You have white shoes.
Daddy will button your shirt.
Here's your coat.

At mealtime parents can say:

Here's your cereal.
Oh, the cereal is hot.
Now eat your toast.
Do you want an egg?

Singing, vocal play, and fun with speech sounds are important also. Nursery rhymes, bedtime stories, and talk about pictures are gradually added to the vocal input. More important than the sound waves is their content. Above all the function of language has first priority. With a parent of an infant, the function of language is to communicate love, so that is where we start.

Parents are asked to note how the child responds affectively, both to the intonational pattern of what he "hears" and to the situation in which he hears it. This is the beginning of auditory training and puts the child well into the *exposure* level of comprehension. If it appears to be a passive period, it is because all the child is doing is whining to be changed, crying to be held, cooing to be played with. These vocalizations must be treated as communication and promptly reinforced. If any vocal activity on the part of the parent elicits response from the child, the parent must continue it. However, if the child gives no differentiated response, teacher/counselor and parents may have to tune in more sharply. These strategies range from simply stopping and waiting for the child's eyes to come to the lips and show attending behavior to providing some overt parent response every time the child does attend.

Difficulties do arise in children who, for reasons other than hearing impairment, fail to respond to sound. The effects of such things as sound deprivation, deprivation of meaningful interaction, illness, and retardation need to be carefully observed and understood in a diagnostic look at the child. Again, individual sessions give the teacher/counselor an opportunity to analyze the case carefully.

Several stages of development follow the exposure level, the first of which is *awareness*—a necessary step before comprehension takes place when the child seems to attend and appears conscious of communication. He may do something and then look to the mother's face as if he expects her to tell about it.

At this time he may turn to the parent's voice. He may quiet to rhythmic speech. He may smile and coo at endearing vocalizations. He seems aware of communication. Language should continue to surround him, but now more effort is extended to give him the names for things. Simple sentences with the particular word stressed become the pattern.

Here's your Teddy Bear.
Poor Teddy Bear.
Don't throw Teddy Bear.
Pat Teddy Bear.
Or just Teddy Bear.

Parents use reiteration and segmentation in their interactions with their infant in a fascinating way. For example, if mother wishes to direct the child to give her the red truck, she says, "Give me the red truck. The red truck. Red truck." In other words, the mother segments the fairly complex sentence for the child.

Thus the child is embarked on vocabulary learning. Things have names. Only when he comprehends this can we check for performance, but even at this stage of awareness baby must see what parent is doing in order for the baby to understand. So before we ask the child to identify "shoe" in the sentence, "Get your shoe," we must give the child the exposure and the awareness we have been talking about.

Parents will probably have to give the instructions and help the baby find the shoes long before they can expect an independent response. When that is possible, we then guide the parent to turn her head away and give only the one word "shoe," out of the child's line of vision, and thus we begin to train his listening ability.

Alert to the child's interest, parents can continue to strive for responses to names of toys, clothing, foods, and activities, but always in context. As the repertoire of nursery rhymes increases, parents can easily obtain pictures and play auditory games with their child in which he is asked to identify the particular rhyme given. They can prepare a scrapbook about their experiences and it can be the object of the auditory game. They may elect to speak to the side, cover their mouth, or talk behind the child, but always in the natural setting.

Parents need assistance in learning strategies of time to be spent on this type of activity, of motivation, and of reinforcement. They need to know about distance and volume, about masking noises, about single speaker, about signal-to-noise ratio, and about attenuation. But above all, they must learn about hearing aids:

> about what they can do, but also what they cannot do; that batteries need regular monitoring; that the cord shouldn't be knotted or chewed; that the earmolds must be kept clean and tight; that cereal doesn't improve microphones, and that an adult should calibrate the power before putting it on the child. (Simmons-Martin, 1975a)

An informal global approach that addresses the learning of auditory perception as a tool to learning speech requires structure on the part of the team, but not on the part of the "teachers," the child's parents.

SUMMARY

There is substantial evidence that effective parenting during the child's early years determines the quality of his life. As the first and most fundamental educational delivery system, parents must provide the necessary experiences if their child is to realize his potential. These useful and beneficial experiences influence the child's intellectual and academic achievement, but more important, they have an impact upon the child's language development, the key to all intellectual, emotional, and social growth.

Parent education is not new, but the increasing awareness of the role of the parent during the child's early development has led to intensive programming for parents during the child's very young life. Recall Schaefer's (1972) conclusion that these types of programs provide an effective alternative for preschool education. Such parental involvement is even more essential for the development of children with a handicap.

In parents of a child with a handicapping condition, we often find an emotional disorganization accompanying the recognition of the problem. Some parents cope with the handicap in a constructive manner with a minimum of counseling assistance. Most parents, however, need help over a period in which they are experiencing grief patterns that, while they may seem irrational, unreasonable, or inappropriate, do exist intensely in almost all cases.

While most parents, as reported by White and Watts (1973) and a substantial number of others, are not being properly prepared for parenthood, parents of a handicapped child are also not prepared for their child's condition. In addition to needing support, they need guidance to help their child develop his full range of human abilities. They need to know about children and child growth and about language and cognitive development. But most important, they need to know how these areas are affected by a hearing impairment. They need to know how amplification, acoustics, and audition relate to the language development. Also important is their need to learn strategies for providing the necessary experiences without sacrificing the important parental role for one that is primarily pedagogical.

The clinical audiologist and the teacher/counselor need to work as a team in educating the parent of the hearing-impaired child. The program, appropriate to the particular family's level, needs to include practical experience with their own child. The person doing habilitative audiology needs to explain language and cognitive development and to assist parents in understanding the effects of hearing impairment.

Management, child care, language input, and the use of the hearing aid are part of the realistic practicum. Along with guiding the parents in getting attending behavior, the teacher/counselor helps the parent learn stages of auditory perception based upon the global aspect of language. Working together, the team assists parents to set realistic goals and to work toward achieving them.

RESEARCH NEEDS

As indicated in the context of the chapter, there is still much research needed in language behavior. While there is some information about language per se, much more needs to be known about how children, especially children deprived of hearing, learn the *function* and *content* as well as the form of language. Most of the work in language development concerns itself only with language form or structure. Far too few researchers have explored *language behavior* and there is an appalling dearth of developmental studies with children who have a hearing impairment.

The effectiveness of the social milieu and parents in particular needs considerably more attention. Research on social factors affecting language development has so far dealt with differences in rate of acquisition, linguistic rules, and differences in frequency of use of the optimal linguistic structures; however, there has been little interest in the social factors which affect the acquisition and maintenance of different language functions and content. Conditions for producing behavioral changes need to be clearly delineated.

That there is an urgent need to understand the handicapped child himself as well as his interaction with his environment was documented by a recent conference, Research Needs of Early Childhood Education for the Handicapped (U.S. Office of Education, 1975). The major themes that emerged from the conference were:

1. Great concern for improved early diagnosis.
2. Appropriate intervention that will lead to optimum development.
3. The need for comprehensive research on programs and agencies (institutions) to develop models for total service to the handicapped and their families.
4. Improved preparation of all personnel who work with the handicapped child by the identification of necessary competencies and the design of effective strategies to develop these competencies.

It is hoped that in the immediate future, research-oriented personnel will join the team of clinical audiologists, educational audiologists, teachers, and parents to effect substantive changes in the management of the child with a hearing impairment.

REFERENCES

Allen, D.V., "Modality Aspect of Mediation in Children With Normal and Impaired Hearing Ability," Final Report, Project No. 7-0837, Bureau of Education for the Handicapped, Wayne State University, Detroit, 1969.

Alschuler, I.N., "An Experimental Study of the Effects of a Parent Education Intervention Program Designed to Increase Young Children's Sustained Attention to Verbal Stimuli." Doctoral dissertation, State University of New York at Albany, 1972.

Ambrose, J.A., "The Development of the Smiling Response in Early Infancy," in *Determinants of Infant Behavior,* edited by B.M. Foss. New York: John Wiley & Sons, 1961.

Bellugi, U., "Studies in Sign Language," in *Psycholinguistics and Total Communication: The State of the Art,* edited by T.J. O'Rourke. American Annals of the Deaf, 1972.

Bernstein, B., "A Sociolinguistic Approach to Socialization: With Some References to Educability," in *Directions in Sociolinguistics,* edited by D. Hymes and J. Gumperz. New York: Holt, Rinehart & Winston, 1971.

Blesser, B., "Speech Perception Under Conditions of Spectral Transformation: I. Phonetic Characteristics," *Journal of Speech and Hearing Research,* 15 (1972), 5–41.

Boothroyd, A., and S. Cawkwell, "Vibrotactile Thresholds in Pure-Tone Audiometry," *Acta Oto-Laryngologica,* 69 (1970), 381–387.

Bronfenbrenner, U., *A Report on Longitudinal Evaluations of Preschool Programs, Vol. II, Is Early Intervention Effective?* U.S. Dept. of Health, Education and Welfare Publication No. (OHD) 75-25, 1974.

Brown, R., and U. Bellugi, "Three Processes in the Child's Acquisition of Syntax," *Harvard Educational Review,* 34 (1964), 131–151.

Calvert, D., "Communication Practices: Aural/Oral and Visual/Oral," *A Bicentennial Monograph of Hearing Impaired: Trends in the USA.* Washington, D.C.: *Volta Bureau,* 78 (1976), 76–81.

Calvert, D., "Speech Sound Duration and the Surd-Sonnant Error," *Volta Review,* 64 (1962), 401–422.

Calvert, D., and S.R. Silverman, *Speech & Deafness.* Washington, D.C.: A.G. Bell Association, 1975.

Clark, E.V., "Some Aspects of the Conceptual Basis for First Language Acquisition," in *Language Perspectives—Acquisition, Retardation and Intervention,* edited by R.L. Schiefelbush and L.L. Lloyd. Baltimore: University Park Press, 1974, pp. 105–128.

Clark, M., "Hearing: A Link to IQ?" *Newsweek,* 87 (June 14, 1976), p. 97.

Dennis, W., and P. Najarian, "Infant Development Under Environmental Handicap," *Psychological Monographs,* 71:7, No. 436, 1957.

Downs, M., "The Deafness Management Quotient," *Hearing and Speech News,* 21 (1974).

Erber, N.P., "Amplification and the Development of Communication Skills by Deaf Children." Paper presented at a Conference on Extended Low Frequency Amplification and the Deaf Child, White Haven, Penna., 1974.

Erber, N.P., "Audiologic Evaluation of Deaf Children," *Journal of Speech and Hearing Disorders,* 41 (1976), 256–267.

Erber, N.P., "Body Baffle and Real-Ear Effects in the Selection of Hearing Aids for Deaf Children," *Journal of Speech and Hearing Disorders,* 38 (1973), 224–231.

Erber, N.P., "Evaluation of Special Hearing Aids for Deaf Children," *Journal of Speech and Hearing Disorders,* 36 (1971), 527–537.

Erber, N.P. "Speech-Envelope Cues as an Acoustic Aid to Lipreading for Profoundly Deaf Children," *Journal of the Acoustical Society of America,* 51 (1972), 1224–1227.

Erber, N., and Alencewicz, C., "Audiologic Evaluation of Deaf Children," *Journal of Speech and Hearing Disorders,* 41 (1976), 256–267.

Ervin-Tripp, S. "Some Strategies for the First Two Years," in *Cognitive Development and the Acquisition of Language,* edited by T.E. Moore. New York: Academic Press, 1973, 183–191.

Friedlander, B.Z., "Receptive Language Development in Infancy: Issues and Problems," *Merrill-Palmer Quarterly,* 16 (1970), 7–51.

Fry, D.B., "Speech," *Report of the Proceedings of International Congress on Education of the Deaf,* 1963, 183–191.

Furth, H., Participant in *Sensory Capabilities of Hearing Impaired Children,* edited by R.E. Start. Baltimore: University Park Press, 1974.

Gengel, R.W., D. Pascoe, and **I. Shore**, "A Frequency-Response Procedure for Evaluating and Selecting Hearing Aids for Severely Hearing-Impaired Children," *Journal of Speech and Hearing Disorders,* 36 (1971), 341–353.

Giattino, J., and **J.G. Hogan**, "Analysis of a Father's Speech to His Language-Learning Child," *Journal of Speech and Hearing Disorders,* 40 (1975), 524–538.

Gilmer, R., J.O. Miller, and **S.W. Gray**, *Intervention With Mothers and Young Children: Study of Intra-Family Effects.* Nashville: Darcee, 1970.

Gordon, I.J., "Parenting, Teaching, and Child Development," *Young Children,* 31 (1976), 173–184.

Gordon, I.J., *Research Reports: The Florida Parent Education Early Intervention Projects: A Longitudinal Look.* Gainsville, Fla.: Institute for Development of Human Resources, University of Florida, 1973.

Grammatico, L.F., discussion in *Hearing Aids, Current Developments and Concepts,* edited by M. Rubin. Baltimore: University Park Press, 1976, 123–137.

Greenstein, J.M., B.B. Greenstein, K. McConville, and **L. Stellini**, *Mother-Infant Communication and Language Acquisition in Deaf Infants.* New York: Lexington School for the Deaf, 1976.

Hanners, B.A., "The Audiologist as Educator: The Ultimate Hearing Aide," in *Mainstream Education for Hearing Impaired Children and Youth,* edited by G.W. Nix. New York: Grune & Stratton, 1976.

Hess, R.D., "Early Education as Socialization," in *Early Education,* edited by R.D. Hess and R.M. Bear. Chicago: Aldine Publishing Company, 1968.

Hess, R. and **V.C. Shipman**, "Early Experience and the Socialization of Cognitive Modes in Children," *Child Development,* 36 (1965), 869–886.

Hoffmeyer, B.E., "And Finally . . .," *Gallaudet Today* (Winter 1976), 33.

Lewis, M., *Language, Thought and Personality.* London: George G. Harrap, 1963.

Ling, D., and **A.H. Ling**, "Communication Development in the First Three Years of Life," *Journal of Speech and Hearing Research,* 17 (1974), 146–159.

Lloyd, L.L., "Mental Retardation and Hearing Impairment," *Deafness Annual,* Vol. 3. Silver Spring, Md.: Professional Rehabilitation Workers with the Adult Deaf (1973), 45–67.

MacNamara, J., "Cognitive Basis of Language Learning in Infants," *Psychological Review,* 79 (1972), 1–13.

McNeill, D., "The Capacity for Language Acquisition," *Volta Review*, 68 (1966), 17–33.

Madell, J.R., "Hearing Aid Evaluation Procedures with Children," in *Hearing Aids, Current Developments and Concepts*, edited by M. Rubin. Baltimore: University Park Press, 1976.

Malkin, S., R.D. Freeman, and J.O. Hastings, "Psychosocial Problems of Deaf Children and Their Families: A Comparative Study," *Audiology and Hearing Education*, 2 (1966), 21–29.

Menyuk, P., Participant in *Sensory Capabilities of Hearing Impaired Children*, edited by R.E. Stark. Baltimore: University Park Press, 1974.

Phillips, J.R., "Syntax and Vocabulary of Mothers' Speech to Young Children: Age and Sex Comparison," *Child Development*, 44 (1973), 182–185.

Radin, N., "Three Degrees of Maternal Involvement in a Preschool Program: Impact on Mother and Children," *Child Development*, 43 (1972), 1355–1364.

Read, K., *The Nursery School*. Philadelphia: W.B. Saunders, 1960.

Rhodes, M.J., "From a Parent's Point of View," *The Deaf American* (1972), 20.

Rintelmann, W.F., "Effects of Overamplification on Hearing." Paper presented at the International Symposium on Childhood Deafness, Central Michigan University, Mount Pleasant, Michigan, June, 1976.

Ross, M., "Hearing Aid Selection for the Preverbal Hearing-Impaired Child," in *Amplification for the Hearing Impaired*, edited by M.C. Pollack. New York: Grune & Stratton, 1975.

Ross, M., "Introduction and Review of Hearing Aid Evaluation Procedures," in *Hearing Aids, Current Developments and Concepts*, edited by M. Rubin. Baltimore: University Park Press, 1976a.

Ross, M., "Summary and Review," in *Hearing Aids, Current Developments and Concepts*, edited by M. Rubin. Baltimore: University Park Press, 1976b.

Rubenstein, J., "Maternal Attentiveness and Subsequent Exploratory Behavior in the Infant," *Child Development*, 38 (1967), 1089–1100.

Rubin, M.E., "Hearing Aids for Infants and Toddlers," in *Hearing Aids, Current Developments and Concepts*, edited by M. Rubin. Baltimore: University Park Press, 1976.

Ruland, M.A., "A Longitudinal Demographic Study of a Parent-Infant Program for Hearing Impaired Children." Independent study, Washington University, St. Louis, May 1976.

Sanders, D.A., "Residual Hearing—The Yeast of Communication," in *Mainstream Education for Hearing Impaired Children and Youth*, edited by G.W. Nix. New York: Grune & Stratton, 1976.

Schaefer, E.S., "Parents as Educators: Evidence from Cross-Sectional Longitudinal and Intervention Research," *Young Children*, 27 (1972), 227–239.

Schreiber, F.C., "and the Cons." *Gallaudet Today* (Winter 1974/75), 5–6.

Simmons, A.A., "Language and Hearing," *Speech for the Deaf Child*, edited by L.E. Connor. Washington, D.C.: A.G. Bell Association, 1971.

Simmons-Martin, A.A., *Chats With Johnny's Parents.* Washington, D.C.: A.G. Bell Association, 1975b.

Simmons-Martin, A.A., "A Demonstration Home Approach With Hearing Impaired Children," in *Professionals Approach Parents of Handicapped Children,* edited by E.J. Webster. Springfield, Ill.: Charles C. Thomas, 1976.

Simmons-Martin, A.A., "Facilitating Parent-Child Interaction Through the Education of Parents," in *Journal of Research and Development in Education,* 8 (1975a), pp. 96–102, edited by P.G. Adkins.

Sinclair-de-Zwart, H., "Developmental Psycholinguistics," in *Studies in Cognitive Development: Essays in Honor of Jean Piaget,* edited by D. Elkind and J.H. Flanell. New York: Oxford University Press, 1969.

Slobin, D.I., "Cognitive Prerequisites for the Development of Grammar," in *Studies of Child Language Development,* edited by C.Z. Ferguson and D.I. Slobin. New York: Holt, Rinehart and Winston, 1973.

Snow, C.E., "Mothers' Speech to Children Learning Language," *Child Development,* 43 (1972), 549–565.

Sommers, R.K., W.J. Meyer, and A.K. Furlong, "Pitch Discrimination and Speech Sound Discrimination in Articulatory Defective and Normal Speaking Children, *Journal of Auditory Research,* 9 (1969), 45–50.

Trevoort, B.T., "Development of Language and the Deaf." Paper given at International Congress on Education of the Deaf, Tokyo, 1975.

U.S. Office of Education, *Proceedings of the Conference on Research Needs Related to Early Childhood Education for the Handicapped.* Washington, D.C.: Bureau of Education for the Handicapped, 1975.

Van Uden, A., "New Realizations in the Light of the Pure Oral Method," *Volta Review,* (1970) 524–527.

Watson, T.J., "The Use of Hearing Aids by Hearing-Impaired Pupils in Ordinary Schools," *Volta Review,* 66 (1964), 741–744.

White, B.L., *The First Three Years of Life.* Englewood Cliffs, N.J.: Prentice-Hall, 1975.

White, B.L., and J.C. Watts, *Experience and Environment: Major Influences on the Development of the Young Child.* Englewood Cliffs, N.J.: Prentice-Hall, 1973.

Zink, G.D., "Hearing Aids Children Wear: A Longitudinal Study of Performance," *Volta Review,* 74 (1972), 41–51.

SUGGESTED READING

Matkin, N., "Hearing Aids for Children," in *Hearing Aid Assessment and Use in Audiologic Habilitation,* edited by W. Hodgson and P. Skinner. Baltimore: Williams and Wilkins, 1977, pp. 145–169.

The Public Schools

The focus in the preceding chapter of this book has been on the very young child. As the final two chapters reveal, the responsibilities of the pediatric audiologist continue well into the school years. These responsibilities involve the identification of hearing-impaired children as well as appropriate remediation.

In Chapter 11, Drs. Wilson and Walton present both historical and modern approaches to identification audiometry in the public schools. Procedures to locate children with ear conditions requiring medical attention, or with hearing impairments which can interfere with normal progress in the classroom are given. Dr. Garwood, in Chapter 12, details the audiologist's responsibilities to students with a hearing loss. He then illustrates a variety of ways to meet the challenge of public school audiology.

CHAPTER ELEVEN

Public School Audiometry

WESLEY R. WILSON, WENDEL K. WALTON

INTRODUCTION

The assessment of auditory function of school-age children is an important responsibility in the schools today. Although public school audiometry can be defined as the assessment of hearing of school-age children, the fact that it takes place in a school environment suggests that a major component of such a program should be identification. Identification, or screening, audiometry defines a subgroup of a total population that needs detailed audiometric assessment. The detailed assessment should facilitate appropriate intervention, complemented by continued assessment. Screening tests do not attempt to define type of problem, severity of problem, or such; rather, their sole purpose is to identify children in need of more detailed audiologic assessment.

Within the organizational framework of this book, the intervention components of a complete school hearing program are detailed in other chapters. Thus, although we firmly believe that the hearing program in a public school setting must include identification, assessment, and intervention components, the primary focus of this chapter will be on identification. Discussions and procedural considerations for intervention are contained in Chapter 12. Numerous detailed treatments of assessment procedures exist elsewhere (for example, Martin, 1975) and will not be duplicated here.

CHAPTER OBJECTIVES

The purpose of this chapter is to describe briefly the philosophic bases for providing an audiology program in the schools, then to cover in detail the topic of identification audiometry including the available research literature. Emphasis is given to administrative organization, methodologies, personnel, equipment, funding, and laws govering identification audiometry programs and hearing conservation.

390

HISTORY OF IDENTIFICATION AUDIOMETRY IN SCHOOLS

Public school audiometry had its origin approximately 50 years ago with the development of equipment (Fowler and Fletcher, 1926) that led to the first widely accepted audiometric screening test—the Western Electric 4A Test (named after the company that developed the equipment) or, more popularly, the Fading Numbers Test. This group speech test involved a recording of a woman saying pairs of one-digit numbers. Up to 40 individuals were tested at once. It required that the persons being tested be able to write down their responses. The test started 30dB above a "normal" threshold (no calibration standard existed at that time) and each pair of digits was repeated at a level 3dB lower than the preceding pair; the complete test included four series of attenuation for each ear. This test had a variety of defects, the most notable being the use of speech as a test stimulus. Children with hearing losses at frequencies above 500 Hz often successfully passed this screening test. Other weaknesses included the fact that a written response, requiring knowledge of numbers, precluded the use of this test with young school-age children. In addition, the problems in providing calibrated earphones for up to 40 listening positions were difficult. Finally, the opportunity for children to pass by simply copying their neighbor's score sheet was hard to control and scoring each of the answer sheets was time-consuming.

Following the development of the pure-tone audiometer, group pure-tone screening tests became popular. Examples included the Massachusetts Test (Johnston, 1948). It provided test stations for up to 40 individuals and sampled at four frequencies—512, 1024, 4096, and 11584 Hz. A single sound-pressure level, different for each frequency, was used. Again a written response, on this test the circling of the word *yes* or *no,* was required. Children scored their own test sheets by counting the number of *no* responses. Some of the same difficulties described for the Fading Numbers Test applied to this test—namely, the limitations placed on any test using a written response and the problems associated with group administration. In addition, finding and maintaining an adequate test environment in terms of ambient noise for pure-tone testing of 40 children was a serious problem.

The difficulties with group tests led many to consider the individual pure-tone sweep frequency screening test as the test of choice. Considerable detail concerning this procedure is contained in later sections of this chapter. Briefly, this screening procedure involves testing each child individually with a pure-tone audiometer and sampling at a single intensity across discrete octave frequencies. Since each child is tested individually, any response mode appropriate to the age and abilities of the child can be used. The claimed advantages of the procedure include its ability to detect frequency-sensitive losses that were not detected with standard speech screening tests, the apparently greater accuracy possible in a one-to-one test situation, and, because a written response is not required, its applicability to a younger population. Its apparent disadvantage, contrasted to the group procedures, is obviously one of time spent per test. However, when the equipment for a group test is not permanently installed (for example, in a mobile unit), the time spent in setting up and taking down the group test equipment and in checking calibration of the multiple headsets often more than offsets the time saved by testing more than one individual at a time.

Most recently impedance audiometry, particularly tympanometry, has been suggested for or included in the screening procedures in some school districts. As we shall see later, the primary impetus for including this procedure comes from a desire to increase the accuracy of the screening audiometry in predicting cases of otopathology. Certainly the evidence is clear that pure-tone screening is not an effective predictor of middle-ear problems, and inclusion of impedance audiometry is a logical step for screening programs that set as a primary goal the detection of such pathology.

In briefly tracing the history of identification audiometry, it is also interesting to consider the scope of such programs in the United States today. Perhaps the best source of such demographic information is contained in a report issued in 1972 entitled the *National Survey of State Identification Audiometry Programs and Special Educational Services for Hearing-Impaired Children and Youth,* prepared by the Office of Demographic Studies of Gallaudet College (Murphy, 1972). In this report, detailing a survey completed in 1971, we find that approximately half of the states have legislation mandating the screening of hearing of school-age children. Virtually all of the remaining states have some type of screening program, even though it is not mandated by state law. In addition, we find that within 35 states responding to a question concerning numbers of children screened during the past academic year, over 9 million children had been tested. If we project this information to the total 50 states and District of Columbia, it is likely that over 13 million children were screened during that academic year. (For comparison, the United States Census Bureau figures indicate a population of approximately 40 million children between the ages of 4 and 14 for the same year.)

Certainly, these data make it easy to appreciate the scope and magnitude of identification audiometry programs in the schools as well as the tremendous growth that has taken place during the 50-year history of such activity. However, our enthusiasm should not allow us to infer that simply because a large number of children are being screened, the programs are all necessarily efficient or appropriate. In fact, one of the primary purposes of this chapter is to suggest means of evaluating the effectiveness of screening programs so as to allow for continued improvement in the future.

SCOPE OF IDENTIFICATION AUDIOMETRY

The issues surrounding identification audiometry in the schools are primarily of two types: (1) the philosophic base of such programs; (2) methodological and logistical considerations in implementing such programs. These two issues interrelate in that the philosophic base of an identification program within a specific school district should dictate the methodology selected. However, such has not always been the case. Certainly, when one realizes the district resources (personnel time and equipment money) that will be expended and the large number of children who will be tested, we should realize the importance of developing fully the philosophic base of the identification audiometry effort before setting out to solve methodological questions and problems.

The first issue is the purpose of identification audiometry programs in the school setting. Is it to identify children with educationally handicapping hearing problems, or is it to identify children with ear pathology, regardless of whether or not the pathology is causing a handicapping hearing loss? Certainly, the issue is not polar, and many programs identify one as the primary purpose of the program and the other as a secondary purpose. However, in surveying much of the literature concerned with methodology, one is impressed with the fact that many authors either explicitly or implicitly take the position that the validity criterion of a specific procedure should be its effectiveness in defining otopathology. Conversely, almost no literature has been developed detailing the specific characteristics of what constitutes an "educationally significant" loss. One is left with the impression that, although many programs claim their primary purpose is that of defining educationally significant losses, it has been far easier to attempt to identify losses as they relate to otopathology and, in effect, the actual purpose of the program has often been shifted to such definition.

A district's philosophic stance as to the purpose of its identification audiometry program has important implications in terms of the methodology selected for completing the program. Likewise, the methodology or methodologies selected dictate in large part the cost and necessary personnel. For example, if the primary purpose of the screening program is to identify educationally significant losses, then such a program best would be supervised by persons responsible for the educational management of hearing-impaired children. On the other hand, if the primary purpose is to identify all children with medically significant pathology, the program more properly would be supervised and developed by health personnel within a school district. In terms of test procedures to be employed in the screening audiometry, the traditional pure-tone screening test is reasonably accurate in identifying educationally significant shifts in hearing sensitivity; however, it is highly inaccurate in identifying otopathology. On the other hand, otoscopic inspection and/or impedance audiometry are efficient in defining middle-ear pathology, but are not efficient in defining all educationally significant losses. Furthermore, if the primary purpose of the hearing screening program is to determine which children have educationally significant hearing problems, one would question whether or not screening of hearing sensitivity alone is adequate. Almost no literature exists on the wide-scale application of screening procedures for determining difficulties in auditory or speech perception. As is apparent, careful consideration must be given to determining the philosophic bases of an identification program within a specific school district before one attempts to determine the specific methodologies to be employed. Certainly, political and social decisions play on this issue, and over the next decade, as society determines the extent to which the educational system is to be involved in health-delivery serivces, solutions in keeping with such decisions will be required of the identification audiometry effort.

It seems to us that the primary goals in the public-school audiometry program must always emphasize identifying educationally significant hearing problems. With such an emphasis in mind, it is important to consider the role of the audiologist and speech pathologist. Ideally, such a program will be coordinated so that identification is only the first step in an overall process that includes adequate on-going assessment and educational management of hearing problems. As professionals uniquely qualified to deal with communication problems, the audiologist or speech pathologist, or both, should be responsible for the overall organization and management of such a program. When the identification effort is viewed within the broader framework of habilitation for those with educationally significant loss, it is easy to see the need for coordination of the on-going management program of such children. Situations in which identification is isolated from assessment and management often do not provide optimum programming because of breakdowns in communication and coordination.

Practical Considerations

This chapter emphasizes the pragmatics of conducting identification audiometry programs in schools. To be effective, any such program must take cognizance of the issues, attitudes, facilities, and budgets existing in the school system generally and the schools to be included particularly. For example, few would debate the desirability of using special hearing testing booths for hearing screening and testing, but to insist that they are essential is to ignore the need for a program that will be obtainable in low socioeconomic, densely populated, urban communities as well as in affluent, sprawling suburbs.

Another consideration is that all too frequently those participating in the identification audiometry program in the schools may be doing so for all the wrong reasons. Even though laws may mandate the identification of the hearing impaired and the administrators may order the programs invested, such directives hardly provide the kind of motivation needed to inspire the participants for an effective and accurate identification of those with impairments. Today, teachers are frequently burdened with a host of extra activities, each justifiable in its own right. Many times the teachers will appropriately question when they have the time to provide the basic instruction society demands. A clear sensitivity to the needs of all professionals in the schools must be demonstrated by the designers and administrators of the identification effort.

The addition of new procedures to existing screening programs involves other practical considerations. For example, research on impedance audiometry (Walton, 1975b) and with automated pure-tone procedures (Wood, Wittich, and Mahaffey, 1973) has demonstrated their viability for use in identification audiometry programs. However, a decision to include new procedures must be based on a well-developed philosophic base for the overall hearing program and must involve careful cost-accounting studies. Too often in the past identification efforts have been undertaken without adequate financial support for follow-up, personnel, and equipment. Consequently, the net result has been minimal in terms of improving the educational situation for hearing-impaired children. An identification effort which serves only to produce lists of "identified children" without offering effective referral and follow-up is worse than no program at all. In the first place, valuable district resources have been wasted. These resources might more appropriately have been expended on other aspects of the total educational effort. Second, parents mistakenly believe that monitoring of their children's hearing is taking place in the school and, therefore, may not seek evaluation in the private sector.

When considering the pragmatics of identification programs, it is important to appreciate the dilemma of over versus under referral (that is, "false positive" and "false negative" results). Criteria so stringent as to fail a high number of those screened may be philosophically justified on the basis that it is better to provide attention for as many potentially handicapped individuals as possible rather than to neglect a single real problem. This solution, however, can be very expensive in terms of the staff time necessary to assess all of the children overreferred. On the other hand, too liberal a set of criteria would pass many who should legitimately be referred for educational and medical attention.

The dilemma of establishing appropriate pass-fail criteria becomes most apparent for those who have borderline hearing impairments. Severe impairments are rather easily identified by the most crude procedure; yet, for children in elementary grades, research provides evidence (for example, see Eagles, 1973) that losses in hearing sensitivity are most likely to be conductive in nature and, therefore, most likely to be transient. This transiency will mean that frequently, when there is a prolonged time lapse between the screening and threshold evaluation and the referral, the children either do not receive appropriate educational management or, when medical attention is finally available, the problem is no longer evident. It cannot be stressed too strongly that the child with the mild-to-moderate conductive impairment is the child most likely to suffer educationally because of the transient nature of his loss and because of the possibility, if not probability, that his hearing needs will be overlooked by both his parents and educators.

Finally, consideration must be given to providing the time necessary to follow audiometrically the hearing status of those who have failed the screening. This follow-up testing is not only for possible referral for special testing and/or medical attention, but also to allow for educational management and possible amplification. Frequently there is an inordinate time lapse between the completion of the screening program and completion of the threshold testing before the child can be referred for necessary medical attention. Meanwhile, the child remains in the same educational environment. Certainly the educational personnel should be informed as soon as possible of the questionable nature of the child's hearing and of procedures that may be used in assisting the child to function optimally.

INADEQUACIES OF IDENTIFICATION AUDIOMETRY PROGRAMS

The accuracy of identification audiometry is stated in terms of the number of correct identifications. Incorrect identifications take two forms: children who fail the procedure, but actually have normal hearing (false positives or overreferrals); children who pass the procedure, but have educationally significant hearing losses (false negatives or underreferrals). To determine either false positives or false negatives, one must first define what is to be used as the validity criterion or "truth." For pure-tone screening, pure-tone threshold tests can serve as the validity criterion if certain assumptions are met: (1) the threshold test occurs in close time proximity to the screen test; independent testers accomplish each test in blind design (no knowledge of other test results); and standard test procedures are used with each child. To determine both false positives *and* false negatives it is necessary to threshold test a substantial number of children, including both those who have failed and those who have passed the screening test. Since the percentage of true failures is relatively small, as is the percentage of false results of either type, it is necessary to complete threshold tests on a large sample if meaningful data are to be developed.

In service programs, determination of false positives is easy: all children who fail the first screen should be scheduled for a rescreen. Children who pass the rescreen represent most of the false positives from the first screen. Children who "pass" a threshold test—hearing levels lower than screening level—represent the remainder of the screening false positives. Determination of false negatives is much more difficult since it necessitates the retesting of a large number of children who pass the first screen, a procedure not normally carried out. However, determination of false negatives is crucial to the evaluation of a methodology, since they represent "fatal" errors in the identification process—children with hearing loss who pass the screen.

Two studies have looked at the accuracy of individual pure-tone screening procedures. Melnick, Eagles, and Levine (1964) studied the accuracy of the identification audiometry procedures developed in 1960 by the National Conference on Identification Audiometry, Baltimore (Darley, 1961), and Wilson and Walton (1974). Both studies found overall accuracy based on results following the rescreen to be about 95%. The inaccuracies ranged from 2% to 3%, depending on whether the validity criterion was restricted to screening frequencies only or included some frequencies not screened.

An important factor related to validity determination is that as the number of actual identified losses declines as a result of a successful hearing conservation program, the number of false negatives seems to remain constant. In such cases, the relative accuracy of the method appears to have declined. Research is badly needed on how to reduce false negatives in present screening paradigms. For example, Wilson and Walton (1974) found that first-graders without exception presented the highest inaccuracy figures when compared to kindergarten children and second-, third- and fifth-graders. One might predict that while the tester expects the kindergarten child to need special attention and instructions for the task, he might expect the first-grade child to remember the task from his kindergarten test period. Our results suggest that the first-grade child needs the same attention typically provided to the kindergarten child if we are to expect equivalent accuracy; this question should be studied in terms of instructional set, possible change of test from constant vigilance task to a detection paradigm, etc., since serious effort must be devoted to finding efficient means of reducing the false negative results of any screening procedure.

If the accuracy of pure-tone screening audiometry is defined by success in the detection of otopathology, any number of studies have shown the lack of validity of the method for such purposes. In such cases, otoscopy has usually become the validity criterion. The publications from the Pittsburgh Study (e.g., Eagles, 1961, 1972, 1973; Eagles et al., 1963; Jordan, 1972; Jordan and Eagles, 1961; and Melnick, Eagles, and Levine, 1964) stand out as classics on this topic.

CLINICAL METHODS AND INTERPRETATIONS

Bases of an Effective Identification Audiometry Program

Early attention must be paid to establishing the roles and responsibilities of each individual to be involved in the identification audiometry program, no matter how minimal the actual involvement might be. Who will test? Who will interpret, refer, recommend? Who will follow up, counsel? All responsibilities must be agreed upon in advance. Close alliances among the speech pathology and audiology staff, administration, instructional personnel, and other school professionals such as psychologists, social workers, counselors, nurses, and reading specialists must be developed to meet the educational needs of the children in a comprehensive manner. Each person to be involved must be identified and his respective responsibilities delineated *in writing* to reduce confusion and concern for professional "territories."

Administrative Organization. A cost-effective identification audiometry program is built on the efficient and effective use of the time of all the testing and support personnel. This requires an organized screening team. We suggest that the basic team consist of an administrator and a professional and two assistants for screening. Ideally, the administrator should be an ASHA-certified audiologist who has thorough knowledge of pure-tone audiometric screening procedures and the many subtleties of screening and testing school children, as well as a thorough knowledge of educational programming for the hearing-impaired. The administrator's responsibilities include designing the entire identification effort, securing suitable facilities and equipment, selecting and training personnel, obtaining the necessary clearances, and monitoring the screening while it is in progress.

Experienced personnel who have been involved in audiometric testing may not welcome supervision and counsel regarding their screening techniques. Nevertheless, in our experience all persons—even certified audiologists—do on occasion need counsel with respect to improving their screening and threshold-testing techniques. The administrator should be cognizant of all details affecting the screening effort and, in particular, should allow adequate time to observe the screening techniques of each tester. Because most students want to pass every test—including a hearing test—they are consciously searching for cues as to when the stimuli are present. When errors are made on the part of the testers and cues are inadvertently provided, the students are assisted in passing the test when perhaps they ought not—a false-negative identification. In such cases, the student with true loss of hearing sensitivity may be unintentionally passed—a serious error in the identification process since he will not be reassessed. Concern for the false-negative identification must always be uppermost in the minds of the administrator and those performing the testing.

Administrative Support. Laws, both federal and state, may mandate the identification and treatment of the hearing-impaired, and prevalence statistics on hearing impairment may sensitize the local education administration to the need for an identification effort; yet, administrative support will be predicated on the preparation of a comprehensive identification and remediation program. A carefully conceived and detailed plan that includes all aspects of the program, particularly the follow-up, is essential for effective support from the superintendent, principals, board of education, and especially the classroom teachers. Consideration should be given to sponsoring workshops to explain the purposes of the identification effort and to outline the responsibilities of all personnel. Such workshops should focus on plans for future maintenance of the program to ensure proper follow-through for those identified.

Plans should be formulated for securing the support of the local director of nursing and the local medical consultants and physicians. The program should never be promoted as a means for locating all children with medically significant middle-ear conditions; nevertheless, those whom the program does identify need medical examination, and the support of the medical profession is critical to an effective effort. Consideration should be given to involving the medical practitioners in planning the program and to inviting their observation of the testing and referral processes when they are actually in progress in order to benefit from their suggestions. It is particularly important to be aware of any local referral criteria that may have been adopted by the health personnel so that acceptable referrals can be made.

Personnel. Responsible to the administrator of the identification program is a professional audiologist, speech pathologist, or nurse who has been designated to do the screening. This person must also be thoroughly familiar with the procedures to be employed. While the professional concentrates on the screening, assistants expedite the process by preparing the students for screening, controlling the student traffic, and recording results. Nurses' aides, responsible high school students, and volunteers recruited from parent-teacher or community service organizations can be used as assistants. Overall efficiency may be increased even more and disruption of classroom activities reduced further by increasing the number of persons screening and recording. We strongly recommend that a minimum of two screening stations operate simultaneously in a school.

When bilingual students are included, provision must be made for adequate translation of the instructions into the student's native language. Other personnel whose participation is essential to the success of the program are secretaries and clerks. Their responsibilities include preparing lists of the names of the students to be screened and notifying the teachers of the screening schedule. School custodians are needed to arrange furniture and to see that the rooms are comfortably lighted, heated, and ventilated. Using those persons competent to screen for screening while others prepare the students, record results, manage traffic, prepare lists, and arrange facilities will significantly enhance the efficiency and effectiveness of the screening activity.

Training and Preparation. Provision should be made for the training and preparation of all personnel to be involved in the program. Concern should be given to the training and preparation of those directly involved in the testing and referral processes and also to the training of the teachers, psychologists, social workers, counselors, and reading specialists who have professional contact with hearing-impaired students. The particular responsibilities of each individual involved in the program should be addressed in workshops. Workshops in which the professionals have direct exposure to the problems of the hearing-impaired students would enhance the significance of the training and increase the likelihood that the material will be incorporated into their own daily contacts with the students.

Confidentiality. The Family Educational Rights and Privacy Act (Federal Register, Volume 41, No. 118, June 17, 1976, 24662-24675) details the procedures to be followed in protecting confidentiality, describes the rights of the individuals to know what is being retained about them, provides for challenge to the information, establishes procedures for altering or eliminating the information, provides for safeguards as to the storage and disclosure of information, details procedures respecting the transmission of information to a third party, and details procedures for the destruction of data.

In conducting an identification audiometry program, the law requires that notice be given to the parents or guardians of those involved. Ordinarily this is accomplished by what is called "informed consent": notices are sent home with the student and the parents are given the opportunity to comment or to exclude their children from participation. Particular problems arise in defining what constitutes "informed consent." If the parent does not receive the notice sent home, through no negligence of school personnel, has the intent of the law been satisfied? It is clear from the law that the burden is on the agency initiating the activity to make certain that consent is obtained. The law also requires that the notification shall be in such a style and language as to be understandable to the responsible adults. In addition public awareness of the identification effort must be assured through appropriate announcements in the local newspaper or public service announcements on radio or television.

Although this chapter recommends the use of aides and volunteers, we appreciate the difficulty of protecting against unauthorized divulgence of personal information by nonprofessionals. Professional expectations regarding confidentiality may not be fully appreciated by nonprofessionals. Nevertheless, they must be clearly and forthrightly counseled on this matter by the program administrator. Consideration should be given to having the volunteers and paraprofessionals serve at schools other than those their children attend.

Target Population. Public law 94-142 requires that the educational needs of all handicapped children from birth through age 21 (up to their twenty-second birthday) be provided for. Most likely those of primary concern to the schools will be between the ages of 5 and 18, although provisions should be made to accommodate children between the ages of 3 and 21. Local statutes may restrict the overall age range to something less.

The ideal screening audiometry program would allow different schedules for different children, depending on history, past screening results, diseases suffered, and such. Such a system would require a data storage and retrieval system not widely available at present; moreover, funding for such idealism is rare. Nonetheless, annual mass screening of all school children is wasteful of personnel time; what is needed is a means by which children in need of more frequent screening can be seen on a flexible schedule.

At present, most programs focus their annual screening efforts on the first three or four grades. After grade three, children may be followed at three- to four-year intervals. Downs, Doster, and Wever (1965) have suggested that routine screening beyond grade three is not justified on a cost versus benefit analysis. The time saved in a program emphasizing the lower grades can be used to follow-up more adequately those children at risk—screening test failures, chronic illness, and teacher referrals, for example. A sample set of guidelines for pure-tone identification audiometry programs in schools is included in Appendix A of this chapter and provides a suggested set of criteria for the selection of children.

Equipment—Caveat Emptor! Even for the most seasoned clinical audiologist, caution in the selection of audiometric equipment makes good sense. Daily, it seems, a new manufacturer offers audiometric equipment designed for use in schools. Since the acquisition of such equipment may constitute the single largest equipment purchase by the professionals involved, thoughtful consideration should be given to the choice. All audiometric equipment used in the schools should meet the current *American National Standard Specifications for Audiometers* of the American National Standards Institute (ANSI, 1970). In addition, counsel should be obtained from other professionals who have used the equipment in similar circumstances.

Although it would be surprising to find an audiometer that is not advertised as meeting all of the specifications of the ANSI, more factors are included in the ANSI specification than are ordinarly rigorously controlled by the manufacturers or rigorously checked by most calibration laboratories. In a study on the stability of routinely serviced audiometers, Walton and Williams (1972) reported on the accuracy with which 50 routinely serviced audiometers used in public schools met all of the calibration requirements of the ANSI. The performance of the audiometers was determined for each of the 13 factors detailed by the Institute. Of the audiometers 82% had one or more of the 13 types of errors evaluated. The six most frequently encountered, in decreasing order of occurrence, were problems with: (1) mechanical conditions; (2) extraneous noise; (3) intensity; (4) rise time; (5) linearity; and (6) frequency. The authors recommended that these factors be assessed on every audiometer at least once a year. Full evaluation of the other factors detailed by the Institute should be completed at least every two years.

Intensity is the single most critical factor affecting the accuracy of an audiometric test; however, any parameter that does not meet the specification of the Institute *can* adversely affect the testing results. For example, Walton and Wilson (1974a) in a study on the relationship between audiometer rise time and pass/fail ratios in identification audiometry, observed that significantly more children passed a screening test when screened with an audiometer having excessively fast rise time as compared to their performance on an audiometer having rise time meeting the specifications of the Institute.

Walton and Wilson (1974b) have reported on the stability of pure-tone audiometers during periods of heavy use in identification audiometry. Fifteen audiometers that were being used in a school screening program received daily electro-acoustic calibration checks on the six factors found critical by Walton and Williams (1972). Some audiometers required circuit modifications to meet calibration requirements initially, but it was observed that once calibrated, all but 1 of the 15 audiometers held to specifications over the course of the screening program. The authors concluded that the stability of the audiometers was good. Perhaps what had been at issue in the generally condemnatory reports on audiometer calibration, such as those by Thomas et al. (1969) and Walton and Williams (1972), was the possibility that the audiometers previously assessed may never have met specifications. Eagles and Doerfler (1961) also have reported that audiometers labeled as meeting specifications did not, in fact, meet all specifications when delivered new and required actual circuit modifications to allow them to satisfy calibration standards.

This fact suggests that when ordering audiometric test equipment, the audiologist should stipulate that the equipment must meet all current ANSI specifications in the as-delivered condition. Then, the audiologist must be prepared to check the equipment or have someone else check the equipment at delivery to determine that this requirement has been met. Likewise, the administrator of a hearing screening program should require that laboratories providing calibration services for his equipment be prepared to provide full-scale calibration on all factors of the ANSI specifications. This is not to imply that those persons calibrating audiometers have been negligent, but rather to suggest that the responsibility rests with those requesting the service. They should specify how their audiometers are to be calibrated and be willing to bear the expense. A calibrated audiometer is one that meets all of the requirements of the current specifications. Those who believe that some of the factors included in the specifications are of no consequence and can therefore be ignored should cite evidence to support their position.

Walton and Wilson (1974b) recommended that weekly intensity assessments of audiometers by sound-level meter as well as daily performance checks and the monitoring of sequential test results should be carried out. Wilber (1972) has provided detailed suggestions for performance checks the clinician can easily conduct on an audiometer, and Walton (1975a), in a narrated film strip, demonstrates such procedures. Finally, Walton and Wilson conclude it is essential that spare audiometers be available during the conduct of an identification audiometry program and recommend that a reserve of approximately one audiometer for every five in use be provided. It is a false economy not to provide such spare equipment since audiometer malfunction will halt the identification audiometry effort, causing serious disruptions in programming and necessitating rescheduling. Furthermore, substantial staff time is usually wasted when such malfunctions occur.

Audiometric equipment manufactured today is more rugged and stable than that of five years ago. With more attention being paid to electrical and mechanical stability, the audiometers can be expected to sustain more abuse. Nevertheless, operators should recognize that the equipment is still somewhat fragile and caution should be exercised in transporting and operating it.

A final cautionary note about the purchase of equipment for which calibration standards do not exist: Unfortunately, some manufacturers provide audiometric test equipment with earphones and/or bone oscillators for which no calibration standard has been promulgated. In such cases, the purchaser is left with equipment that cannot be calibrated by the calibration lab. Although loudness-balance procedures can be used with such equipment, the procedures are time-consuming and therefore expensive. It is far more economical in the long run for the purchaser to be sure that the equipment is supplied with standard transducer units for which calibration values currently exist.

Timing. Walton (1975b), in a study of identification audiometry procedures conducted in six Connecticut communities during the winter and spring of 1973/ 74, observed that the pass-fail ratios for the pure-tone screening results were essentially unaffected by the seasonal variation. Eagles et al. (1963), in a 22-month study in Pittsburgh, also found no consistent seasonal trend in pure-tone hearing sensitivity measurements. They did find periods of reduced sensitivity that coincided with epidemics of acute respiratory infections; however, the epidemics did not occur consistently in the same month each year. With regard to tympanometry test results, Walton (1975b) did find consistent group mean results showing poorer compliance and higher negative air pressure in the winter as compared to the spring. Accordingly, more tympanometry screening failures occurred in the winter.

Ideally, the necessary screening and follow-up testing would be conducted during the summer, prior to the beginning of the school year. Realistically, however, scheduling screening for the early fall is probably the most desirable. A program carefully developed and coordinated during the preceding spring should be operational within the first few weeks of the school year. Concluding the program before the middle of November will allow sufficient time for appropriate referral and follow-up testing so that the child will receive the maximum benefits available from the educational experience. In cases where initial screening testing is scheduled over the entire school year, many children are identified too late in the year to receive appropriate intervention to maximize their educational experience. Classroom teachers should be informed of the screening results early in the school year if a student's hearing is in doubt. Following threshold assessment, consultation with the teacher about classroom management is required.

One might question how staff personnel can be deployed so as to be involved in the intensive screening aspects of the program and still have an appropriate work load throughout the remainder of the year. However, in the hearing program suggested in this chapter, the mass screening is simply the first step. Follow-up testing, referral, and continued testing of those identified as well as educational management of children with irreversible hearing losses, are the primary functions of the audiology staff during the remainder of the school year.

Many school systems conduct prekindergarten screening programs in the spring, prior to a child's entrance into school. Inclusion of hearing screening within the total screening program is strongly recommended so that, when necessary, appropriate medical intervention and educational planning can be provided before the child starts school.

Record-Keeping. Record-keeping should serve two basic purposes: (1) to document the hearing status of each individual student; and (2) to facilitate administration of the program by providing a data base for program modifications. Administration of the program from the viewpoint of cost necessitates keeping records that provide a time base for each of the procedures. Records should identify student, grade, school, sex, time of day, equipment used, test procedure, and tester as well as test results. Coding of this detailed information facilitates administrative planning. For example, determination of pass-fail data by audiometer will often suggest calibration needs; likewise, pass-fail data as a function of tester may suggest the need for more detailed instruction. The data to be kept on each individual student are dictated by the particular record-keeping systems employed in a district, community, or state. As previously noted, data systems must be consistent with laws concerning confidentiality.

Simple computer programs are available to automate the data-keeping suggested in this section. For example, mark-sense record sheets (see example in Appendix B) can provide automated scoring and analysis. With appropriate algorithms, the computer program can provide outputs appropriate for transmittal of information to parents, school health records, and student educational records and can provide schedules for rescreening and follow-up testing. Where such systems are not available, volunteers can be trained to record and tally such data if appropriate forms are developed. We cannot overemphasize the importance of appropriate data-keeping for both purposes described in this section. Far too often, screening service programs have kept data only on an individual student basis and have not been able to provide the documentation appropriate for designing changes in screening strategies. When one considers the large numbers of children who are screened each year, it is interesting to note how few studies have appeared in the literature which describe modifications in existing screening programs based on data collected as a part of the service program.

Facilities. Careful selection of the facilities to be employed in the identification program is essential. Excess noise is the single most important factor to consider.

The ASHA *Guidelines for Identification Audiometry* (1975) provide approximate allowable octave-band ambient noise levels for screening testing. Since many school programs will need a sound-level meter to check audiometer intensity calibration, prospective screening sites can be checked against the ASHA suggested values if the sound-level meter purchased is selected with octave-band measurement capabilities. The *American Standard Criteria for Background Noise In Audiometer Rooms* (1960)[1] provides maximum allowable noise values that can be applied to threshold testing sites.

Our experience has been that the allowable noise values presented in the ASHA document must be considered the maximum allowable ambient noise. In an unpublished study relating screening test results to measured ambient noise levels, we found that even though all schools evaluated had maximum noise levels within acceptable limits, the pass/fail ratio varied systematically as a function of noise levels. In fact, three times as many children failed the initial screening test in the school with the highest noise level compared to the school with the lowest noise level even though both schools were within the limits suggested in the ASHA document. Thus, we were led to conclude that although a test space may be adequately quiet in that it does not provide masking of the test signal, attention factors are equally important. Children asked to accomplish a listening task in a quieter environment with fewer noise distractions will show a lower percentage of failures on a screening task.

These data suggest that perhaps sound isolation in school test sites would be justified from the point of view of program efficiency. When a screening program can present data detailing the specific number of overreferrals produced by having to carry out the screening programs in environments with higher levels of noise, it may well be possible to convince district administration that provision of additional sound isolation is cost-effective. For example, if a given school environment annually produces 40 children who fail the screening and rescreening sequence because of noise levels, the cost of providing threshold evaluation for those 40 children each year will be substantial. Given this approach to description of sound isolation needs, it may be far easier to justify the provision of sound isolation where *required*. Without supporting documentation, the school administration will generally react negatively to arguments that each school should be provided with a sound-isolated space.

Where sound-level measurement equipment is not available, a test site can be analyzed for noise in a different manner. By determining threshold for a normal-hearing individual, using a low frequency pure-tone in different possible test locations, one can infer the best site by choosing the one that produced the lowest threshold value. If, in the site selected, ambient noise prohibits a person with normal hearing from responding to a tone of 1000 Hz at a level of 15dB

---

[1] This ANSI document is undergoing revision at the time of this writing (December, 1976); a new document on allowable background noise should be available soon.

HL, the room must not be used for screening until the noise levels are reduced. Screening levels must never be raised to accommodate the noise in a particular room. Raising the screening level invalidates the screening effort. Sometimes it is possible to reduce the noise level in a test environment by providing portable incandescent lighting to replace fluorescent lighting, temporarily turning off the heating or cooling system, and controlling the movement of students in halls near the test room.

The facility should also be checked for availability of electrical power, room furniture arrangement for traffic flow, heating or cooling, and other physical arrangements. The comfort and safety of the testers who will be working in the test room should be considered. Moreover, sound-isolated test environments must provide visual and/or auditory hookup to the building alarm system to provide warning in case of fire or civil disaster.

Funding. In determining the cost of the identification audiometry program, a fundamental responsibility of the program administrator, all expenses should be included: personnel, equipment depreciated over life expectancy, maintenance-calibration, forms, secretaries and custodial personnel, telephone, stationery supplies, computer time, and printing. Total costs as well as the cost per child served should be recorded. Per-child accounting necessitates keeping records on the average number screened per hour, the time required for re-screening, threshold testing, and referral and follow-up activities.

Given the limited financial resources ordinarily available, cost factors must be considered in determining program policy. Any tendency of the administrator to mask true costs is inappropriate. The true costs should be presented as accurately and as completely as possible so that adequate funding can be found to meet the statutory and professional responsibilities to identify and serve the hearing impaired.

It is our opinion that the basic personnel costs should be borne by the particular agency. In addition, consideration should be given to securing financial support from private service organizations, which are often willing to contribute money to purchase audiometers, pay for their maintenance and upkeep, and even supply volunteer help. Program administrators should be aware that Public Law 94-142 provides that a certain portion of the federal support for special education must pass through the State Education Agency to the local education agencies for building their respective programs. Where a district finds itself without sufficient equipment, consideration should be given to applying for federal funds through the state agency.

The thorough program administrator will be knowledgeable concerning the total cost of the program, will be firm in his rationale for supporting the program, will be able to defend each of the costs on a time/effort basis, and will be diligent in seeking both school district as well as private, not-for-profit, funding. Extreme care should be exercised in accepting funding from those who stand to benefit financially from the identification effort. Potential conflicts of interest should be scrupulously avoided.

Conducting the Identification Audiometry Program

Screen-to-Reevaluation Sequence. The first step in the sequence is the pure-tone screening test, followed by a rescreen for all children failing the initial test. It is essential that the rescreen phase be included. Melnick, Eagles, and Levine (1964) found that 27% of the children who failed the first screen passed a second screen, even when the first screen was given in a sound-treated room. Wilson and Walton (1974) found that 52% of the children who failed the first screen passed the rescreen and Walton (1975b) found a 51% reduction in failures. While each of these studies dealt with school-age children, Seidemann and Laguaite (1973) reported a 54% screen-rescreen reduction in a population of 900 inner-city pre-school children.

When tympanometry is included in the screening battery, the audiologist likewise should be aware that rescreen or multiple test sessions are advisable. For example, Walton (1975b) reported a 30% reduction in false-positive identifications by retesting tympanometry. Although a number of authors (for example, Brooks, 1971; Liden, Peterson, and Bjorkman, 1970) have demonstrated highly repeatable test-retest tympanometry data for normal ears, Lewis et al. (1975) reported on the day-to-day variability of tympanograms obtained from children with active pathology. Because of the variability, which they believe reflects change in middle-ear status, they feel that referral should be based on successive-day screening with criteria for referral being based on the pattern of results. Other authors (Orchik and Herdman, 1974; Cooper et al., 1975) have also commented on the high overreferral rate which occurs with a single tympanometry screening.

Collectively, these data suggest that failure of either pure-tone initial screen or tympanometry initial screen should result in a rescreen test for referral. In this chapter, we have strongly recommended that screening audiometry be followed by audiometric assessment with referral for either educational or medical management based on such assessment. One might question why we recommend the step of rescreen if assessment is to follow the initial screening effort. The answer is one of economics. It is far less expensive to rescreen a child than it is to schedule him for assessment. For example, a school district in which 8000 children are screened in a year might have 600 to 800 children who would fail the initial pure-tone screen and pass a rescreen. If those children were referred for audiometric assessment based on the results of the initial screen, the man-hours involved would be overwhelming. On the other hand, the simple act of rescreening all children who fail the initial screen takes far less time and therefore is much more cost efficient. Similar results would occur with tympanometry.

We feel, then, that inclusion of the rescreen procedure in the sequence of testing is mandatory. In fact, we feel it most appropriate to talk about screening test results based on the results following the second, or rescreen, test, since the group that fails both screens more properly represents the yield from the screening effort. Finally, we should note that identification audiometry programs that base medical referral on the results of the first pure-tone screening test will have a serious source of error in the large number of overreferrals, often producing a "credibility gap" with the medical community.

Threshold testing follows the screening effort. As a minimum, threshold assessment is strongly recommended prior to medical referral; more detailed evaluation is preferred. Where possible, it is highly recommended that threshold testing be part of a total audiometric assessment. It is essential that detailed information about each child with hearing impairment be obtained if appropriate educational management is to occur. In districts that cannot provide such assessment, it is essential that children be referred for full-scale audiometric appraisal. Air-conduction threshold testing does not provide an adequate base for developing a program of educational management for the child who is hearing-impaired. Thus, educational management must be based on the results of more detailed testing.

After audiometric assessment, appropriate personnel should confer about the management of the child in question. Conferences and/or referrals for medical management should be handled through the health personnel in the school. Conferences on educational programming should include all interested professionals—speech and hearing personnel, teacher, counselors. The parents should be informed of the results of the screening and evaluative procedures and included in the planning for educational management of their child. It is often beneficial if a single person assumes responsibility for follow-through on management of the child—the audiologist may be the appropriate person to assume such a role. This person monitors the status of referrals, reviews incoming reports detailing the results of such referrals, and reconvenes the management team when new information indicates a need to change the child's programming. Periodic rescreening and reevaluation are integral parts of this program.

In many districts, it is not presently possible to follow children throughout the year with periodic rescreens. We need additional research to allow us to find adequate predictors of children needing such assessment. However, we would recommend that, as a minimum, each child who is referred for medical therapy be either rescreened or reevaluated periodically throughout the school year until consecutive tests show no fluctuation in his hearing levels. This research of Holm and Kunze (1969) and Kaplan et al. (1973) suggests a need for additional concern over the effect of even very mild conductive losses on the academic achievement of children. A program to monitor these "high risk" children much more frequently than the present annual test is desirable.

Pass-Fail Criteria. For pure-tone screening tests, it is recommended that failure to respond satisfactorily at any test frequency in either ear is the basis for failure of the screening test. We would emphasize that use of the word failure here is restricted to results of the test and does not necessarily imply hearing loss. Likewise, we would point out that multiple presentations of a signal at a single frequency/ear setting can be used with this procedure. The tester must satisfy himself that the child does in fact hear the signal at each of the frequencies for both ears if the child is to be scored as having passed the screening test. We recommend use of the same pass-fail criteria for the rescreening test.

Any child failing the second screening evaluation (rescreen) should be seen for threshold testing. As noted above, we consider air-conduction threshold assessment as a minimum prior to referral for medical evaluation. Any child showing thresholds greater than 20dB at frequencies up through and including 2000 Hz or 25dB at frequencies above 2000 Hz should be considered for referral. Specific criteria for either medical referral or consideration of educational programming cannot be based only on air-conduction threshold scores, but rather, must be based on the collective information available on the child.

Pass-fail criteria for tympanometry screening are not standardized at this time; nor is the instrumentation used. Results are even obtained in different measurement units. Thus, the clinician must develop his own criteria, based on the instrument used and the available data base for that instrument and procedure.

Reevaluation should be scheduled regularly for all children with known hearing loss. In particular, children undergoing medical therapy for such losses should be evaluated on a regular basis either by the schools or as a part of the medical treatment.

Screening Techniques and Procedures. A set of general guidelines for individual pure-tone identification audiometry was developed in 1970 by the National Conference on Identification Audiometry (Darley, 1961). These guidelines called for the screening test to take place in a sound-treated test room, and included screening at the frequencies of 1000, 2000, 4000, and 6000 Hz. The recommendation as to inclusion of 500 Hz was ambiguous. The applicability of the guidelines to most identification audiometry programs was limited by the fact that screening testing was to be conducted in sound-treated test rooms. Most school districts do not have sound-treated rooms in each school building and very few have mobile test vans for moving the test environment from school to school. Consequently, identification audiometry usually is conducted at best in a quiet part of the school building.

Recognition that sound-treated rooms generally are not available led to the development and acceptance of a new set of procedures for identification audiometry by ASHA, entitled *Guidelines for Identification Audiometry* (1975).

The main points are as follows:

1. Test frequencies shall be 1000, 2000, and 4000 Hz.
2. Screening levels shall be 20dB HL (ANSI, 1969) at 1000 and 2000 Hz and 25dB at 4000 Hz.
3. Failure criterion shall be failure to respond at the recommended screening level at one or more frequencies in either ear.
4. Mandatory rescreening shall occur within one week for all screen failures.
5. Audiologic evaluations are to be accomplished for individuals failing the rescreening.
6. Medical referrals should be based on the results of audiologic evaluations.
7. Screening personnel should have professional preparation in screening young children.

These recommendations differ from those suggested by the National Conference on Identification Audiometry in the following ways: (1) there is no recommendation that testing be conducted in acoustically treated test rooms; (2) the frequencies of 500 and 6000 Hz are excluded; and (3) rescreening of all failures is mandatory.

The ASHA techniques were evaluated by Wilson and Walton (1974) in a field experiment conducted in the Renton, Washington, School District and involving over 7,800 students. With threshold test results obtained in a blind experiment as the reference data, the ASHA screening techniques were found to be better than 95% accurate in terms of correct identifications. Walton (1975a), in a set of three filmstrips on identification audiometry in the schools intended for instructing paraprofessionals, has in a simple manner presented the essential features of the ASHA recommendations.

Special comment is warranted relative to the screening frequencies included in the ASHA guidelines—1000 Hz and above. Screening at frequencies below 1000 Hz can be included in the program *if* an adequate test environment in terms of ambient noise is available. However, ambient noise generally has its greatest energy in the low frequencies and accordingly most affects testing of 250 and 500 Hz. Few school test sites that do not have special sound treatment will provide an adequate test environment for these low frequencies. Inclusion of these frequencies without an adequate test environment will greatly increase the overreferrals from the screening program. Proponents of screening at low frequencies point out that certain otopathologies will be better detected by so doing. However, use of tympanometry as a part of the screening program can accomplish the same goal more accurately at perhaps less expense than providing sound-treated test rooms.

Considerable interest has been shown during the last few years in the possibility of combining tympanometry and pure-tone screening techniques to develop a composite model that might serve both educational and medical referral needs. Walton (1975b) investigated the feasibility of using such a combined model in a total of 32 elementary schools located in 6 Connecticut towns. In all, 7,928 children received both tympanometry and pure-tone screening testing. It was concluded by the author that the routine inclusion of tympanometry in hearing conservation programs for schools is practicable and desirable. Nursing and speech and hearing personnel were quickly taught to operate the equipment and obtain reliable data. The slight additional time required for such testing was found to be more than offset by the valuable information obtained on the status of the middle ear. The author advised that abnormal tympanometry results, suggesting otopathology, should be monitored over time to establish whether the condition is chronic or transient and used as supportive evidence of the need for referral.

Using volunteers for data recording and traffic management, Walton (1975b) found that an average of 1.5 minutes was required for tympanometric testing and 1.0 minutes for pure-tone screening. Walton found further that usable tympanometric data were obtained from 99.94% of the cases—indicating the utility of tympanometry in elementary schools.

Hygiene in Testing. Too little attention has been paid to this topic in most public school audiometry programs. For pure-tone assessment, the audiologist should have available spare sets of earphone cushions so that the cushions can be exchanged when a child shows evidence of active pathology in the external canal or pinna area. Cushions can easily be sterilized by ultraviolet light (Talbott, 1969) with inexpensive equipment. Where impedance audiometry is part of the screening or assessment test battery, the clinician must be equipped to sterilize the ear tips. This can present logistical problems in large-scale screening programs, since many tips are needed in the course of one day. Walton (1975b) has described his solutions to these problems.

Efficiency in Screening. Efficiency in screening involves consideration of time: disruption time, action time, and staff time. Screening procedures inevitably disrupt the normal curricular schedules, affecting students, teachers, administrators, aides, custodians, clerical and secretarial personnel, and volunteers. Those involved in screening must be sensitive to the needs and feelings of those affected by the screening and do everything possible to minimize the effects of the disruption.

A cost-effective identification audiometry program is built on efficient and effective use of the time of all testing and support personnel. This requires an organized screening team as has been described above. A screening schedule for each school and class must be developed and agreed to well in advance (see Appendix B for sample forms). Allowances should be made for special school programs, bus schedules, group achievement testing, lunch and recess schedules, and so forth. The administrator of the program should know in advance the planned activity for each period of each class on the days scheduled for screening. Efficiency is generally enhanced by attention to detail.

Careful attention must be paid to the physical details of conducting the screening. The room arrangements should accommodate at least two screening stations with minimal interference from the flow of traffic. The audiometers should be positioned, checked, and allowed to warm up prior to use. Power cords should be taped in place to reduce any hazard to the students. "Quiet" signs in corridors and screenings areas and announcements in the classrooms will help keep the noise at acceptable levels.

To prepare the students, class lessons on hearing might be scheduled prior to the days of the screening. Study materials, filmstrips, and talks from members of the speech pathology and audiology staff, nurses, and local physicians will help the students appreciate the importance of hearing and of noise control during the screening and testing period. Persons who familiarize the students with the screening procedures must be thoroughly familiar with these procedures themselves and follow the techniques agreed to in the particular identification audiometry program. Familiarizing the students with the task will reduce anxiety and increase the efficiency of the screening. The screening administrator should monitor periodically the preparatory activities.

To minimize disruption, an entire class of 25 to 30 students should be taken at one time. The adults accompanying the class maintain order and remind the students of the necessity of being quiet. Each student must be easily identifiable so that those doing the screening will not waste time guessing names. With the students identified and in a predetermined order, between 6 and 8 can be admitted to the screening area at a time. An assistant will maintain order within the area and direct the students to the desired screening station.

Those persons assigned to screening should restrict their activities to this; their assistants record the results and monitor traffic. The person recording must be certain that the student is identified correctly and the results recorded accurately. Test personnel should not have to wait for a student to screen; a steady flow of students to the screening stations and a steady testing pace permit the screening of approximately one student per minute per station. The administrator of the screening operation should monitor frequently the performance at each screening station.

Threshold Testing. Threshold testing as well as more detailed audiometric assessment should be accomplished by a certified audiologist. Although air-conduction threshold testing can be completed at the screening site if testing is limited to the frequencies screened, the requirements for facilities and equipment usually will be somewhat higher to allow an adequate test environment for this more detailed assessment. Therefore, it is recommended that a district provide a single location—either a central location or a mobile test unit—for such evaluations. This may require that transportation be provided for the child to the assessment site.

It is urgent that such assessment occur as soon as possible after the screening so that appropriate referrals can be expeditiously carried out. In some districts, it may be more efficient to divide the assessment procedure into threshold assessment and more detailed assessment and to make medical referrals on the basis of the threshold assessment. Then, following medical evaluation, more thorough evaluation can take place. However, we would hasten to note that it is equally urgent that the necessary test data be developed for educational planning; any delay in such planning may harm the child's education. Specific procedures for threshold testing with children are given in other chapters of this book and in a number of other sources (for example, Martin, 1975) and will not be repeated here.

The school program must be prepared to deal with questions concerning appropriate amplification for children with hearing loss. These questions include selection and maintenance of wearable amplification as well as selection and maintenance of classroom amplification systems. A number of studies (for example, Gaeth and Lounsbury, 1966; Zink, 1972) have shown that the use of amplification by hearing-impaired children in the schools has not been optimal even in terms of simple working conditions of the amplfying devices themselves. It is beyond the scope of this chapter to deal with this issue; however, we wish to state very strongly that it is the responsibility of the school program to determine that decision points are reached and management strategies carried out in the area of amplification (see Chap. 12 for more detail). If the school district does not have appropriate staff or equipment for evaluation, it must see that the parents receive appropriate recommendations for acquiring such information.

Special Cases. Inclusion of preschool children in a public school identification audiometry effort is highly recommended where funding is available. We have found that the standard pure-tone screening procedure recommended in this chapter is applicable to preschool children as young as 3½ years of age, and have routinely used it in screening 300 preschool children each year. For a small percentage of the children, we must go to a play response (stacking toy); however, most children can complete the test easily if the instruction is modified to fit their age level. Likewise, tympanometry procedures are easily used on children of any age.

For those younger than 3 and for the developmentally delayed, some modifications in test procedure, ranging from a simple change in response mode to more elaborate modifications, may be necessary. In such cases, we favor use of operant test procedures similar to those described by Dr. Fulton, in Chapter 6 of this book. For example, Wilson, Moore, and Thompson (1977) and Moore et al. (unpublished manuscript) have shown that the head-turn response coupled with visual reinforcement can be used to satisfactorily develop auditory thresholds for infants as young as 6 months of age both in sound field and under earphones. Greenberg et al. (unpublished manuscript) and Decker and Wilson (1977) have shown that these procedures can be applied successfully to a high percentage of severely retarded children. For screening purposes, this procedure can be quickly accomplished and sampling can occur with several types of signals in both the sound field and under an earphone. When coupled with impedance audiometry, such evaluation allows an appropriate base for referral.

Since these procedures require more elaborate equipment than could easily be used on a portable basis, testing is usually carried out in a soundroom. Also, such testing requires the skills of a certified audiologist, since decisions must be made concerning the most appropriate approach to each individual.

Typical Findings. Fig. 11-1 presents the results obtained from one controlled study conducted in Connecticut during 1974 which utilized the recommendations in this chapter (Walton, 1975b). Over 8,000 students received initial and, where necessary, rescreenings. The students, kindergarten through fifth grade, were drawn from six towns representing diverse socioeconomic, racial/ethnic, and urban/suburban populations. As shown, 77.9% passed the initial pure-tone screening and 71.0% passed the initial tympanometry screening. The number failing initially but passing the rescreening was 11.3% of the total for pure-tone screening and 8.7% for tymanometry. Almost twice as many (20.3%) failed two tympanometry screenings as failed the two pure-tone screenings (10.8%). Two-ear failures were more than twice as common for tympanometry (11.9%) as they were for pure-tone testing (4.6%).

Performance by grade on the respective tests is shown in Fig. 11-2. Improved performance with increased grade is evident for all three tests, but most pronounced for tympanometry. From kindergarten through grade five, those failing pure-tone screening decreased from 17.2% to 6.6%. Similar results are shown for tympanometry where the slope of the curve approaches that for pure-tone screening but appears to asymptote somewhere beyond the fifth grade.

The importance of conducting a rescreening is illustrated by Fig. 11-3, where the reduction in false-positive identifications is shown as a function of grade level. As illustrated, approximately 50% of the children who failed the initial pure-tone screening passed the rescreening; 30% of those who failed the initial tympanometry passed the rescreen.

Pure-tone screening performance by frequency and grade was examined by combining the results for the two ears and then computing the respective pass/fail ratios. Fig. 11-4 presents the percentage failing each of the test frequencies as a function of grade level. Consistently, more children failed at 1000 Hz than at any of the other frequencies; failure at 4000 Hz was the second most frequent. Inasmuch as the ambient noise levels were monitored and found to be insufficient for masking at the screening frequencies, it is possible that the increase in failures at 1000 Hz was due primarily to conductive losses while the increase in failures at 4000 Hz was due primarily to sensorineural losses.

Caution should be exercised in using the percentage figures provided in this

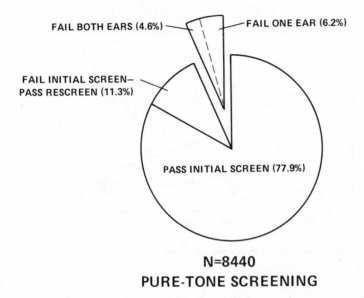

FAIL INITIAL & RESCREEN (10.8%)

FAIL BOTH EARS (4.6%)

FAIL ONE EAR (6.2%)

FAIL INITIAL SCREEN—
PASS RESCREEN (11.3%)

PASS INITIAL SCREEN (77.9%)

N=8440
PURE-TONE SCREENING

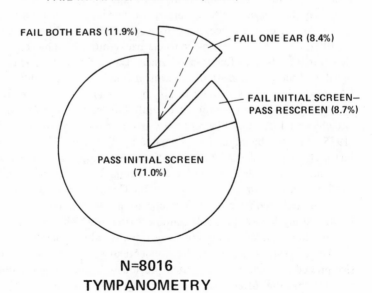

FAIL INITIAL & RESCREEN (20.3%)

FAIL BOTH EARS (11.9%)

FAIL ONE EAR (8.4%)

FAIL INITIAL SCREEN—
PASS RESCREEN (8.7%)

PASS INITIAL SCREEN
(71.0%)

N=8016
TYMPANOMETRY

Fig. 11-1. Screen-Rescreen Results for Pure-Tone Screening and Tympanometry.

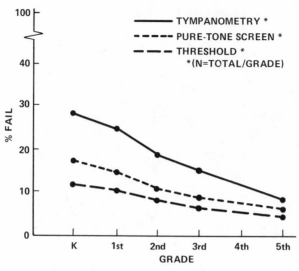

*Values based on results of screen - rescreen

Fig. 11-2. Test Performance by Grade.

section as absolute values for prediction of results in other programs. In reviewing pass-fail ratio figures from reports in the literature, one finds reported screening failure rates ranging from less than 10% to 20% or higher. The difference may be assignable to a variety of factors: (1) methodology employed; (2) use of rescreening procedure before considering a child to have failed; (3) the age of subjects; (4) the socio-economic background of subjects, to name a few. However, results as a function of grade, type of test, frequency of pure-tone signal, and such, are consistent in terms of trends across the studies. For example, Fig. 11-5 illustrates screening results by frequency and grade for two studies which used the same pure-tone procedure but were accomplished in two different physical locations. Figure 11-5A is that developed from the Walton study (1975); 11-5B is based on data generated by Wilson and Walton in Renton, Washington, during the 1972/73 academic year. As is apparent, the overall percentage of children who failed the pure-tone screening in the Renton data is somewhat smaller than the number who failed in the Connecticut data: however, the trend by grade and frequency of test is consistent. It is important to note that the Renton study involved a single school district in which a comprehensive hearing conservation program, using the same test procedures, had been underway for a number of years. In contrast, the Connecticut study involved more comprehensive procedures than had been used previously in these communities. Thus, it is possible that the differences in results may reflect not only differences in population but also the effectiveness of an on-going program—that is, during the second and third years of operation, a hearing conservation program will identify fewer children.

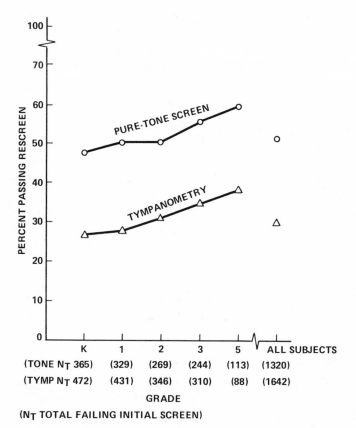

Fig. 11-3. Reduction of False-Positive Identifications.

Alternative Strategies. This chapter has emphasized an individual test procedure rather than a group test procedure. We do not feel that group procedures are inherently less accurate; however, we do believe that if equipment to be used must be set up and dismantled at each test site, calibration problems and time spent setting up *may* make the procedure more time-consuming and potentially less accurate. Logistically speaking, if a mobile unit permanently equipped with multiple test stations can be provided, then time can be saved with group testing. For example, Hollien and Thompson (1968) and Hull (1973) have suggested that three times as many children can be tested per hour once the equipment is set up. Maintenance and calibration of equipment should present fewer problems in a permanent installation. Before considering such a program, the person in charge would be wise to contact other individuals in his area who have attempted such strategies. In many districts, it is difficult to find a location at each school where such equipment can be used. In addition, movement of children to and from the test van can create other difficulties. Finally, movement of the van itself may require special personnel and/or special licensing. Obviously, such

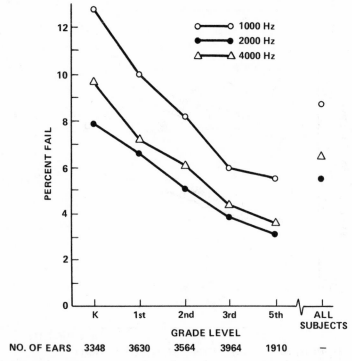

Fig. 11-4. Pure-Tone Screening Results by Frequency and Grade.

questions demand careful consideration. For readers interested in use of a mobile unit, Rower and Carlin (1976) have described a program using a van.

In group screening procedures, a variable of considerable importance is the method of response. If a written response is required, the procedure may be limited to children somewhat older than low elementary grades. If the procedure is a pointing response—for example, identifying a picture among four foils—a monitor must be provided for each child being tested to score responses. If the response is hand-raising, as used in individual pure-tone screening, some means must be provided for excluding the signal to certain headsets and the children must be aware that they will not always hear the tone when their neighbors do. Examples of group screening tests using each of these response modes have been developed.

A group pure-tone screening test that uses a written response is the pulse-counting procedure. It was first described by Reger and Newby (1947). During the test procedure, a signal light comes on alerting all persons being tested to listen. A stimulus is presented, consisting of one, two, three, or four pulses. The subject marks his answer sheet, indicating the number of pulses. In a series of articles, Hollien and Thompson (1961, 1967, 1968) report on modifications to this procedure for use with school-age children and young adults ranging from

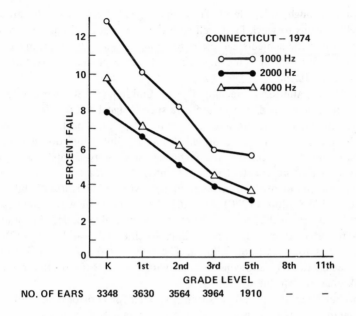

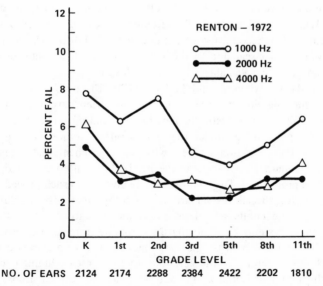

Fig. 11-5. Comparative Results for Pure-Tone screening with Similar Methodology in Two Locations

first grade through college level. They report good success with the procedure, although it seems to work least well with the youngest children. For a screening program where the subjects can easily be brought to a single location (for example, a university hearing screening program) such a procedure may prove both effective and efficient.

The Verbal Auditory Screening Test for Children (VASC) was developed for testing young children. It makes use of a speech signal and requires the child to point to the correct picture among a group of pictures positioned in front of him. Multiple test stations are provided and an adult monitors two children's responses and records correct and incorrect answers by comparing the child's responses to a score sheet. The VASC procedure was evaluated in terms of effectiveness in identification audiometry with kindergarten children by Mencher and McCullogh (1970). Although their sample size was extremely small, the results suggested the VASC to be relatively insensitive in defining mild losses that were detected by pure-tone testing. Ritchie and Marklein (1972) report similar results for preschool children. The fact that the VASC makes use of a speech signal, thereby allowing children with certain loss patterns to complete the task, may explain these findings.

Another alternative strategy, often suggested for control of noise in screening programs, is that of using special "noise-excluding" circumaural earphone enclosures. We would caution against such use for a number of reasons. First, several studies have cast doubt on the efficacy of some models of such devices (Martin, Williams, and Lodge, 1971; Roeser and Glorig, 1975; Roeser, Seidel, and Glorig, 1975). Second, use of the circumaural phones with young children may prevent proper seal due to the size of their heads, thereby removing any attenuation generally available with the enclosures (see Copeland and Mowry, 1971; and Martin, Williams, and Lodge, 1971). Third, no calibration standard exists for such earphones since no coupler has been developed that provides adequate stability for acoustically measuring sound output of such earphones. Thus, as we pointed out under the section on calibration of equipment, the purchaser of these earphones is left with test equipment that cannot be calibrated by standard electroacoustic means. The only alternative is one of loudness balance procedures. The amount of time involved in such procedures as well as the need for special test environments means that such a solution is not practicable in the public school setting. Some laboratories have attempted to calibrate these systems by removing the earphone from the enclosure and calibrating the audiometer with the earphone coupled to a standard calibration cavity. However, return of the earphone to the noise-excluding enclosure will change the values delivered to the subject's ear. For these reasons, we do not suggest the use of noise-excluding earphones as part of the standard screening program. Rather, we feel it is necessary to find test sites that allow an adequate noise environment for screening.

Another alternative strategy for provision of the hearing screening program within the public school setting is that of contracting for all service. In such a case, the district personnel should be responsible for detailing the overall goals of the program, the extent of testing to be included and the time lines to be met by the contractor.

A similar concept involves having several school districts combine to form a larger structure for provision of special services. Advantages include the ability to hire specialists and provide more appropriate instrumentation, since the costs can be spread among the cooperating districts. For example, provision of calibration services for a group of districts with personnel hired and managed by the collective organization might prove cost-efficient. Likewise, provision of administrative skills by a person devoting his total effort to a single area may well be more advantageous than an administrator who must split his efforts among several programs within a smaller district.

Hearing Conservation Among School-Age Children

Although not the focus of this chapter, we feel it important to note the need for an active hearing conservation program in the schools and community. Considerable effort should be expended, in cooperation with school and community health professionals, to provide educational materials and programming in an attempt to *prevent* hearing loss rather than devoting all efforts to identifying and managing loss. Materials which can be integrated into the curriculum of the district concerning proper hearing conservation from the point of view of disease should be developed, as should information about the possible detrimental effects of noise exposure. Expansion of these educational efforts might well include community groups as there is rising concern about the effect of noise on hearing and the right to live a life relatively free of pollutants, including noise. Average noise levels in our cities have increased throughout the past twenty years, with much larger increases in the most recent few years. Likewise, many of the avocational interests of children and young adults have included exposures to higher levels of noise. A hearing conservation program within a school district should educate children and adults on these matters.

Finally, the public school audiometry program must consider to what extent it should and can become involved in a service program for district personnel. In many districts, requests from administration to insure compliance with federal and state occupational and safety health requirements may be directed to the auidologist. The overall efforts of the educational hearing conservation program will often be heightened if an actual service program is in effect for district personnel.

SUMMARY

This chapter has described the philosophic bases that must be considered in developing a public school audiometry program. After detailing alternative rationales for such programs, focus has been given to methods of identifying children with educationally significant hearing loss. Specific procedures for a pure-tone screening test have been covered along with logistical and administrative considerations necessary for successfully implementing such an identification effort. In addition, inclusion of tympanometry as a part of a screening battery is considered from the point of view of rationale, methodology, and results. Sample data are provided that illustrate the results of such an identification battery and allow the reader a comparative data base.

Although the primary focus of the chapter is on identification audiometry, we feel strongly than an identification effort is of little or no value unless it is a part of a comprehensive hearing program in a school district. Considerations for a total hearing program within a school district are covered, including personnel, scope of program, and administrative structure. Finally, the chapter provides alternative strategies that individuals may consider for particular situations as well as research needs for continuing to improve hearing services in the public school setting.

RESEARCH NEEDS

Throughout this chapter we have attempted to emphasize the need for ongoing data collection in an identification audiometry program. We feel that a primary research need is for service programs to be involved in effectiveness/efficiency analysis. Unfortunately, many methodological decisions have been reached with only impressionistic information, not a solid data base, as a guide. The simple addition of systematic data collection, reduction, analysis, and publication of results could bring about substantial improvement in the delivery of services to hearing-impaired children. Although some may argue that funding is not available, we would argue that such analysis is essential to proper program planning. To do any less serves only to perpetuate past myths by cloaking them in the respectability of "tradition."

A second general research topic, badly in need of study, has to do with the types of tests to be included in a hearing screening program. If one believes the purpose of an identification program is to locate children with potential auditory deficits, we must expand our thinking to include deficits other than those related to middle-ear pathology and/or shifts in hearing sensitivity. We are not aware of any large-scale studies on the possible application of screening procedures for detecting auditory perceptual difficulties. It is our opinion that audiologists and speech pathologists must be concerned with the definition of such deficits and must be involved in research efforts within service programs to determine potential avenues of identification and assessment.

Within each of the broad areas suggested above, a number of specific research efforts can be identified. For example, studies attempting to relate threshold sensitivity to academic performance to define when hearing is at risk for educational purposes would be welcomed. Likewise, very little data exist on the effect of ambient noise levels on screening and threshold test results as a function of distraction rather than as a function of masking. Preliminary work suggests that viewing the effect of ambient noise only in terms of masking is too limited to explain the results obtained with school-age children. Further, many teachers and administrators are interested in the issue of ambient noise levels within classrooms and their possible effect on learning. As the audiologist assumes a broader role in educational management of hearing-impaired children, he will also be turned to for consultative services on such questions.

Within the area of impedance procedures, work at present suggests that tympanometry can be effectively incorporated in a hearing screening battery. A number of methodological studies and cost-effectiveness studies remain to be completed. In addition, prototyping of instrumentation which combines the pure-tone test function with the impedance test function is needed, since such equipment is now being designed. Calibration studies on impedance audiometry equipment as used in large service programs are nonexistent at present.

The above suggestions are not intended to detail all of the research needs in the area of identification audiometry. Instead, they are simply to suggest the types of studies that can be and need to be accomplished if we are to see improvements. Collaborative efforts between public school systems, state education and/or health agencies, and universities seem particularly suited to answering some of the questions suggested above.

REFERENCES

American National Standards Institute, Inc., *American National Standard Specifications for Audiometers* (ANSI S3.6–1969). New York, 1970.

American National Standards Institute, Inc., *American Standard Criteria for Background Noise in Audiometer Rooms* (ANSI S3.1–1960). New York, 1960.

American Speech and Hearing Association, *Guidelines for Identification Audiometry*. Washington, D.C.: 1975.

American Speech and Hearing Association, *Standards and Guidelines for Comprehensive Language, Speech, and Hearing Programs in the Schools*. Washington, D.C.: 1973/1974.

Brooks, D.N., "Electroacoustic Impedance Bridge Studies on Normal Ears of Children," *Journal of Speech and Hearing Research,* 14 (1971), 247–253.

Cooper, J.C., G.A. Gates, J.H. Owen, and H.D. Dickson, "An Abbreviated Impedance Bridge Technique for School Screening," *Journal of Speech and Hearing Disorders,* 40 (1975), 260–269.

Copeland, A.B., and H.J. Mowry, "Real-Ear Attenuation Characteristics of Selected Noise—Excluding Audiometric Receiver Enclosures," *Journal of the Acoustical Society of America*, 49 (1971), 1757–1761.

Darley, F.L., editor, "Identification Audiometry," *Journal of Speech and Hearing Disorders*, Monograph Supplement 9, 1961.

Decker, T.N., and W.R. Wilson, "The Use of Visual Reinforcement Audiometry (VRA) with Profoundly Retarded Residents," *Mental Retardation*, 15 (1977), 40–41.

Downs, M.P., M.E. Doster, and M. Wever, "Dilemmas in Identification Audiometry," *Journal of Speech and Hearing Disorders*, 30 (1965), 360–364.

Eagles, E.L., "Hearing Levels in Children and Audiometer Performance," Appendix B in *Journal of Speech and Hearing Disorders*, Monograph Supplement No. 9, 1961, 52–62.

Eagles, E.L., "A Longitudinal Study of Ear Disease and Hearing Sensitivity in Children," *Audiology*, 12 (1973), 438–445.

Eagles, E.L., "Selected Findings from the Pittsburgh Study," *Transactions of the American Academy of Ophthalmology and Otolaryngology*, 76 (1972), 343–348.

Eagles, E.L., and L.G. Doerfler, "Hearing in Children: Acoustic Environment and Audiometer Performance," *Journal of Speech and Hearing Research*, 4 (1961), 149–163.

Eagles, E.L., S.M. Wishik, L.G. Doerfler, W. Melnick, and H.S. Levine, *Hearing Sensitivity and Related Factors in Children*. St. Louis: Laryngoscope, 1963.

Fowler, E.P., and H. Fletcher, "Three Million Deafened School Children: Their Detection and Treatment," *Journal of American Medical Association*, 87 (1926), 1877–1922.

Gaeth, J.H., and E. Lounsbury, "Hearing Aids and Children in Elementary Schools," *Journal of Speech and Hearing Disorders*, 31 (1966), 283–289.

Greenberg, D.B., W.R. Wilson, J.M. Moore, and G. Thompson, "Visual Reinforcement Audiometry (VRA) with Young Down's Syndrome Children." Unpublished manuscript.

Hollien, H., and C.L. Thompson, "An Evaluation of the Reger-Newby Group Hearing Test Administered Manually," *Journal of Auditory Research* 1 (1961), 294–305.

Hollien, H., and C.L. Thompson, "Forms C and D of the Hollien-Thompson Group Screening Test of Hearing," *Journal of Auditory Research*, 8 (1968), 143–150.

Hollien, H., and C.L. Thompson, "A Group Screening Test of Hearing," *Journal of Auditory Research*, 7 (1967), 85–92.

Holm, V.A., and L.H. Kunze, "Effect of Chronic Otitis Media on Language and Speech Development," *Pediatrics*, 43 (1969), 833–839.

Hull, R.H., "Group vs. Individual Screening in Public School Audiometry," *Colorado Journal of Educational Research*, 13 (1973), 6–9.

Johnston, P.W., "The Massachusetts Hearing Test," *Journal of the Acoustical Society of America,* 20 (1948), 697–703.

Jordan, R.E., "Symposium: Conservation of Hearing in Children. Introduction," *Transactions of the American Academy of Ophthalmology and Otolaryngology,* 76 (1972), 340–342.

Jordan, R.E., and E.L. Eagles, "The Relation of Air Conduction Audiometry to Otological Abnormalities," *Annals of Otology, Rhinology and Laryngology,* 70 (1961), 819–827.

Kaplan, G.J., J.K. Fleshman, T.R. Bender, C. Baum, and P.S. Clark, "Long-Term Effects of Otitis Media—A Ten-Year Cohort Study of Alaskan Eskimo Children," *Pediatrics,* 52 (1973), 577–585.

Lewis, N., A. Dugdale, A. Comty, and J. Jerger, "Open-ended Tympanometric Screening: A New Concept," *Archives of Otolaryngology,* 101 (1975), 722–725.

Liden, G., J. Peterson, and G. Bjorkman, "Tympanometry," *Archives of Atolaryngology,* 92 (1970), 248–257.

Martin, F.N., *Introduction to Audiology.* Englewood Cliffs, N.J.: Prentice-Hall, 1975.

Martin, M.C., V. Williams, and J.J. Lodge, "An Evaluation of Noise Excluding Enclosures for Audiometric Earphones," *Sound,* 5 (1971), 90–93.

Melnick, W., E.L. Eagles, and H.S. Levine, "Evaluation of a Recommended Program of Identification Audiometry with School-age Children," *Journal of Speech and Hearing Disorders,* 29 (1964), 3–13.

Mencher, G.T., and B.F. McCulloch, "Auditory Screening for Kindergarten Children Using the VASC," *Journal of Speech and Hearing Disorders,* 35 (1970), 241–247.

Moore, J.M., W.R. Wilson, and G. Thompson, "Visual Reinforcement of Head-Turn Responses in Infants Under 12 Months of Age," *Journal of Speech and Hearing Disorders,* 42, (1977), 328–334.

Moore, J.M., W.R. Wilson, K.E. Lillis, and S.A. Talbott, "Earphone Auditory Thresholds of Infants Utilizing Visual Reinforcement Audiometry (VRA)." Unpublished manuscript.

Murphy, N.J., *National Survey of State Identification Audiometry Programs and Special Educational Services for Hearing Impaired Children and Youth.* Washington, D.C.: Gallaudet College, Office of Demographic Studies, 1972.

Orchik, D.J., and S. Herdman, "Impedance Audiometry as a Screening Device with School-Age Children," *Journal of Auditory Research,* 14 (1974), 283–286.

Reger, S., and H.A. Newby, "A Group Pure-Tone Hearing Test," *Journal of Speech and Hearing Disorders,* 12 (1947), 61–66.

Ritchie, B.C., and R.A. Merklein, "An Evaluation of the Efficiency of the

Verbal Auditory Screening for Children (VASC)," *Journal of Speech and Hearing Research,* 15 (1972), 280–286.

Roeser, R.J., and A. Glorig, "Pure-tone Audiometry in Noise with Auraldomes," *Audiology,* 14 (1975), 144–151.

Roeser, R.J., J. Seidel, and A. Glorig, "Performance of Earphone Enclosures for Threshold Audiometry," *Sound and Vibration* (Sept. 1975), 22–25.

Roberts, J., and J.V. Federico, *Hearing Sensitivity and Related Medical Findings Among Children,* Vital and Health Statistics, Series 11–No. 114, U.S. Dept. of Health, Education and Welfare Publication, 1972.

Rower, M., and T.W. Carlin, "Identification Audiometry on the Move," *Audiology and Hearing Education,* 2 (1976), 13–15.

Seidemann, M.F., and J.K. Laguaite, "The Incidence of Hearing Impairments in 900 Inner-City Preschool Children." A paper read at 1973 ASHA Convention, Detroit, 1973.

Talbott, R.E., "Bacteriology of Earphone Contamination," *Journal of Speech and Hearing Research,* 12 (1969) 326–329.

Thomas, W.G., M.J. Preslar, R.R. Summers, and J.L. Stewart, "Calibration and Working Condition of 100 Audiometers," *Public Health Reports,* 84 (1969), 311–327.

Walton, W.K., *Procedures for Identification Audiometry* (three narrated filmstrips). Hartford: Special Education Resource Center, 275 Windsor St., Hartford, Conn. 06120 (1975a).

Walton, W.K., *Project TAMI–A Tympanometry-ASHA Model for Identification of the Hearing Impaired.* Windsor, Conn.: Capitol Region Education Council, 1975b.

Walton, W.K., and P.S. Williams, "Stability of Routinely Serviced Portable Audiometers," *Language, Speech and Hearing Services in the Schools,* 3 (1972), 36–43.

Walton, W.K., and W.R. Wilson, "Pass-Fail Ratios in Identification Audiometry as a Function of Audiometer Rise Times," *Journal of the Acoustical Society of America,* 56 (1974a), 601–604.

Walton, W.K., and W.R. Wilson, "Stability of Pure-Tone Audiometers During Periods of Heavy Use in Identification Audiometry," *Language, Speech and Hearing Services in Schools,* 5 (1974b), 8–12.

Wilber, L.A., "Calibration: Pure-Tone Speech and Noise Signals," in *Handbook of Clinical Audiology,* edited by J. Katz. Baltimore: Williams and Wilkins, 1972, 11–35.

Wilson, W.K. J.M. Moore, and G. Thompson, "Auditory Thresholds of Infants Utilizing Visual Reinforcement Audiometry." Unpublished manuscript.

Wilson, W.R., and W.K. Walton, "Identification Audiometry Accuracy: Evalua tion of a Recommended Program for School-Age Children," *Language, Speech and Hearing Services in Schools,* 5 (1974), 132–142.

Wood, T.J., W.W. Wittich, and R.B. Mahaffey, "Computerized Pure-Tone Audiometric Procedures," *Journal of Speech and Hearing Research,* 16 (1973), 676–684.

Zink, G.D., "Hearing Aids Children Wear: A Longitudinal Study of Performance," *Volta Review* (1972), 41–51.

SUGGESTED READINGS

American Speech and Hearing Association, *Guidelines for Identification Audiometry.* Washington, D.C., 1975.

American Speech and Hearing Association, *Standards and Guidelines for Comprehensive Language, Speech, and Hearing Programs in the Schools.* Washington, D.C., 1973–74.

Melnick, W., E.L. Eagles, and H.S. Levine, "Evaluation of a Recommended Program of Identification Audiometry with School-Age Children," *Journal of Speech and Hearing Disorders,* 29 (1964), 3–13.

Roberts, J., and J.V. Federico, *Hearing Sensitivity and Related Medical Findings among Children,* Vital and Health Statistics, Series 11–No. 114, U.S. Department of Health, Education & Welfare Publication, 1972.

Walton, W.K., *Project TAMI–A Tympanometry-ASHA Model for Identification of the Hearing Impaired.* Windsor, Connecticut: Capitol Region Education Council, 1975.

Wilson, W.R., and W.K. Walton, "Identification Audiometry Accuracy: Evaluation of a Recommended Program for School-Age Children," *Language, Speech and Hearing Services in Schools,* 5 (1974), 132–142.

Appendix

SAMPLE GUIDELINES FOR PURE-TONE IDENTIFICATION AUDIOMETRY PROGRAMS IN SCHOOLS

1. Definitions

identification audiometry The process by which individuals are identified whose hearing sensitivity differs significantly from the normal (also known as hearing screening and auditory screening). For purposes of these guidelines, identification audiometry is restricted to the use of pure-tone, air-conducted stimuli for the identification of those whose hearing sensitivity exceeds 20dB at 1000 Hz, 20dB at 2000 Hz, and 25dB at 4000 Hz in either ear (all values in Hearing Level).

licensed audiologist An individual who, pursuant to Public Act_____, is duly authorized to practice audiology in _____(state).

licensed speech pathologist An individual who, pursuant to Public Act _____ , is duly authorized to practice speech pathology in_____ (state).

threshold evaluation The process by which an individual's response thresholds for pure-tone stimuli are determined. The definition is herein restricted to the use of pure-tone air-conducted stimuli at 250, 500, 1000, 2000, 4000, and 6000 or 8000 Hz.

threshold evaluation failure Failure of an individual to respond appropriately to pure-tone stimuli at designated hearing levels. For purposes of this guideline, hearing threshold failure, per frequency, is defined as hearing levels equal to or greater than 20dB at 250, 500, 1000, and 2000 Hz; and 25dB at 4000 Hz and 6000 or 8000 Hz. Nothing shall prohibit more strict criteria from being established by local school personnel. Decision regarding whom to refer to the School Planning and Placement Team shall be the responsibility of the licensed audiologist or speech pathologist performing the threshold evaluation.

2. Criteria for Selection of Children for Screening

Children are to be selected for auditory screening according to the following minimal criteria:

1. All children in kindergarten through the first three elementary grades and in grades five, eight, and eleven shall be screened annually.
2. All children in ungraded schools or classes shall be screened annually during their fifth, sixth, seventh, eighth, tenth, thirteenth, and sixteenth year of age.

428

3. All new students in a district, regardless of grade level, shall be screened within three months of admission.

4. Kindergarten children (or those 5 years of age in ungraded schools) shall be screened within three months of admission to school.

5. All children referred to the district by parents or guardians, or by teachers, nurses, or other school personnel as having a possible loss of auditory sensitivity shall be screened within 14 calendar days of referral.

6. All children referred to the School Planning and Placement Team because of possible speech, language, learning, and/or behavioral problems shall be screened within 30 calendar days of referral.

3. Equipment for Screening

Instruments utilized for auditory screening shall provide calibrated pure-tone stimuli at each of the following frequencies: 1000, 2000, and 4000 Hz. An attenuator providing hearing levels at 20 and 25dB re: current American National Standards Institute (ANSI) Specifications for audiometers, as measured at the earphones, shall be utilized for each of the frequencies provided.

4. Screening Methods

Screening shall be done on an individual basis.

5. Screening Frequencies

Each child shall be screened at least at 1000, 2000, and 4000 Hz.

6. Screening Levels

Stimuli shall be presented at a hearing level of 20dB based on current ANSI standards at 1000 and 2000 Hz and at 25dB at 4000 Hz. If 500 Hz is utilized, the screening level shall be 20dB.

7. Screening Environment

Auditory screening shall take place in an environment sufficiently quiet for a subject with normal hearing sensitivity to hear the test stimuli at the screening levels.

8. Calibration

Audiometers used in identification audiometry programs shall meet the current ANSI Specifications for Audiometers. At least annual assessment and, where necessary, correction of the following factors shall be considered minimal for adequate calibration: mechanical and electrical integrity, extraneous noise, intensity, rise time, attenuator linearity, and frequency. A statement showing the date of last calibration, and the results thereof, shall be kept with each audiometer.

9. Screening Failure

A child who fails to respond to one or more of the three required screening frequencies in either ear shall be rescreened within one week of the original screening procedure. A child who fails to respond at one or more frequencies in either ear at the second screening shall receive at least a complete air-conduction threshold evaluation by a licensed audiologist or speech pathologist using appropriate test environments and equipment. Diagnosed exceptional children presenting unusual audiometric testing problems (such as the mentally retarded, emotionally disturbed, and neurologically impaired) shall receive a threshold evaluation from a licensed audiologist only.

10. Parent Notification

Parents or guardians of a child failing an audiometric rescreening examination or a threshold evaluation shall be notified, in writing, of the child's performance within seven calendar days of such testing.

11. PPT Referral

All children failing an audiometric threshold evaluation shall be referred to the School Planning and Placement Team for decision regarding appropriate management. No more than 30 calendar days shall elapse between the first pure-tone screening procedure, and, where necessary, review by the School Planning and Placement Team.

12. Teacher Notification

All school personnel responsible for the education of a child failing an audiometric rescreening or a threshold evaluation shall be notified of the child's performance within seven calendar days of such testing.

13. Reports

Data shall be retained identifying the student by name and/or student identification number, school, grade, and sex. Information on the type of audiometric test and results, by ear and frequency, shall also be retained. Reports documenting the results of identification audiometry programs, and the names of the person responsible for said program, shall be submitted on request to the State Department of Education.

SAMPLE FORMS FOR IDENTIFICATION
AUDIOMETRY PROGRAM

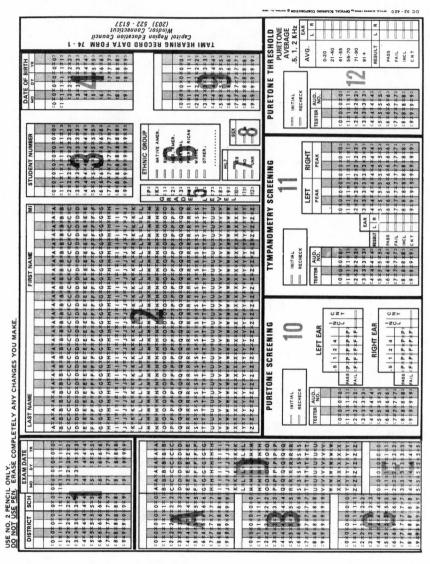

Fig. 11-A-1. Hearing Record Data Form

PROCEDURES FOR COMPLETING FORM 74-1

Use only a <u>dull</u>, number 2 pencil. Erase any error completely; smudges will be misinterpreted by the computer.

Complete the heading blocks first.

Blacken the designated area to the printed bracket, being certain to cover the number (or letter) completely. If necessary, go over the number (letter) several times to insure a fully blackened area.

Stay in the correct columns.

A. Section 1

1. Heading: Complete the heading to the following subsections:

   a. District number
   b. School code

2. Sense-mark areas: Fill in sense-mark areas for the above subsections.

3. Exam date will be completed by volunteers on the date of examination.

B. Section 2

1. Heading: Enter as many letters of the child's last and first names as space allows. Enter the middle initial.

2. Sense-mark areas: Starting in the first column for the last name, blacken the appropriate box beneath the letter of the name. Be careful to stay in the correct column and to blacken the areas completely.

C. Section 3

1. Heading: Student numbers have been provided by the ____ Project. If unnumbered forms are used, student numbers will be provided at the time of examination.

2. Sense-mark areas: Where numbers are provided, blacken sense-mark numerals. The right-most digit in the number (i.e., the digit in the "units" position) must be entered in the right-most column.

D. Section 4

1. Heading: Enter child's birthdate using numerals. Example: If the child's birthdate is June 9, 1964, enter 060964.

Fig. 11-A-2. Procedures for Completing Hearing Record Data Form 74-1

2. Sense-mark area: Blacken appropriate numbers.

E. Section 5

Blacken the child's equivalent grade level. Be certain to fill in the area completely for grade.

F. Section 6

Blacken the box corresponding to the child's most representative ethnic group. Native American is the same as American Indian.

G. Section 7

Mark YES if the child is known to have a hearing loss;
Mark NO if he does not have a hearing loss;
Mark UNK if the child's hearing status is unknown.

H. Section 8

Blacken the box corresponding to the child's sex.

I. Section 9

1. Two left most columns: Enter the number of absences which the student has accumulated since school began in September.

2. Middle two columns: Enter the child's equivalent grade level for READING. Use two digits. Example: For a child reading on the 4th grade level, enter "04." Record "90" for children reading below the first-grade level.

3. Two right-most columns: Enter the child's equivalent level for ARITHMETIC. Use two digits. Example: For the child functioning at 5th grade level in arithmetic, record "05." Record "90" for children functioning below the first-grade level.

Many thanks for your help! You are making it possible to test far more children in a limited time than would otherwise be possible.

Fig. 11-A-2. Continued

School _____

District _____

Name _____

Date of Screening _____

Dear Dr. _____

The above-named child participated in our hearing screening program.
We refer him to you for medical examination. Test results were as follows:

(1) Puretone Screening

      Right Ear   Left Ear

      _____   Pass   _____

      _____   Fail   _____

(2) Puretone Threshold

      Right Ear   Left Ear

      _____   Within normal range   _____
                   (0–20db HTL)

      _____   Mild Loss   _____
                   (20–40db HTL)

      _____   Moderate loss   _____
                   (41–55db HTL)

      _____   Severe loss   _____
                   (56–70db HTL)

(3) Tympanometry

      Right Ear   Left Ear

_____ Normal middle ear pressure; normal middle ear compliance _____

_____ Negative middle ear pressure; normal middle ear compliance _____

_____ Normal middle ear pressure; reduced middle ear compliance _____

_____ Negative middle ear pressure; reduced middle ear compliance _____

Fig. 11-A-3. Hearing Screening Referral Form

MANAGEMENT SERVICES RECORD

Name of child _____

ID # _____

Date of report _____

Date identified _____

School _____

City _____

Professional respondent(s) completing this form: _____

(Complete all applicable items in each section)

I. Results of Hearing Screening

____ Passed puretone Screening   ____ Failed puretone threshold

____ Passed tympanometry   ____ Failed tympanometry

II. Referral Statement Recommended

____ Educational management

____ Medical management

____ Both

____ Notify parents

III. Status of Referral

Notification of Findings Made to

____ Physician

____ School nurse

____ Lang., Speech and Hear. Clinician

____ School principal

____ Classroom Teacher

____ Parents

____ Other (specify) _____

Fig. 11-A-4. Management Services Record

Medical Management and Intervention

    ___ Physician's management ___ in process ___ completed ___ continuing

    ___ Otologist's management ___ in process ___ completed ___ continuing

Recommended Medical Intervention

    Record Procedures Used (i.e., wax removal, surgery, etc.)

    _____

    _____

    _____

    Date _____ M.D. _____

Medical Findings

    ___ Confirm results of hearing testing

    ___ Do not confirm results of hearing testing

Recommended Medical Follow-up

    ___ Recheck by managing M.D.   Date _____

    ___ Surgery by managing M.D.   Date _____

    ___ Referral to _____   Date _____

    ___ Other _____   Date _____

Audiological Management and Intervention

    ___ Audiologist   ___ in process ___ completed ___ continuing

    ___ Nurse   ___ in process ___ completed ___ continuing

    ___ Lang., Speech and Hear.
          Clinician   ___ in process ___ completed ___ continuing

    ___ Rescreen   Date _____
          Results

		Audiological	Tympanometric
Pass:		RE ___ LE ___	RE ___ LE ___
Fail:		RE ___ LE ___	RE ___ LE ___

Fig. 11-A-4. Continued

Complete Evaluation   Date _____

Results

    Type of loss: ___ Sensori-neural ___ Conductive

    Degree of loss: RE   LE

    Comments: _____ _____ normal   _____

    _____ _____ moderate _____

    _____ _____ severe   _____

Recommended Audiological Follow-up

  ___ Hearing aid management

  ___ Referral to _____ Date _____

  ___ Hearing recheck

                        Audiological   Tympanometric

    bi-monthly   _____   _____

    monthly   _____   _____

    quarterly   _____   _____

    annually   _____   _____

  ___ Other (Specify _____)

Audiological Findings

  ___ Confirm results of   hearing screening

  ___ Do not confirm results of   hearing screening

Educational Management and Intervention

  ___ Lang., Speech and Hear.
      Clinician   ___ in process ___ completed ___ continuing

  ___ Audiologist   ___ in process ___ completed ___ continuing

  ___ Classroom Teacher   ___ in process ___ completed ___ continuing

Fig. 11-A-4. Continued

Recommended Educational Intervention

    ___ Preferential seating

    ___ Hearing aid

    ___ Language and speech services

    ___ PPT conference

    ___ Classroom teacher conference

    ___ Parent conference

    ___ Tutorial help

    ___ Special class placement (title and location _____)

    ___ No further management

    ___ Other (specify _____)

Recommended Educational Follow-up

    ___ Preferential seating

    ___ Hearing aid assessment

    ___ PPT referral

    ___ Classroom teacher conference

    ___ Parent conference

    ___ Hearing rechecks ___ bi-monthly ___ monthly ___ quarterly ___ annually

Fig. 11-A-4. Continued

AUDIOMETER CALIBRATION WORKSHEET

IDENTIFICATION INFORMATION:

DATE _____
EXAMINER
NAME _____
_____

Owner _____

Model _____

Year _____

Serial No. _____

Physical Characteristics (Mechanical Condition)

Dials, (Loose, malaligned, clicks?)   _____

Knobs (Loose, noisy?)   _____

Earphone cushions (Split, deteriorated?)_____

Cords, (Split, frayed?)   _____

Noise During Test (Extraneous noise)

Attenuator hum (dirty?)   _____

Radiation from chassis (oscillating?
                        components)   _____

Power supply hum   _____

Clicks when changing int. or freq.   _____

Other _____

GROSS AUDITORY TEST

_____ Cords   – Set at 1000 Hz, 70db, HTL, tone on. Jiggle earphone
                     cords back and forth one half turn. If tone is inter-
                     mittent, either the cord is loose or defective. First
                     try to tighten screws. If there is no change, replace
                     cord.

_____ Power hums   – Set audiometer at 40db HL and increase intensity;
                     listen for any random signals.

_____ Rise time   – More dials (attenuator and frequency) and interrupter
                     switch. Judge if there are any audible clicks above
                     threshold levels.

_____ Linearity   – Set at 2000 Hz and increase intensity in 5db steps.
                     Give gross estimate of uniformity.

Fig. 11–A–5. Audiometer Calibration Worksheet 1

AUDIOMETER CALIBRATION WORKSHEET

DISTRICT _____   MAKE _____   EXAMINER NAME _____

SERIAL # _____   MODEL _____   EXAMINER # _____   DATE _____

FREQUENCY (Hz)	MIC. #439403 REF. SPL (TDH 39)	INTENSITY CALIBRATION TOLERANCE (± dB)	FREQUENCY (Hz) CALIBRATION TOLERANCE (± dB)
125	114.5	5	4
250	95.0	3	2
500	81.0	3	15
750	78.0	3	23
1000	77.0	3	30
1500	76.5	3	45
2000	79.0	3	60
3000	81.0	3	90
4000	80.5	4	120
6000	86.5	5	180
8000	80.5	5	240

INTENSITY CALIBRATION — LEFT PHONE (**SPL, dB ERROR), RIGHT PHONE (**SPL, dB ERROR)

FREQUENCY (Hz) CALIBRATION — MEASURED FREQUENCY, ERROR

PURITY OF TONES (dB) — LEFT PHONE (FREQ. OF LGST. HARM., SPL OF LGST. HARM), COMMENTS; RIGHT PHONE (FREQ. OF LGST. HARM, SPL OF LGST. HARM), COMMENTS

RISE/DECAY TIME CAL. (msec) — LEFT PHONE (RISE TIME 20-100, DECAY TIME 5-100), RIGHT PHONE (RISE TIME 20-100, DECAY TIME 5-100)

*Includes corrections for using B&K microphone Type 4144 (SN439403) with protecting cover.
**Measured with 70 dB input.

Fig. 11–A–6. Audiometer Calibration Worksheet 2

ATTENUATOR LINEARITY

TEST FREQ. _____ Hz   DATE _____

PHONE _____

DIAL SETTING Hz	MEASURED LEVEL SPL	LINEARITY VALUE
110		
105		
100		
95		
90		
85		
80		
75		
70		
65		
60		
55		
50		
45		
40		
35		
30		
25		
20		
15		
10		
5		
0		

(3.5-6.5 dB TOTAL RANGE)

OVERALL LINEARITY

MAX. SPL _____

MIN. SPL _____   _____ dB

($\pm$ 5 dB TOLERANCE)

Fig. 11-A-7. Audiometer Calibration Worksheet 3

ENVIRONMENTAL NOISE RECORD

DATE _____

SLM # _____

DISTRICT _____

SCHOOL _____

OPERATOR NAME	PISTON PHONE LEVEL	ROOM	LOCATION WITHIN ROOM	TIME	TEST TYPE (1) PTS (2) TPS (3) PTT	LINEAR	dBC	dBA	500 Hz OCTAVE BAND	COMMENTS

Fig. 11-A-8. Environmental Noise Record

TESTING FACILITIES AND SCHEDULES

District _____   Principal _____

School _____   Nurse _____

Initial Test Date _____   Speech Clinician _____

Rescreen Test Date _____

Testing Rooms: Names and/or numbers _____

_____

Schedules

Num. Chn. in:	Num. Classes for:	Room Nos.:	Times Available:
KAM _____	_____	_____	_____
KPM _____	_____	_____	_____
1st _____	_____	_____	_____
2nd _____	_____	_____	_____
3rd _____	_____	_____	_____
4th _____	_____	_____	_____
5th _____	_____	_____	_____
Other ____	_____	_____	_____

Arrival/Dismissal times:	Recess times:		Lunch times:
KAM _____	_____	_____	_____
KPM _____	_____	_____	_____
1st _____	_____	_____	_____
2nd _____	_____	_____	_____
3rd _____	_____	_____	_____
5th _____	_____	_____	_____
Other ____	_____	_____	_____

Other times not available for testing: _____

Fig. 11-A-9. Testing Facilities and Schedules

ORDER OF TESTING

PRINCIPAL _____
NURSE _____
CLINICIAN _____

DATE _____
SCHOOL _____
DISTRICT _____

TEST SCHEDULE	GRADE	TEACHER & ROOM NO.	TOTAL CLASS ENROLLMENT	NO. CHILDREN TO BE TESTED	NO. CHILDREN ABSENT	NO. CHILDREN W/O PARENTAL CONSENT	NO. CHILDREN TO BE RETESTED
9:00							
9:15							
9:30							
9:45							
10:00							
10:15							
10:30							
10:45							
11:00							
LUNCH							
12:45							
1:00							
1:15							
1:30							
1:45							
2:00							
2:15							

Fig. 11–A–10. Order of Testing Worksheet

CHAPTER TWELVE

Audiological Management of the Hearing-Impaired Child in the Public Schools

VICTOR P. GARWOOD

INTRODUCTION

Full-time audiologists in public schools have become a reality only within the past decade. A recent ASHA survey has shown that about 700 out of an approximate 3,500 certificated audiologists are engaged in school-related activities. Currently, the Academy of Rehabilitative Audiology (ARA) is attempting to determine more exact counts of audiologists in schools.

It became apparent to me, as a practicing school audiologist, that in large urban areas, children with hearing impairments require far more attention than the intermittent audiologic management presently offered by external agencies, hospitals, and private practitioners. A new federal law, Public Law 94–142, designed to provide education for all handicapped children, is currently being implemented and will undoubtedly result in a significant increase in services to the handicapped child, and consequently, an increase in manpower in the public schools.

School administrators have assumed that teachers of the hearing-impaired have sufficient time to deal with audiologic issues, not realizing that a standard teaching load is a full-time responsibility. Training institutions with audiologic curricula have made similar assumptions, stating that their training programs will adequately prepare students for entry into the public schools. In my experience, such statements are unrealistic. As a former full-time audiologist in a large public school system, I have also observed the absolute need for continuous observation and monitoring procedures by audiologic personnel within the school system. Generally speaking, schools are reluctant to exchange information with outside agencies—a consequence of new legislation relating to the privacy of school records. Parents are reluctant to take their children out of school for clinical treatment while school is in session.

I would like to acknowledge Celeste A. Baker, principal of the Mary E. Bennett Elementary School for Hearing Impaired Children; and Joan C. Nassberg, audiologist, Los Angeles Unified School District, for their assistance.

One of the first impressions of the new school audiologist is the enormous range of hearing impairments ranging from mild unilateral to severely handicapping losses accompained by a multiplicity of other problems. The audiologist will find (1) children whose hearing aids will not work, (2) children who don't need hearing aids wearing them, (3) children who reject body for ear level aids, (4) children with minimal impairment who are fitted with high-power aids, and (5) children whose only exposure to amplification is with school-purchased training units—used only when school is in session. The audiologist will be shocked, and understandably so, by the poverty and ignorance as evidenced by a high incidence of middle ear infections overlying severe sensorineural impairment, parental neglect, and generally poor hygiene. With regard to proper program placement, the audiologist will be startled by the lack of prior otoaudiologic evaluative data, which should, of course, be of paramount importance.

When knowledge of the availability of audiologic services filters down to the teachers, the audiologist is bombarded with requests to "see" their pupils, generally because of an amplification problem. One of the most disruptive problems and chronic concerns of the audiologist is the development of a priority system that will satisfy not only the teachers but the counselors, nurses, and principals as well.

The rewards for conscientious clinicians become apparent when, because of their intervention, the child begins to succeed as an active participant in the educative process. The time is always right to serve, despite the current wave of financial conservatism in most schools. It may well be, however, that as they do their jobs the relatively small force of audiologists presently employed by public schools will prove to be in an area where the requirements will far surpass all present clinical opportunities for employment.

Because the majority of school audiologists will be employed by large school districts, the thrust of this chapter will be aimed accordingly. Smaller districts will undoubtedly join forces to hire audiologists on a shared-time basis. Certainly all school districts share one area of concern—they all have hearing-impaired children and few audiologists to serve them. The author will, by using the Los Angeles city school district as an example, attempt to describe responsibilities, problems, and satisfactions of school audiologists at a moment in history that is characterized by significant changes in the management of handicapped children.

CHAPTER OBJECTIVES

This chapter describes the responsibilities, techniques, and relationships of audiologists in public schools. Emphasis is placed on amplification practices, school procedures, relations with other school specialists, and educational regulations.

REVIEW OF THE LITERATURE

This review will not cover general literature of hearing aids for children, but will be restricted to references to public school audiology.

The Role of the Audiologist in Schools

The importance of audiologic management of hearing-impaired children in schools has been recognized by ASHA with its 1976 position paper, of suggested guidelines for personnel, equipment, and job description, and its accompanying excellent bibliography. The reader should view these suggested guidelines as a model for future attainment, not as the status of audiologists in the schools today. By extrapolating from the statistics presented by Jensema (1974), the basis for the ASHA position is obvious—there are an estimated 17,000 to 22,000 hearing-impaired children enrolled in special classes, of whom 40% have severe impairments.

To relate this population to the number of audiologists available for service, Garstecki (1976) sent out questionnaires to ASHA-certified audiologists identified as being associated with the schools. The questionnaire solicited information about specified duties and preparatory academic training. The results of the survey should be available late in 1977 as a position paper in the *Journal of the Academy of Rehabilitative Audiology.*

Siegenthaler[1] has pinpointed one of the truly significant (and controversial) issues dealing with the noneducational management of the hearing-impaired child in the schools. Who is responsible, the audiologist or the "hearing clinician"? (For further information, see the section on Auditory Training.)

Audiology and the Law

Since the practice of any specialty in the public sector closely relates to the law, Caccamo (1974) reported various cases of litigation relating to children's rights. He points out the need for legislation relating to communicative disorders. Funding, a partial answer to this need, is provided for under Public Law 94-142, the Education for All Handicapped Children Act. This law supports the practice of audiology within the school system and should provide an impetus toward a significant number of job openings.

Related to this general topic, the reader may be well informed about the legal status of the handicapped by subscribing to *Amicus,* a free-of-charge journal distributed on an infrequent basis (see Suggested Readings).

[1] Personal communication with Dr. B. Siegenthaler, 1976.

School Audiology as a Profession

Educational audiology as a speciality within the general area of audiology has been reported by Garwood et al. (1973), Garwood (1975), Jones (1973), Zink (1973), O'Neill (1974), Sheeley and Hannah (1974), and Johnson and Forbes (1975). Perhaps the most extensive study of the audiologic services needed by the schools and the competencies required of audiologists to perform those services has been provided by Jeffers (1973). This study utilized the RAND-Delphi method of consensus to solicit best opinions by the correspondents. The evidence presented by this project was an important factor in the construction and final approval of a school audiology credential in California. In a unique interview by the editor of Audiology and Hearing Education (1975), Berg described the background, philosophy, and execution of the training program in Educational Audiology at Utah State University. Berg (1976) has formalized his approach in book form.

Amplification

Auditory Training Units. The first significant study on types of classroom units and their characteristics was accomplished by Griffing and Hayes (1968). Unfortunately, no study of current auditory training units has followed. Olsen and Matkin (1971), Ross (1973), and Staab and O'Gara (1974) describe typical classroom systems and point out the need for expert assistance within the schools.

Personal Hearing Aids. The importance of monitoring performance of hearing aids has occupied the largest segment of the literature in recent years. Coleman (1975), Grammatico (1975), and Hanners and Sitton (1974) have cited the need for such programs and have specified procedures to accomplish this objective. Schell (1976) has described a program in the Cincinnati schools covering not only the need for routine monitoring but the costs involved in maintaining such procedures. Bess (1976) and Chial (1976) have presented results on a study of electroacoustic assessment of personal hearing aids with a sample of children enrolled in the deaf and hard-of-hearing program in the Los Angeles city schools. The study was unique in that the sample was tested at the local schools, and later a portion of this sample was retested under laboratory conditions. Results of the study once again indicated the relatively high percentage of malfunctioning aids and the marked discrepancy between factory specifications and later field tests. Of specific importance to audiologists were suggested differences between field and laboratory test results and the need for monitoring by personnel within the schools. Ross (1976) traced the history of publications relating to hearing-aid function and the need for informed involvement of parents and school professionals. He also defined hearing amplification for children in contrast with the total population of hearing aid users.

Classroom Acoustics

Ross and Giolas (1971) commented on the acute need for a rigidly controlled acoustic environment in regular classrooms. More important, however, was the need for such control in classrooms occupied by the hearing-impaired child enrolled in special classes. Crum and Matkin (1976) measured the noise and reverberation levels of eleven classrooms, only one of which met their noise-level criterion. They also described the measures necessary to modify classroom acoustics.

Special Devices

Damashek (1976) presented the circuit and description of a visual reinforcement unit to auditory training that can be utilized in the schools at a very low cost. Mecham (1976) developed a relatively simple system for verbal repetition and feedback reinforcement. He accomplished this by combining a portable FM radio equipped with a tape recorder, the personal hearing aid, a "mini-loop," microphone, and transmitter for use during auditory training periods in the classroom. Randolph (1976) described a simple procedure for recording the output of personal hearing aids through a low-cost coupler to a cassette recorder.

SCHOOL PROCEDURES

A new audiology program in the schools can produce considerable confusion at all levels of the school hierarchy. Personnel should be informed at an early stage that there are differences as well as similarities between audiologists and audiometrists.

The sole functions of audiometrists in the Los Angeles City School System are to identify the hearing-impaired child by conventional pure-tone test methods, and report such findings to the school administration. The audiometrist's academic preparation is specified by California law and consists of the successful completion of six units of undergraduate preparation in audiometry and "hearing conservation," with the additional specification of a valid credential. This credential may be earned in an area of health and development—for example, teaching exceptional children. This program is highly restrictive and involves no clinical management.

In theory, the audiologist picks up where the audiometrist leaves off. His concern is the management of those children whose pure-tone screening results are above a normative threshold criterion specified by law. Children with unilateral losses, however, should be rated with a relatively low priority when compared to children possessing equal or greater bilateral losses. The actual priority differential may be directly related to regulation by third-party payees, such as the Crippled Children program and Medicaid, who do not supply hearing aids to children with unilateral losses. At this stage, the school audiologist may have to assume the role of a "clinical" or "diagnostic" audiologist, performing additional diagnostic tests on individuals. Because the audiometer furnished the audiometrist is generally the portable pure-tone type, speech tests in sound-treated quarters are required.

In a sense then, the school audiologist is a diagnostician, although he is generally restricted to those speech tests designated as conventional—that is, Speech Awareness Threshold, Speech Discrimination Score, Speech Reception Threshold under earphones and in a sound field. The so-called special tests should be performed in quarters where medical support is immediately available. Practically speaking, the testing program, although necessary, should be second-ary to the audiologist's other responsibilities, which will shortly be explained. If the pupil has a personal hearing aid, the schools may request a reassessment, both aided and unaided, even though the child has been tested in a clinic. It is at this point that a conflict may be generated between the school and the clinic regarding this retest procedure.

In my experience, clinics have been most cooperative, particularly if the parents were unable to bring the child in for a re-evaluation. The basic responsi-bilities of the school audiologist in contrast with the clinical audiologist may be delineated operationally by the procedures that follow: (1) day-to-day, or week-to-week, monitoring of hearing-aid usage, (2) hearing-aid performance checks, (3) conducting auditory training as a part of the school curriculum, (4) frequent and consistent conferences with classroom teachers, and (5) monitoring the acoustic characteristics of the classroom and the school in general. It may well be that in the future, the "clinical" pediatric audiologist will restrict his function to diagnostic procedures, leaving the entire hearing-aid evaluation and follow-up procedures to the school audiologist. Furthermore, the entire evaluation proce-dure, which consists of testing, earmold impressions, and subsequent hearing-aid fitting, would be performed in the schools. Such procedures for ocular problems are presently being implemented in the Los Angeles city school district. Prece-dents have already been established in the fitting of eyeglasses in one of the Parent-Teacher Association clinics in the district. Concurrently, the same should hold true for the dispensing of hearing aids to the hearing impaired. California's Crippled Service program has shown a supportive attitude toward this concept.

Tests and Equipment

The requisites for adequate testing are expensive, whether the testing is done in permanent environments or in mobile units. In districts where agencies and

454   VICTOR P. GARWOOD

hospitals are plentiful, it is unnecessary to purchase the sophisticated equipment available at such clinics. Purchases should be restricted to the level required for conventional pure-tone and speech testing. Such equipment should contain booster amplifiers and loudspeakers for hearing aid checks and evaluations. Required and not optional is an impedance measuring device with an X-Y plotter. A simple circuit with suitable toy stimuli for conditioned orienting response audiometry has proved most helpful. The test room should conform to ANSI specifications, and be large enough to hold at least two people—the child and a second audiologist or aide for testing "difficult-to-test" children. An inexpensive and useful device to aid the test room assistant is a simple circuit containing a battery-charged amplifier-microphone for use by the control room audiologist. This, fed through the wall to a monaural headset, enables the tester to instruct the assistant without going through the master control panel of the audiometer. This device more than pays for itself in just one test session with a "difficult" child.

Earphone Calibration—Sound-Level Meter

In the long run, it will pay a district to invest in a sound-level meter—artificial ear kit with a sufficient number of extras to calibrate earphones as well as evaluate noise levels in the classroom. An octave or one-third octave-band filter accessory is desirable, since the audiologist may be called on to take measurements at locations where complaints are common: classrooms, cafeterias, hallways, playgrounds, and secondary school auditoriums.

Hearing Aid Analyzer

Devices for measuring the electroacoustic characteristics of amplification systems have undergone many changes over the years. Instead of an instrument rack composed of four or five expensive laboratory components at a fixed location, a limited array of portable units is now available. Such equipment may yield the type of information required for an overall estimate of hearing-aid performance. These units have also proved to be an essential adjunct to the understanding of amplification at the school level by personnel other than the audiologist who can gain some insight into the role played by the hearing aid. The anechoic chamber should be large enough to test both personal aids and auditory training units.

Although the school personnel involved in purchasing the equipment cited above may be appalled by the expense, none of the foregoing equipment is superfluous and the cost is actually small when compared to equipment required for other programs for physically handicapped children. The justification for these expenses should be augmented by the recent passage of Public Law 94-142, mentioned previously.

Amplification

Hearing Aids. Within the varying legal definitions specifying hearing loss levels, the crucial task of the audiologist in the public schools is to be assured that the hearing-impaired child wears suitable amplification. If audiologic services are new to the district, a position paper on amplification should be presented to the schools explaining concisely the role of the audiologist as a member of the team skilled in the use of auditory amplification.

The school audiologist may have little to say about the prior otoaudiologic evaluation and the hearing aid fitting, but is in the position to comment about the fitting as a positive factor in the educative process. There is nothing more discouraging than to find that the child with a beatific expression on his face has no battery in the case or that the volume control has not been turned on. Then there is the child who enters the classroom with the hearing aid in its box, not having used it since school was over the day before. Even more pathetic is the child who comes to school without the hearing aid because the parent "forgot." These examples, common experiences of school audiologists, are a reflection on prior care. The assumption is made that the child is "responsible." Hearing-impaired children, like all children, have to learn responsibility. The occasional trips to the otologist and the audiologist must be reinforced in the school. It is imperative that the school audiologist be trained for such a task.

Accomplishing this objective is not at all simple. The audiologist must work closely with the school principal to inform parents of their role in this situation. Parents should not only be notified of their responsibility to see that the hearing aid is working before the child goes off to school in the morning, but also be encouraged, if not coerced, into attending both individual and group information and guidance sessions at the school. Home visits may be required, but should be made only with the advice and approval of the principal. Often parents feel that once their child has completed a specialized preschool program their responsibility is over and the school will take charge. Other parents have had their child in a residential school where presumably such needs were met.

When the child walks into the classroom, however, the legal responsibility for that child is vested in the classroom teacher, whether it is a special school, integrated class, or regular classroom. It then becomes the responsibility of the audiologist as a resource specialist to render such services as will augment the teacher's role, services that are mutually decided on by both parties. Oftentimes the role of resource personnel in the schools is not clearly defined. The classroom teacher working with handicapped children is confronted by such a formidable array of consultants that continuity in the educative process is almost impossible. It is essential that the audiologist assure the principal and the classroom teachers collectively that individual service is integral to the learning process and must occur at times of mutual convenience. The "old" criticism of "speech teachers yanking children out of the classroom" may well be leveled at the audiologist unless an intervention program is carefully planned in advance. By learning in advance of the teacher's lesson plans and working around them, both the audiologist and the teacher will achieve their own objectives, with the child receiving a continuity of service appropriate to his needs.

The method of providing services will vary with the educational setting. In the regular school, the audiologist may begin the year with a demonstration of the function of hearing aids, charts of the ear, and simple explanations of hearing impairment. By using the child's own hearing aid as an example, the audiologist can check its performance. Subsequent monitoring can be more direct and probably more acceptable to the child, the rest of the class, and the teacher. In the integrated class and at special schools, a period of time scheduled for checking both personal hearing aids and classroom units is beneficial so that the educative process is not disrupted.

The above discussion presupposes that the audiologic work load will allow for such individualized attention. It is most unlikely, however, that the audiologist can afford this much time, especially if four or five schools must be served. In one special school, the audiologist trained an aide to perform such tasks as battery, earmold, tube, and cord continuity checks.

In other settings, audiologists have arranged in-service sessions for the teacher. This technique, however, produces varying levels of success. Many teachers, knowing that an audiologist has been assigned to the school, prefer to assume that the monitoring task must be performed by the audiologist, and will be inclined to "forget" or pass over the responsibility. Others (often those who have taken introductory courses in audiology) may be eager to check personal aids and are generally most helpful. Ancient prejudices against "mechanical things" must also be recognized and, therefore, a charitable attitude should be extended toward teachers who show this train of thought.

After the school audiologist has had a chance to visit the pupils in their classroom and observe their performance, a very disquieting thought appears and is intensified with further observation. The hearing aid model and type are apparently satisfactory for the type of loss, but the child is not attentive and may actually be failing in the classroom. Other resource specialists may have no other constructive information bearing on achievement, health, or learning. It has been demonstrated that the hearing aid itself may be the crucial factor. Studies already cited have shown that up to 30% of hearing aids tested in the schools are not up to specifications designated by the manufacturer and that some 50% of the hearing aids are malfunctioning. These studies suggest a high-priority need for the coordinating role of the school audiologist and the necessity for hearing aid test equipment in the schools.

Classroom Training Units

Auditory training units (ATUs) over the years have evolved into fairly sophisticated electronic systems. Although some districts may still prefer the portable desk units, the general trend in the past 10 years has been toward high-powered frequency-modulated-radio frequency (FM–RF) body units. These units operate as a one-way wireless system on a radio frequency band approved by the Federal Communications Commission. The pupil wears the receiver unit and the teacher a microphone transmitter antenna unit. These units appear either as combined units (regular body type aid with a snap-on FM unit), closed loop FM units, or the open RF unit that may be switched either to a conventional hearing aid circuit or to the RF circuit.

The loop and the open RF type employ chargeable batteries that must be put into a charger overnight or for the weekend. Obviously both the teacher's microphone and the student's receiver must be compatible for frequency. Nearby classrooms, of course, must be on different frequency bands.

The school district will be well advised to secure audiologic consultation during the purchasing negotiations for this type of equipment. The district must also know the guarantee terms and maintenance contract conditions in advance of the purchase. The school purchasing agent must be adequately familiar with the philosophy of the program so that the contract will specify suitable amplification without interruption during the school year. These facts must be known, as local hearing aid repair depots will usually not touch this type of equipment. Audiologists should closely examine the contracts to avoid future problems related to repair time, loaner ATUs, replacement of straps, and exchange of frequency modules. As motivation for sales often exceeds facilities for maintenance and repair, the audiologist must coach the school staff to see that units are repaired on schedule and that the pick-ups are made at times suitable to the school. School districts should be encouraged to purchase extra units and modules for emergencies. It is a matter of great importance that the audiologist meet with the repair technician to learn basic circuitry, lower-echelon trouble shooting, and adjustment of internal controls (especially for low-frequency and maximum power modification). It is advisable to set the output at 130dB SPL as a safety precaution. This setting should be verified, however, by an analyzer. Performance characteristics are sometimes not supplied with the ATU nor is it always possible to secure them from the factory.

Encouraging the use of units in programs whose philosophy is based on "total communication" can be an exhausting and futile task, especially if the classroom teacher's orientation is more "manual" than "oral-aural." If the school policy is avowedly dedicated to "total communication," the audiologist has no recourse other than to dig in and ferret out those children who can profit by amplification and demand its consistent usage—a formidable task!

Hearing Aids vs. Classroom Units

The discussion of classroom units is not complete until mention is made of their value in comparison with personal hearing aids. The audiologist must make decisions regarding the relative merits of ATUs with earphones or earmolds. If the latter coupling is preferred, the problem is diminished. However, if the child has standard body type molds for his personal hearing aid, the internal ATU volume control will have to be adjusted to avoid blasting.

The matter of hearing aids vs. trainers arises chiefly in cases where children have severe losses. Shall the child with a personal aid or aids wear the classroom unit only during school hours? Only during special speech classes? Not at all? Regardless of size, bulk, and placement of the unit, the child's ears are only 6 to 8 inches from the teacher's mouth when RF units are employed. This intimacy or "presence" is not available to the child wearing personal hearing aids. Despite this advantage, pupils at the upper elementary, junior high, and senior high levels resent the conspicuousness of the training unit—a body type aid. A practical solution may be to restrict the use of this equipment to speech and language classes. Utilization of their personal aids during the remaining hours of the school day may be a compromise acceptable to the teen-ager.

Recently, these arguments have been complicated by more extensive use of ear level aids for severe losses. Undoubtedly, the microphone at ear level is far more effective than at chest level. The rationale for both types is defensible, but the human variable has yet to be satisfactorily explained. The task, then, for the audiologist is clearly defined; both types must be investigated against the criteria of wearability, communication skill, and educational achievement. Unfortunately, the problem cannot be solved in a single sentence; its solution still rests on the shoulders of the school audiologist. It is the audiologist who must spearhead a team approach, consisting of the otologist, audiologist, hearing aid dispenser, parents, child, educational resource personnel members, and often public agencies providing hearing aids.

Experience with this matter leads one to believe that the question of body vs. ear level aids for the child with severe sensorineural hearing loss is one of the most crucial issues confronting the pediatric audiologist today. The audiologist must exert considerable caution when confronted by irate parents who have been subjected to a sales pitch on ear level aids by teachers and hearing dispensers.

It is logical to assume that the best amplification should provide the best educational results. Undoubtedly, children with mild to moderate losses, when subjected to tests of educational and communication skills, can show success with ear level instruments. However, such definitive results for children with only low-frequency residual hearing are hard to come by. At the present, we have only a vague idea of what the severely impaired child must hear. We have yet to develop an electronic filter that can simulate the severe loss. Currently, audiologists have tended to maximize the results of running tests of performance, frequency response, maximum power output, and harmonic analysis as a positive indicator of wearability. Such nonsense will continue as long as ignorance regarding true parameters of human hearing loss prevails. As a check on manufacturers' quality control, performance analyzers yield results that may provide useful data. How many of these analyzers, though, utilize new coupler designs? What happens to the ear when signals come through the human system at 130dB SPL? Such questions may be answered in the future, to be sure, but our strategy for the present must consist of elements of time, patience, and creative observation that are often avoided due to the exigencies of the occasion.

Auditory Training

It is truly unfortunate that audiologists have been associated more with hardware than with the rehabilitative-educative process. Perhaps some find it is more rewarding to deal with electronic "things" than with people. Whatever the reason, the fact remains that the majority of audiologists prefer to work as diagnosticians; they are somewhat reluctant to take on the role of rehabilitators. The diagnostic process is neat and relatively quick.

In the short history of the study of human communicative disorders, the therapeutic aspects of the field have historically been the domain of the speech pathologist—this because audiology, as a separate discipline, is new and its re-habilitative aspects generally untried. When cornered, audiologists protest (mightily) that the hearing aid evaluation is rehabilitative and patients are "followed up."

According to the California Speech and Hearing Association directory, only a handful of clinics engage in aural rehabilitation. In the California schools, there are presently approximately 25 school audiologists—not all of them full-time—and approximately 3,000 speech pathologists. In addition, there are some 1,000 teachers of the hearing-impaired. It becomes apparent that speech pathologists and teachers of the hearing-impaired must be the pediatric rehabilitators.

School audiologists resist their role as rehabilitators and generally explain that their other duties are so great that they have no time left for this activity. On the surface, the alibi sounds satisfactory. In the Los Angeles City School District there simply are not enough audiologists to accommodate the needs of the hearing-impaired. Presently 1,000 children are enrolled in the deaf and hard-of-hearing program and some 500 suspected hearing-impaired children in other special education programs: 1,500 cases and 4 audiologists. Even if there were 1 audiologist for every 75 to 100 hearing-impaired children, aural rehabilitation would still play a minor role, since this function is stated as one of the responsibilities of the teacher of the hearing-impaired. These teachers are doing a tremendous job and many incorporate communication skills in every subject area, especially in oral-aural schools for deaf children.

Although the new audiologist may have received only 300 to 500 hours of practice in clinical audiology as a student, some of the training should have engendered a feeling for basic principles of the rehabilitative process. Having already tested the child and investigated the efficiency of the amplification utilized, the audiologist is in the unique position of advising the teacher of the child's potential to apprehend certain sounds and suggest techniques for incorporating them into speech. A simple template or overlay showing energy levels of speech sounds as a function of frequency on the audiogram may illustrate this point. Sound-level data collected during classroom activity may modify the teacher's approach to speech, language, and environmental sounds. Although the audiologist may regard this role as assistive, it may prove to be one of dominance.

The fact remains that after the otolaryngologist, the audiologist, and the hearing aid dispenser have completed their evaluative examinations and fittings, it may be six months to a year before a child is again evaluated, and then the results are measured only in terms of a few hours observations. Such relatively infrequent visits do not provide the continuous evaluation required for growing children. What then? It is an interesting commentary on our philosophy of child care in a culture that specifies a brief evaluative period on one hand, but expects continuity of academic education on the other. Intimately related to this problem are supplementary rehabilitative programs offered to selected children by community and hospital clinics. The selection is primarily based on economic consideration, since current federal subsidies cannot be applied to children of the poor. The basis for this determination is that it is the mandate of the public schools to provide such services to school-age children. The legislation is discriminative, in that children in private schools are already eligible for such services. This applies particularly in the State of California where Medi-Cal (state Medicaid) regulations specifically exclude children in the public schools from supplementary speech and hearing rehabilitation.

For those who can afford this extra training, it is effective only if communication is open and continuous between the public school and the clinic. This communication must not occur just at the specialist level, but at the administrative level as well. Audiologists must understand that the legal responsibility for a child enrolled in the public schools rests with the schools. Aural rehabilitation is a technique for facilitating the educative process, wherever it takes place.

The question of whether teachers of the deaf or audiologists are better prepared to work with hard-of-hearing children is being approached in Pennsylvania by a proposal to the legislature that a new classification, the "Hearing Clinician," be formed.

'Hearing Clinician' means a person who offers habilitative and rehabilitative services to hearing impaired persons, including speech reading, auditory training, remediation of speech and language development problems due to hearing disorders, and consultation about auditory training and speech reading (Siegenthaler, 1976).

The justification for this addition to the speech and hearing licensing bill is based on the following premises (Siegenthaler, 1976):

1. Hearing clinicians exist.

2. Hearing clinicians deliver a valuable service to the communicatively impaired, different from the service delivered by teachers of the deaf.

3. Hearing clinicians have competencies and make contributions different from those of audiologists and speech pathologists.

4. Ethical, responsible, and competent professional people deserve to be and should be recognized when they have contributions to make to the welfare of the hearing-impaired.

This new category, separatist as it may be, reveals a thoughtful approach that may well solve some of the bothersome relations among specialists whose present roles are not operationally well defined in the schools today.

Reports and Forms

The school audiologist, like other public servants, is caught up in a paper explosion that inevitably consumes time that could more valuably be spent with children. Audiologists should accept this fact only with great reluctance. A partial solution may rest with the now ubiquitous technique of assigning priorities. The chief priority relates to the child and should always take precedence over other matters of importance to the system. To save time, report forms should be designed so that with a minimum of time a maximum amount of pertinent information can be stated.

Evaluation Report. This important report should clearly state the findings of the audiologic evaluation. The results of the evaluation should appear on a printed form (Sample Form 1).

By exercising some ingenuity, most items may be reduced to numbers, check marks, or very brief, one-line comments. This report is most important for future reference and as support for a recommendation. The crucial elements are the impressions, observations, and recommendations. In these sections the audiologist specifies operationally the child's behavior, procedures to be followed, and personnel to be informed. The findings are then sent to the principal of the child's school. It is his responsibility to then inform both intra- and extra-school personnel of the findings and request subsequent action. A variety of individuals and agencies may be required to fulfill these requests: physicians, school nurses, counselors, teachers, and other resource personnel.

Of equal importance may be the necessity for further testing at some specified date. The last item is self-explanatory if school policy requires only a validating signature. The audiologist may be subjected to the slight indignity of a countersigning supervisor who must be either ASHA-certified, state-licensed, or both.

The original copy of the report should stay in the audiology office. Legible copies should be sent to principals and other administrators. This seemingly minor detail can prove to be major for future retrieval.

A. Identifying Data

    1. Name of pupil
    2. Birth date
    3. School
    4. Evaluation date

B. Audiologist Summary

    1. Type of loss
    2. Degree of loss in dB/HL (PTA)
    3. SAT or SRT
    4. SDS re: SRT
    5. Make, model, type and serial number of Hearing Aid

        a. Ear placement
        b. Type of earmold
        c. Aided speech scores

    6. Impedance

        a. Tympanogram classification
        b. Static compliance
        c. Point of maximum compliance
        d. Reflex
        e. Impression
        f. Comments or remarks

C. Speech intelligibility (*)

D. Lipreading skills (*)

E. Impressions and observations

    1. During evaluation
    2. During prior classroom visits

F. Recommendations

G. Signature of audiologist and date submitted.

(*) These should be brief impressions that are applicable only to the evaluative session.

Sample Form 1. Report Form for Audiologic Evaluation

Along with this form, an audiometric work sheet can be helpful, and can include a graphic display on a standard audiometric form. Often this kind of display can help explain test results to nonaudiologic personnel. According to current regulations in many states, the form must be shown to the parent, if requested. If such is the case, only the audiologist is capable of reviewing test results with the parent, and then only at the school site. The audiogram may be posted on a class bulletin board *only* with parental approval.

Referral for Service Form. The purpose of this form, addressed to the audiologist to request evaluation, is to give signing authority to the referring school principal, whose validating signature and date attest to this fact. This holds true even if the actual referral is requested by a classroom teacher, counselor, or other resource personnel at the school. The form should be relatively simple. (See Sample Form 2.)

The completed form is sent from the child's school to the audiologist for disposition. The audiologist should respond with either a tentative or firm scheduling date for service.

Classroom ATU Monitor Form. With few exceptions, classroom auditory training units are purchased by the district and therefore subject to some form of audit. Responsibility can rest either with a division, a department, or an individual school. The audiologist shares in this responsibility at whatever level by developing a plan to insure that the appropriate instrument is compatible with the child's auditory status. Keeping track of the right instrument for the right child is an arduous task for the audiologist—children move on, instruments require repair and adjustment. Teachers require constant reinforcement regarding

```
A.  Identifying Date

    1.  Student's address, and birth date
    2.  Name of parent or guardian, address, and telephone number (both
        work and home phones)
    3.  School and teacher

B.  Reason for referral

C.  Amplification status

    1.  Factors relating to personal hearing aid
    2.  Factors relating to classroom auditory training unit

D.  Classroom behavior (brief description)

E.  Pertinent physical information

    1.  Prior and current audiologic and medical/surgical consultation
    2.  Hospital patient file number and phone number
    3.  Physician/otolaryngologist (specify) and phone number
    4.  Audiologist and phone number
    5.  Other consultations
    6.  Audiologist's decision
    7.  Validating signatures and dates
    8.  Tentative or firm date for service
```

Sample Form 2. Referral for Service Form

the instrument's value in the educative process. The primary reason for this form is its applicability to a problem. Monitoring forms will supply both the teacher and the audiologist with information regarding the current status of an instrument. (See Sample Form 3.)

Teachers should have a simple but complete description of the unit, microphone, charger and receiver, battery checker, and some simple precautions regarding the maintenance of the system.

Pupil Schedule Form. A posted schedule allows a clerical staff to inform schools of when students are to be tested, by whom, and at what schools. This control is absolutely necessary if more than one audiologist uses the same test facility. The burden may be eased by prior compromises among the audiologists for their choice of test days and times. A major shortcoming is often the lack of a satisfactory solution to the problem of testing the difficult-to-test children. In certain cases two audiologists have been used. A much more efficient solution to this problem would be to train aides to help with this type of child.

Testing Log. This form has proven most effective as a check on the schedule. The form contains names, date of entry, date tested, audiologist's initials, a no-show column, and a space for comments. This form also allows for internal control of personnel as well as for a time lapse between entry and scheduling.

Weekly Activity Report. This was probably the most controversial form developed, and in essence was called "activity" as a more palatable euphemism for time and motion study of the audiologists. The form, developed in conference with a staff, was a weekly report that consisted of two main sections: direct and

---

```
A.  Identifying data

    Date, classroom number, and teacher

B.  Name of child (space should be provided for each student in the class)

C.  ATU Data

    1.  Serial number
    2.  Internal maximum power output (MPO) setting
    3.  Internal tone control setting
    4.  Frequency module designation (with RF units)
    5.  Teacher microphone designation (compatible with student unit)
    6.  Volume control setting(s)
```

Sample Form 3. ATU Monitor Form

other services to children. Indirect services accounted for approximately 70% of the clinician's time. The subheadings are listed below as follows:

Direct Services	*Other Services*
Audiologic evaluation	Parent conferences (individual and group)
Observation in classroom	Teacher conferences (individual and group)
Conferences with pupil	Conference with other personnel (specify)
ATU check	School staff conference
Special projects (specify)	Audiologists staff conference
Other (specify)	Conference with supervisor
	In service (specify)
	Special projects (specify)
	Audiologic reports
	Travel time
	Others (specify)

By breaking down the entries into half-hour segments, a fairly accurate accounting was made that could be utilized internally to compare the efficiency of audiologists. By specifying the similarities and differences, an explanation was made of the business of audiology. Externally, the data were used to negotiate for more space and personnel. After a few months, enough information was accrued to justify the termination of the reports.

Parent Forms. Audiologists often assume that parents are willing to cooperate with the school's requests for information. They soon learn to modify this assumption and be satisfied with a probability model. Parents are flooded with almost as many notices as are school personnel. The audiologist must enter the contest fully equipped as a personnel relations expert, ready to obtain the attention of the parents. One factor emerges: parents are more mindful of directives sent out by the school principal than of those from other school personnel, and some principals are more skillful at this business than others. A notice should go out over the principal's signature, but with the countersignature of the audiologist. Commonly, parents should be notified of the following:

1. A malfunctioning hearing aid
2. A "forgotten" hearing aid
3. Group or individual conferences
4. A guide for daily hearing aid care.

In districts with large non-English-speaking populations, bilingual personnel can be most beneficial. A language barrier is handicap enough, but that compounded with physical impairment is tragic. Most school districts with sizable minority groups have, however, a cadre of translators available for this task. Notices should be simple, clear, concise, and relevant. At the same time they should be so contrived as to contain an amount of redundancy suitable to the importance of the notice. If the notices require a return, the principal should be requested to supply clerical help to facilitate the return and eventual disposition. Although the care and responsibility for personal hearing aids rests with the parents, the audiologist should be in communication with the hearing aid dispenser. He should also be responsible for putting an entry in the pupil's folder specifying the name, facility, and telephone number of the dispenser. Most dispensers are, however, most cooperative and may supply the best entry to the home.

Notices to Teachers. Although teachers of the deaf and hard-of-hearing are relatively sophisticated about the care of hearing aids and earmolds, the development of the following two forms for their use, reinforcing their content through in-service programs and conferences, has been effective. Sample Form 4 is an example of this type of material.

Another form was developed for regular classroom teachers in schools with itinerant programs for deaf and hard-of-hearing children. (See Sample Form 5.)

To supplement the preceding materials, a solicitation of free booklets was made from manufacturers of earmolds, hearing aids, and auditory training units. These were distributed to the teachers with the hope that they would be read. Sometimes they were. . . .

Sound Control of Classrooms

School districts have become increasingly aware of the need for more adequate control of classroom acoustics, not only for special rooms but for regular classrooms as well. Public allocation of funds for schools, however, has been scrutinized much more closely during the seventies. The tendency has been to restore existing buildings rather than to build new structures expressly designed to include acoustic treatment. This fact poses serious problems to the audiologist who may recommend sound treatment of classrooms for hearing-impaired children. In the first place, such improvement is quite expensive; second, the rooms can only be treated partially with carpeted floors and acoustically treated ceiling tile that may extend down to chair rail height. This expense is largely negated by the amount of window space allocated for room brightness and by hard-surfaced hallways and walkways adjacent to the classroom. Administrators question the need for quietness when the pupils have reduced hearing sensitivity. A useful technique for convincing the administration that acoustic treatment is not only desirable but necessary involves two procedures. The audiologist should take overall and band-filtered sound-level readings at peak levels of classroom activity. These results should be presented in a clear, concise form to the principal. Of even more persuasion would be the playing of one of the available tapes made through a hearing aid to school personnel. A most convincing argument to teachers and administrators has been a tape made by Mark Ross and his col-

---

A. Listening Checks for Hearing Aids

1. Use your own individual earmold if you have one.
2. Check the battery to see that it is placed correctly in the case. Clean battery terminals with an eraser if necessary. Terminals of ear level aids are more difficult to clean, so we suggest that you ask the parent to take the aid to their dispenser.
3. Establish a comfortable listening level for each hearing aid and listen daily at this volume setting. If the aid sounds weak, insert a new battery if one is available. If the level is still low, refer to dispenser.
4. Set controls:

   a. "On/Off" switch in "Off" position.
   b. Volume Control at lowest setting.
   c. Switch in "M," or mike, position.
   d. Tone control in setting most frequently used.

5. Place the receiver to your ear. Cover the receiver with the palm of your hand and hold the main part of the hearing aid away from your ear to prevent feedback.
6. Turn the hearing aid to "On." Turn the volume control wheel up and down slowly, listening for scratchiness or dead spots. The volume control should neither be excessively loose, nor bind against the case.
7. Turn the "On/Off" switch back and forth to check for intermittent sound or loose contacts.
8. Establish a comfortable listening level.
9. Roll the cord back and forth between the fingers to check for "cut-outs" with body worn instruments. With ear level aids, check the plastic tubing for possible stiffness, pinholes, or cracks.
10. Check the firmness of cord connections.
11. Gently tap the hearing aid on all sides to check for a reduction of power or loose connections. Check for loose screws in the case.
12. With the aid in the "Off" position and the receiver out of your ear, place your thumb firmly over the opening in the receiver. Turn the hearing aid on and turn the volume all the way up. Listen for a soft whistling sound from the hearing aid case or from the receiver. With ear level aid, put your thumb firmly over the opening of the earmold.
13. Check the earmold for cleanliness. Clean if necessary with soap, water, and a pipe cleaner.

B. Suggestions for Keeping Earmolds Clean - A Classroom Project - We suggest that a weekly classroom project involve cleaning earmolds. In this way the children can learn how to take care of their molds and transfer this knowledge to their home. Schedule a time once a week to thoroughly clean the molds by soaking them in warm soapy water for about 5 minutes. Rinse them with clear water and let them dry on a paper towel until all of the water is out of the canal. A pipe cleaner can be used to dry and to clean the bore of the mold. Do not use the mold until it is completely dry.

Sample Form 4. Suggestions for the Care of Hearing Aids and Accessories

3. Knowledges, skills, abilities, and personal characteristics

   a. Skill in the selection and use of classroom amplification systems, hearing aids, and other audiological equipment.
   b. Ability to evaluate performance characteristics of hearing aids and classroom amplification units.
   c. Skill in interpreting and reporting audio-metric, audiologic, and related behavioral test data.
   d. Ability to recognize needs of individual students in relation to audiological assistance.
   e. Facility in the arts of oral and written expression.
   f. Cleanliness and appropriate personal appearance and manner.
   g. Poise, tact, good judgment, and ability to work effectively with district and community personnel and students.

4. Health: physical and mental fitness to engage in audiological services as evidenced by a certificate from Employee Health Services of the school district.

5. Credential and license: A valid credential authorizing K-12 service must be in force.

   a. A credential authorizing service in audiology as a speech and hearing specialist or as a teacher of the exceptional child with hearing impairment.
   b. A valid license in audiology issued by the responsible state agency.

Sample Form 4. Continued

league, Randolph (1976) illustrating magnificently how noise and distortion are transmitted through high-power hearing aids. They reported a relatively inexpensive evaluation system employing a cassette recorder, a crutch tip for the cavity external microphone, with standard tubing to the hearing aid. A most useful summary of the effects of noise and reverberation on speech intelligibility in the classroom is being reported by Olsen in a forthcoming publication.

Caution should be exercised regarding the importance of sound level recordings at this point. After the survey has been completed, the administration should be cautioned that much more sophisticated noise-level equipment is available and should be performed by a group qualified to not only record levels but to advise amelioration of the noise problem. Architectural firms now employ acoustic consultants who are quite familiar with such problems. The important message here is that the audiologist should initiate the proceedings and convince the administration that sound control in classrooms is important to facilitate learning and to reduce classroom confusion and annoyance factors. The audiologist, in turn, must know the capabilities and shortcomings of instrumentation, impressing heavily upon school personnel the necessity for improving the classroom milieu.

Relations with Community Specialists

The school audiologist also acts as a catalyzing agent and ombudsman. A close relation with children in the schools places the audiologist in a position of

1. Call his name and make sure he is watching you before you begin speaking.

2. Face him all the time while you are talking to him, so he can see your lips.

3. Don't talk to him from another room or while facing the blackboard.

4. Talk slower, and speak from a close distance.

5. Hold your head still while speaking and move around as little as possible.

6. Talk in a formal tone of voice - no shouting and no whispering.

7. Limit speaking to no more than one person at a time.

8. Make sure the light is falling on your lips while you are speaking.

9. If you have a tendency to mumble, practice moving your mouth and lips more when you speak, but do not make exaggerated mouth movements.

10. If he doesn't understand what you are saying, try rewording it. Remember longer and more expressive words are easier to lipread.

11. Keep hands and books away from face so that mouth is not covered while speaking.

12. Never take understanding on the part of the student for granted; only when he answers are you sure he understands. You may have him repeat or demonstrate the instructions.

Sample Form 5. Rules for Communication with Hard-of-Hearing Children

authority among local agencies, physicians, clinical audiologists, hearing aid dispensers, and the schools. This unique position also poses problems that relate to prior diagnosis, medical treatment, and amplification, particularly in urban areas where a high incidence of poverty exists. Areas of poverty demand special consideration as ignornace often accompanies poverty. Some of these children receive competent medical advice and treatment, but the majority are seen by neighborhood general practitioners, not experienced with problems related to ear pathology. Children are often referred directly by the practitioner to hearing aid dispensers, despite regulatory legislation in some states. Someone must take the lead in securing adequate diagnosis, treatment, and amplification for such children. The possibility exists, however, that this population is the one identified with almost continuous expenditure of public funds. Early attention will, in the long run, conserve significant future expense. As children grow and change between annual visits to the physician, the audiologist may, by repeated impedance measurements and hearing aid checks, point out the need for intervention by specialists. The resolution of these problems is a long, hard, and frustrating battle, consuming hours of valuable time and requiring almost endless patience.

Public agencies must be contacted to facilitate treatment for children who have been identified as hearing-impaired but who have not been seen by specialists (or have not been seen at all) and are obviously eligible for care. These

VICTOR P. GARWOOD

children are too often victims of understaffed bureaucratic systems whose responsibilities may be so fragmented as to defy description. These are the children who can be helped by the audiologist, who is, in the final analysis, the "court" of last resort. That this is not an impossible task has been demonstrated repeatedly by the intervention of the school audiologist. Community agencies do want to help the child, but the vital link is often missing. The school audiologist is that "missing link." The work they do is "follow-up" work in the true sense. The rewards are great; the child is served and the community educated.

SCHOOL RELATIONS

Job Description

School audiologists must have a working knowledge of exactly what will be expected of them before accepting a position. Although the preceeding guidelines appear obvious, the facts show that there are very few precendents currently in existence on a national level. In many cases, the audiologist may be the first one in either a district or a state. In my situation, there was no precedent, which meant I created my own job description, namely senior audiologist. In addition, it became necessary to institute positions for those audiologists who, I hoped, would implement my plans. Although I could specify responsibilities in general, I soon found out that the district had somewhat restrictive personnel policies regarding qualifications for both positions. Fortunately, I had already acquired a restricted speech and hearing credential, which the personnel branch assured me was the "clincher" in securing the position. Subsequently, in hiring future audiologists, I specified that they possess a valid credential. This fact alone considerably reduces the available applicants, since most students generally take clinical courses, assuring them of employment in agencies or hospitals only requiring ASHA certification.

There are, fortunately, emergency measures being taken in many states that enable prospective employees to be hired on a temporary basis. As previously stated, the California State Commission on Credentials and Licensing authorized a new credential for audiologists in the public schools. Teacher training institutions are presently in the process of implementing the credential by securing curricula approval.

In the meantime, the chief qualification for the position is ASHA certification and the "old" speech and hearing credential. Although state licensing in audiology is not required in the schools, it is apparent that the prestige of the audiologist is enhanced by the license. Furthermore, if the school audiologist performs any service outside of the school system, a license is mandatory in the state of California. A factor not to be overlooked is the numbers game; the profession must be identified and numbers help. (Unfortunately, in many states licensure laws have been hindered by well-meaning but misinformed legislators.)

As yet, it has not been feasible to secure any positive information on whether the new credential in California will have a "grandfather clause" covering present school audiologists. ASHA-based certification modified to be congruent with the new guidelines specified by the Joint Committee on Audiology and Education of the Deaf would be useful as a model for districts considering audiologic services. Presently, the major problem with the guidelines is an excessive amount of optimism regarding case loads and personnel requirements. The guidelines do, however, point toward an ideal that should be sought.

The class description in Sample Form 6 may act as a guide for students and districts who are considering school audiologic services. Note that the use of the term "audiometry" does not appear in the description.

Job Accountability. The audiology student who has just emerged from a university clinical program enters an environment where, by law, everyone from clerical to certificated personnel must be accountable to an individual in a supervisory capacity. In many states, including California, this is a formal annual or biannual requirement; an evaluation of performance and a statement of goals are contained in a written document signed by both the evaluator and the evaluatee. In many respects this is a redundant procedure, since both the code and local district policy contain clauses relative to job accountability. However, its necessity becomes apparent when promotion or dismissal is under consideration and precise written documentation is absolutely necessary, especially for dismissal. This procedure is extremely valuable because it forces the employee to actually set down on paper his goals and objectives and requires his supervisor to write out his opinions regarding the employee's past and current performances.

This procedure is of equal importance to the new probationary teacher. Since audiology is a new specialty, the probationary period is one that can either encourage or kill a new program. Initially, the newly hired audiologist may resent being put on the spot, particularly if his evaluator is not an audiologist. However, a realization that the experience may be an educative one to both the evaluator and the district may soothe the novice's sense of pride.

To whom an audiology group should be accountable is a moot point. Traditionally, audiologists have been associated with providers of health services. In the schools, however, the power usually rests with the instructional divisions. The prospective audiologist should, therefore, take a long, hard look at the administrative structure before leaping into a division with a low budget and only intermittent contact with pupils. The temptation to be associated with the physician should be tempered by an awareness that education is the name of the game, not medicine!

Speech and Language Specialists

By and large, audiologists are "loners" when they enter the public schools. They are often confronted with a bewildering array of specialists, all of whom

Class Description

A. Primary function: Provides audiologic services to special schools and to integrated or itinerant programs for students with impaired hearing as assigned.

B. Responsible to Senior Audiologist

C. Subordinates: Audiology aide as assigned

D. Responsibilities:

   1. Performs audiological tests of students enrolled in the District's programs for hearing-impaired and of District employees and applicants referred by Employee Health Services.
   2. Discusses audiological findings with school staff, other appropriate personnel, and parents; maintains student records containing audiological information.
   3. Makes recommendations for home and classroom management relating to amplification units and auditory training.
   4. Assists with evaluations relating to the performance characteristics of students' hearing aids, and of wearable auditory training units.
   5. Collects and interprets, from appropriate cooperating agencies, current audiological information about students.
   6. Assists the senior audiologist with in-service education for teachers regarding the effective use of audiological services in the teaching of students with impaired hearing.
   7. Writes audiological reports relating to student assessment as required and special reports as requested.
   8. Assists in evaluating the acoustic environment of classrooms used for students having impaired hearing.
   9. During periods of critical personnel shortage or other emergency situations, shall temporarily perform any duties, as directed, within the authorization of any credentials held by the incumbent, which are registered with the office of the superintendent and which are a part of the class description requirements in effect at the time such duties are performed.
  10. Performs other duties as assigned.

E. Qualifications

   1. Education: Completion of all academic requirements including a supervised clinical practicum, and the clinical fellowship year (CFY) for a Certificate of Clinical Competence in Audiology from the American Speech and Hearing Association.
   2. Experience

     a. Required: none
     b. Desirable: professional experience in the field of public school or clinically based audiology.

Sample Form 6. Job Description for School Audiologists

have specific duties relating to the education of the exceptional child. With the exception of teachers of the deaf and hard of hearing (whose responsibilities have been covered elsewhere in this chapter), the audiologist will be working quite closely with the speech and language specialists. The job description of these specialists generally includes working with children who have speech problems related to hearing loss. They may even carry the title "speech and hearing clinician." Their work may often include responsibilities in special schools that encompass either the total population or special classes. This situation may create some initial confusion that may persist and will subside only when two specialists sit down at the negotiation table and redefine their responsibilities.

The issue of responsibility delegation with regard to the hearing impaired child is not new. Audiologists feel that by virtue of their training, they should be the primary providers of such service. The fact remains, however, that in most systems, speech and language specialists are well entrenched, simply because for years there were no audiologists available to work with these children.

Audiologists, because of their training, may prefer to restrict their activities to evaluation rather than rehabilitation, and by extension of the latter activity, amplification. In small school districts, the audiologist may be called on to handle an entire continuum of oral-aural training. In large districts, the load may be so great that the audiologist may act only as a consultant to both the teacher of the hearing-impaired and the speech specialist.

Schools whose specialists are currently being hired as language and speech specialists but whose credentials are specified as speech, language, and hearing specialists may simply divide their personnel into two categories. By extension, the increase of responsibility regarding the hearing specialist would then include evaluation and amplification procedures. It is interesting to note that in 1975 the California State Board of Education through one of its commissions revised the credential structure by creating two new credentials: specialization in clinical or rehabilitative services in the area of language, speech, and hearing services, and the other, specialization in clinical or rehabilitative services in the area of audiology. The policy and implementation statements regarding these two specialties defy definition and leave one with the impression that some specialists with an audiologic background are better than others. The language is so stilted and so laden with terminology reminiscent of systems research that it is almost unreadable. Undoubtedly other states are burdened with this language preoccupation presumed to be the most efficient language of accountability.

School Psychologists. Another well-entrenched specialty in public education is school psychology. Although the psychologists could logically be close allies to the audiologist, as their evaluation program is important to the total evaluation of the child's psychosocial ability as a function of learning, this is not always the case; their training appears to be negligible in the area of severe hearing loss and deafness. Psychologists are oftentimes at a loss when an evaluation must be made almost solely upon the basis of performance rather than verbal skills. If they were to accept this fact and seek guidance from the audiologist, suitable school placement could be facilitated greatly. Meetings to discuss placement of handicapped children could provide an excellent common meeting ground to resolve differences in opinion, especially if time has been given to observe the child prior to the meeting. (Both parties will complain, with justification, that their other responsibilities are so great that time is rarely available for extended observation.

This complaint is so common to all resource specialists that it must be expected to be a constant.)

School Physicians and Nurses

If a district is fortunate enough to employ an otolaryngologist (even part-time), the audiologist will have a ready ear for consultation, particularly about children with middle-ear problems. The physicians are greatly impressed with the results presently being achieved with impedance tests and may be most helpful with referrals for treatment. The problem is more complicated if the physician is not an ear specialist, and action may be slower unless the audiologist builds a strong case for the consideration of medical or surgical intervention. By and large, most school physicians are pediatricians; they have some knowledge of what transpires behind the eardrum, but it is usually minimal. The Audiology Unit of the Los Angeles city school district was able to provide several lectures a year by local otologists as a component of the district's in-service program. Special invitations were sent to the school physicians and nurses. Fortunately, a large city can support a number of otologists, some of whom are really quite concerned about children and are glad to volunteer their time for such special lectures.

In the last analysis, though, the presence of school nurses is far more valuable. They are in close contact with the children on a day-to-day basis. In addition, their enlightenment was important since nurses generally have the authority to refer the child to an outside physician. Again, the audiologist must come to a meeting of the minds with nurses, who, until an audiologist has been hired, may often serve as amateur audiologists.

School Committee Functions

Admission and Discharge (A & D). Hard-of-hearing and deaf children are not automatically placed in special classes; they are only admitted after the schools conduct formal and legal procedures, generally functions of a committee whose members are specified by law. Audiologists, as a rule, are not specifically recognized as administrators, and experienced special education teachers are. Districts are wise, however, to invite an audiologist, who is the sole member of the committee knowledgeable of diagnostic findings (both medical and audiological) and amplification factors. Often the speech pathologist is an invited member of the committee. In California, a new law specifies that parents must be invited to the committee meeting at which their child will be discussed, and must be notified of the meeting date well in advance.

Of primary concern to the committee is the determination of a child's eligibility for a special program and the determination of whether or not the district has a program capable of meeting the child's needs. Since every state has minimal criteria for admittance into a special program, the audiologist is responsible for checking the child's hearing status against the state criteria. In addition, the audiologist must be able to assure the committee that the medical statement is in general agreement with the state criteria. Generally, otolaryngologists supply excellent reports, often with complete audiologic and hearing aid data. The response from hospital clinics is another matter and the level of their sophistication is generally indicative of the hospital audiologist's ability to secure adequate diagnostic information from a resident staff member.

In the Los Angeles city school district committee meetings were not scheduled until all diagnostic information was available. Occasionally the referring audiologist or physician will present an overzealous recommendation for a child's educational management that accomplishes little more than infuriating the school administrators. Because the parents may be informed of the recommendation, the process can become most uncomfortable. Such recommendations tend to be made in ignorance but, with the aid of a skillful school audiologist who is diplomatically inclined, the situation could possibly be remedied.

The audiologist also contributes to the procedure with his knowledge of hearing aids. He can determine, before a child is actually enrolled in a school, whether the hearing aid is in fact functional. Although parents are requested to see that their child is wearing the aid at the committee meeting, between 25% and 50% of the children arrive without amplification. The aid has either been "forgotten" or "lost"; in many cases it does not even work. In Los Angeles, where the Spanish-speaking population is sizable, parents newly arrived from South and Central America are often accompanied by children who have never been fitted with hearing aids. The recommended procedure then becomes one of trial placement until an aid is purchased or negotiated through state-federal assistance plans.

As much assistance as can be elicited from the parent, some observation of the performance by the child, and a review of the other school data can result in a decision for placement. As part of the decision-making process, the audiologist must exert experience and expertise. Some of the determining questions are: (1) Shall the child be admitted to a special school, and if so, to an oral or a total communications program? (2) Would it be more beneficial to enroll the child in an integrated program within a regular school or in a regular school with itinerant tutoring service?

It is during this discussion that knowledge of the available programs is crucial. Here the audiologist must exercise caution and judgment. The audiologist is not only sending a child out into the world, but into an educational atmosphere that must be conducive to academic growth as well as improved communication skills. If the procedure occurs at the beginning of the school year, the decision can bring about dismissal of a teacher because of low enrollment or perhaps hiring of new personnel because of increased enrollment. The parent may have been advised by the referral source that some schools would better fit the needs of their child than others. It is the function of the referring audiologist to specify the type of treatment, not the location. Despite any number of professional opinions that may be offered, by law it is often the decision of the parent that is final.

The discharge function of the committee occurs when the district determines that a child is eligible for special services that are not available within the district. This is a very tense situation, since the district may have to spend a sizable sum of money to send the child to a private school. A parent, for example, might request that the child be enrolled in a private facility that allegedly supplies better individualized services than those supplied by the district. A state department of education consultant may be appointed to investigate the problem, but even so, the responsibility of the audiologist remains constant regarding admission and discharge procedures, and his contribution must be restricted to audiologic findings.

Placement Review. This function signifies the need for change in placement of a child within the district toward an integrated, or regular, school setting. The school recommends that the committee consider the child for a change in school placement. The usual periods for recommending change are at the end of elementary school and the end of junior high school.

In a city as large as Los Angeles, decisions must rest not only on the basis of the "mainstream" philosophy but also on distance from the home school. In a district of 750 square miles, this can pose quite a problem. In smaller districts with no alternatives, the decision is rather simple; the child moves to an area where programs are available. If the audiologist has been rendering attentive service, his position is generally in agreement with the teacher. However, the procedure, as a rule, is based primarily on "educational" achievement and any information that the audiologist can offer will be seriously considered in the final decision. As the decision is based on current needs, the audiologist may also be called upon to administer further hearing tests and hearing aid evaluations just prior to the meeting, especially if the last evaluation was equivocal. Following the last evaluation, tests might also indicate that the child is making better use of amplification as measured by educational achievement.

The School Principal

Coordinators and supervisors may have a high ranking in the hierarchy of a school system, but in truth the principal runs the school and ranks immediately under the superintendent in level of administration. The new audiologist had best be aware of this fact. Some principals rank higher than others; the secondary principal is not only paid more but has a larger staff. Assuming that the majority of the audiologist's load will be composed of elementary school children, the audiologist should exert considerable effort not only in rendering services to the pupil but in trying to make the job easier for the principal.

One of the first things the new audiologist will notice is the mountain of paper work and the plethora of resource personnel that invade the schools daily. Listen to the principal, who must daily placate the parents, the teachers, and the administration.

In addition to all of this, the principal is now advised that added to this confusion will be yet another resource person, but optimistically, a most necessary one. If he can understand the dilemma faced by the principal in this age of specialists, the audiologist is well on the way to becoming a valuable adjunct to the school team. On one hand, the principal-as-administrator would prefer audiologists to be full-time members of the school staff, but on the other hand, he also realizes that they are employed by a division and, therefore, he must be content with a part-time person. The work week must be planned carefully yet flexibly; schedules must be discussed with each principal. Obviously all principals are not alike and presuppositions must be reduced accordingly. The principal is the audiologist's strongest ally, so successes as well as failures should be shared.

Principals can assist with interpretations of the administrative code, facilitate relations with teachers, and supply important information regarding pupil status.

It might be suggested to teacher trainers that they obtain first-hand experience in public education by following a principal around the school for at least one full school day. In fact, it would be advisable to spend at least one day in a special school, in a school with "integrated" classes, and in a school that provides itinerant services to the hearing-impaired child.

Education Codes and School Policies. Commonly state educational systems have, by law, a set of rules and regulations that insure conformity by the school districts. This law is then transposed into district policy. Several small districts may join forces by consolidating or unifying and may fall under the governance of a county, which in turn is responsible to the state. In California, for example, the state supplies partial funding, according to a formula that, with local revenue, allows the district to stay in business. California also specifies certain programs to be mandatory; it then becomes the responsibility of the district to allocate necessary funding. In the case of special education programs, the school district may be well reimbursed by the state.

In California, speech, hearing, and language programs come under the heading of "physical handicaps." The area of hearing disorders is further divided into subcategories, as follows: the deaf, the severely hard-of-hearing and the moderately hard-of-hearing. The districts are, by law, required to instruct this population between the ages of 3 and 21. Fortunately, the definitions for each are quite broad and extend by decibel level (presumably in hearing level) from over 70dB down to 20dB in the better ear in the "speech range." The language is somewhat quaint regarding the authority to label. As an example, note the extreme diversity in the following corrective measures: A hearing specialist and a qualified educator can recommend special placement for the deaf child; a licensed physician and surgeon can diagnose a severely hard-of-hearing child; and a licensed physician and surgeon, audiologist, or teacher holding a credential in the area of the speech and hearing handicapped can recommend remedial instruction for the moderately hard-of-hearing.

The actual reason for lack of regulations and methods of funding for audiologists is that such functions have been assumed to be accomplished outside the system. It is also presupposed that these functions can be performed, in part, by the teacher of the deaf or the speech and hearing specialist after being identified by the school audiometrist. The school audiometry identification program, incidentally, is mandated in California, and the results of pure-tone threshold tests performed by the audiometrist were considered to be one of the requirements for entrance into the special programs.

The California Code also specifies that an experimental program may be petitioned by a district to the state superintendent of public instruction for deaf and severely hard-of-hearing infants, subject to an annual review for continuance. This program was not mandated, however, and despite our knowledge of optimal ages for instruction, there are few viable programs for very young children in the state. There is nothing in the Code that allows for special instruction of pupils with a unilateral hearing loss unless the child has a speech or language problem; in this case, the child is then eligible for the speech program.

There may be funds available for children who are eligible for "mainstreaming." As a matter of fact, there was one such clause in the California Code that enabled us to hire two audiologists. According to the code, "The Superintendent of Public Schools shall allow to school districts and county superintendents of schools for each unit of average daily attendance an amount of $1,018 for the instruction of physically handicapped minors in regular day classes." This clause was interpreted by the district as authority to hire audiologists to evaluate, not identify, children with hearing losses who did not quality for the hard-of-hearing program. Restrospectively, the acquisition of personnel by this technique may have been somewhat questionable, but the positions were attained.

Of equal importance, the audiologist should systematically research the state code and look for regulations that have even the slightest bearing on hearing handicaps. More to the point, the audiologist should enroll in either college or in-service courses relating to school finance and law. The slight amount of time spent in such "continuing education" will more than pay for itself. One of the remarkable failings with students entering from our field is their apparent lack of interest in educating themselves in these vital areas of school administration.

Not all hearing-handicapped pupils are found in the deaf and hard-of-hearing programs; a sizable number are enrolled in other special programs because the primary disability is other than the hearing handicap. They may be found in the speech, retarded, autistic, aphasic, and orthopedically handicapped programs. The problem of assistance to these other handicapped pupils lies with the philosophy of the programs and the priority system developed by the audiologist. The district may want priority established for those children who are not in the hearing program, based on the assumption that these children are already being instructed by special teachers. However, in my opinion, the audiologist's chief responsibility rests with the severely hard-of-hearing and deaf child. If time is available, the needs of the moderately hard-of-hearing come next. This ordering of priorities, however, may be a trap and can result in more intensive work with fewer children while children with moderate handicaps and higher potential are neglected.

On the other hand, there may be no options. Such was the case in the Los Angeles city school district—enrollment in the deaf and hard-of-hearing programs totalled 1,000 children and there were only 4 audiologists. Despite the efforts of other programs to engage our services, we had little time left over and had to take a firm stand. It was hoped that as the program developed, the district would see how important it was and institute positions for more audiologists. A naive assumption! Perhaps a statement should be made at this moment on the total pupil population—700,000!

Putting our problem into perspective, we soon discovered that our priorities were quite minor when compared to those of the regular instructional program. However, Public Law 94-142 includes programs for audiologists in the near future. Unless professional workers at the local and state levels do not become immediately aggressive, other special services will put in their claims. The law requires that the school file a statement through the district to the state regarding an "Individualized Education Program" (IEP). If audiological care is not included on the IEP, funds will *not* be earmarked for that purpose. Great emphasis should be placed on the importance of pushing particularly hard for preschool services (for children of ages 3 through 5). This should be attractive to the district as they may get a special federal entitlement.

Audiologists need help to interpret the law, to advise on action programs, to assure front-line visibility. They stand on the threshold of one of the greatest stimuli for growth in the field. The facts should be obtained and advertised to potential lawmakers, public figures, state consultants, and school boards. Public school is where the action is!

Aides and Assistants. There are very few professions, regardless of work setting, that do not require the use of supportive personnel. In public schools, precedents have already been set in almost every area of instruction. The audiologist needs two types of assistants, testing and technical:

1. The test assistants are invaluable to the audiologist, particularly with difficult-to-test children. Chiefly, they act as aides in the test room, but they are also needed to assist with the details of arranging schedules and transportation. These tasks are time-consuming and relatively costly to the district when performed by the audiologist.

2. The technical assistant can be of tremendous help in running frequency

curves on hearing aids and auditory training units. In addition, the technical assistant can coordinate the details of repair and maintenance of such units. Technicians, properly trained, can also measure noise levels in classrooms.

For both types of support the chief objective is to have the assistant perform those functions that are subservient to the professional. Relinquishing these functions is often threatening, but in the long run will afford the audiologist time for the principal responsibility, e.g. the face-to-face relations with the hearing-impaired child. The addition of supportive personnel is generally viewed with approval by the administration; providing a carefully designed proposal shows exactly how the district can conserve funds while providing more and better services to the pupil. The audiologist should take the time to get the facts and present them with clarity; the administrators will listen.

Transportation

To an audiologist in a clinical setting, transportation of patients may never become an issue. In schools that must adhere to laws governing the transportation of school children from one place to another during the school day, it certainly is an issue. If the district either has, or has the potential for, a mobile testing unit, the battle is practically won; the tests and evaluations can be performed at the school site. However, in some districts, children may have to be driven to a central test site that could be miles away from their home school.

Preferably, the child should be driven by the parents to the test site. Surprising as it may appear, there are few parents available during the school day and for a variety of reasons: care for preschoolers is not available, the mother does not know how to drive, or the mother is working. Calls to the home, both written and verbal, fail to elicit any response; only a few parents will drive their children for this service. Between them—the audiologist, the classroom teacher, and the principal—a plan must be devised that will accommodate not only district transportation but also suitable scheduling dates. Some schools in large districts have assistants or aides who are bonded to perform such services, but as a rule the children must be driven only in school buses.

Procuring a special bus for such a specific purpose and for such a small group per bus load is a sizable problem of logistics. The bus, for example, may have to be equipped with specialized accessories necessary to transport handicapped children. The buses have to be available only after school starts in the morning and must return the children in time for them to take their regular school bus home. When one works out the transportation problem, time left for testing may total only four hours per day. In order to make the operation minimally efficient, at least one or two children should be scheduled per day. The audiologist may not have an aide at the test site and the home school may have to provide such personnel. If there ever was a single factor that involved more paper work, telephone calls, and teacher conferences than transportation of students, I'll eat my audiometer!

In the regular transportation system in a school district that embraces approximately 750 square miles, the logistics involve servicing a school population of 700,000 children, of which 40,000 are regularly transported and 6,000 are enrolled in special education programs. One thousand buses are involved of which 450 are used for special education alone. Of these children enrolled in the special education program, approximately 35% require more than two hours transportation time to and from school.

Audiologists become further involved in transportation when they should examine noise conditions on the bus. Recently, the Los Angeles district found that the noise level at the driver's seat averaged 94dBA. By sound-treating at high vibration locations, the level was decreased to between 82 and 85dBA at a cost of about $300 per bus. Some 65 buses will have to be so treated. These facts are cited here simply to illustrate a little known area of concern that may prove to be an important one for the school audiologist and also one that should be investigated when a program is initiated.

In-Service Training

For an individual dedicated to a career of helping others, education should never cease. Personal frustration and dissatisfaction are the hallmarks of a successful clinician. School audiologists are in a much better position to observe success in rehabilitation than fellow clinical audiologists because of almost daily contact with the children over an extensive period of time. The proximity and continuity in such a working situation provide constant reminders of success and failure, which, of course, promote professional growth. Growth can be stimulated by perceptive observation and such observations should be reported to others—not only to audiologic colleagues but to other associates involved in the rehabilitative process. Individuals and the community must be served by conducting training sessions that come from such insightful experience. Just as rewarding as informing others is the process of learning how others operate.

In-service training can be divided into two categories: internal and external. Internal sessions are important to fellow audiologists in the district; external sessions benefit resource personnel in the district as well as concerned groups in the community.

Internal Training. Audiologists should know what other services within the district's system can offer in terms of information and cooperation. Directors of personnel, psychology, nursing, audiometry, speech and language, and deaf and hard-of-hearing programs are generally delighted to provide information regarding their responsibilities. Coordinators of other special education programs are also resources that should be tapped. This type of education cannot be secured from colleges and universities in the same intimate fashion that it can be obtained from fellow employees. Inevitably, such sessions promote cross fertilization of ideas that directly improve services.

In-service training provides the necessary experiences not yet generally provided by formal education. As a matter of fact, it may not even be necessary for students in training to be knowledgeable in this area but rather, they can learn while on the job. However, "the American infatuation with mandarin education" (Comfort, 1974) may well defeat this philosophical point of view and the tendency for preservation may be too strong to override such a practical solution. Perhaps we lack the maturity or the opportunity to exercise our talent.

External Training. The value of listening to parents and concerned professionals in the community should never be underestimated. Representatives from social and welfare agencies and hospital clinics, otolaryngologists, and hearing aid dispensers can enable the audiologist to feel the pulse of the community. It is surprising to see how enthusiastically most speakers welcome new activities in the schools. The in-service concept can take other and equally important forms.

One meeting that was organized, for example, was a two-hour afternoon session for hearing aid dispensers in the community. The meeting was not held to inform them of ongoing activities, but rather to show them how the schools were operating in terms of pupil placement procedures in the special education division. The session apparently explained to them for the first time the school's responsibilities and restrictions concerning the handicapped child. Another meeting was held for local audiologists and otologists. Only one otologist attended, but he was the director of resident training in otolaryngology from a large county hospital. Perhaps a future generation of otolaryngologists may benefit from his knowledge.

Of great success was a joint conference offered by our unit and the staff of the Hearing and Speech Clinic, Children's Hospital of Los Angeles. The rationale developed from a community need: the need for better communication between the public school audiology programs of the city and county and private and institutional audiologists in the greater Los Angeles area. By common agreement, the subject that required the most clarification and the most cooperation between these two forces was the general need for discussion of wearable hearing aids and auditory training units. A presentation was made to the participants with 10 proposed areas of discussion at the beginning of the afternoon conference:

1. Coordination and interaction between schools and clinics.
2. Post-auricular vs. body aids.
3. Monaural vs. binaural aids.
4. Procedures for fitting hearing aids to children without oral language.
5. Procedures for fitting hearing-impaired children who have oral language skills.
6. Psychoacoustic characteristics pertinent to fitting hearing aids on children.

7. Fitting hearing aids to children with special problems.
8. Hearing aid delivery.
9. Earmolds.
10. Use of auditory training units vs. personal hearing aids in school.

Participants were divided into 4 groups consisting of 15 members each. Also included in each group were invited principals, teachers, and other related resource personnel over and above the 60 participants. A pair of audiologists was assigned to each group, one from the school, the other from the community. Within the first half hour, the leaders solicited priorities among the 10 items. Discussion then occurred for the following two and one half hours, covering only those items that had been ranked as priority items. Of course, and as one might expect, the discussion could have gone on all night. Of interest may be the priorities selected by each group:

Group I: Items 1,4,2,3.
Group II: Items 4,1,5,7,2,8,9 (and third-party payment)
Group III: Items 4,3,2
Group IV: Items 1,4,2,6

Space does not permit the splendid summarizing statements offered by each group, but it would suffice to say that the experience generated a follow-up conference in the spring of 1977. Such in-service conferences based on the discussion concept, rather than the didactic concept, are well worth the time and effort.

School Organizations, Unions, and Professional Organizations

As an employee of a school district, the audiologist's basic loyalties and obligations are to the district. The division in which one operates may have an organization. If an interest is taken in the status of a division and how it can be improved, the most effective results can be obtained by direct involvement in the organizations. The same may be said for state teachers' associations, which offer worthwhile fringe benefits that certain individuals can ill afford to neglect. Diverse backgrouns have led many people to eschew organizations. If such is the case, a review of their pro's and con's should be considered, especially when contemplating membership in a teacher's union. One can be assured that the administrators are generally well organized, as are the majority of other certificated and classfied personnel.

These organizations have powerful lobbies in state governments. Union organization can be highly beneficial, as representation is often the most efficient way of effecting change.

Although ties may exist to the American Speech and Hearing Association by certification, it will be discovered that their services have been designed to help and not hinder professional growth. The same logic pertains to state speech and hearing associations.

School audiology is a relatively new area and the profession needs constant input. Another organization, The Council for Exceptional Children, through its division for Children with Communication Disorders, welcomes contributions as does the Academy of Rehabilitative Audiology.

It may be found, however, that a district is only interested in releasing an individual for professional meetings if that person is a contributor, which should be a stimulus for participation. The pay received may be nothing more than not being docked for released time. If this is felt to be insufficient, take a look at school taxes. An indifference may be felt because of an apparent anti-intellectual administration, and perhaps rightfully so. Notice should be taken, however, of fringe benefits—these people may be the envy of their colleagues in private practice and community agencies. Besides, professional travel, convention dues, and so forth, are all tax deductible!

SUMMARY

School audiology is an emerging specialty within the board area of pediatric audiology. A chief difference between the "clinical" and the "school" audiologist revolves around the primacy of the rehabilitative-educative role of the latter and the diagnostic function of the former.

Although both pursue the goals of efficient amplification, the school audiologist is in the superior position of being able to monitor, almost daily, performance of both the hearing-impaired children and the hearing aid. The school audiologist is a public servant, working in an environment that is under the public eye and, therefore, more restrictive than other areas of audiology. However, a knowledge of school hierarchies, policies, and administrative codes may alleviate the burden considerably. The school audiologist should realize that the position offers a unique opportunity to observe and share closely the personal growth of the hearing-impaired child.

RESEARCH NEEDS

From a practical standpoint, applied research in the effects of amplification on learning and school achievement occupy a prime position for continuing and future research in the public schools. Also greatly needed are studies regarding school achievement of children with unilateral hearing loss. As a rule, eligibility for special programs and for amplification is restricted to those with bilateral losses. The question of optimal use of classroom training units for children who have personal aids bears investigation, especially for those with severe losses. Although current trends suggest ear level aids, the advisability of their use on very young children with severe losses is still debatable when the variable of learning is considered.

The classroom, not the laboratory, should be the environment of choice for these children. The classroom itself should be further investigated as a vehicle to facilitate learning. Not yet tested are those acoustic variables which are not only necessary, but also practical.

Finally, the question of whether the audiologist should also be a "hearing clinician" should be put to the test—not only for purposes of accountability but also for complete efficiency as well.

REFERENCES

"An Interview with F.S. Berg," *Audiology and Hearing Education,* 1 (1975), 24–26.

Berg, F.S., *Educational Audiology.* New York:Grune and Stratton, 1976.

Bess, F.H., "Characteristics of Children's Hearing Aids in the Public School," mimeographed paper, 1976.

Caccamo, J.M., "Speech, Language and Audiology Services—An Inalienable Right," *Language, Speech and Hearing Services in Schools,* 5 (1974), 173–175.

Chial, M.R., "Electroacoustic Assessment of Children's Hearing Aids: Repeatability of Measurement and Determinations of Merit," mimeographed paper, 1976.

Coleman, R.F., "Is Anyone Listening?" *Language, Speech and Hearing Services in Schools,* 6 (1975), 102–105.

Comfort, A., The American Infatuation with Mandaran Education," *Center Report, Center for the Study of Democratic Institutions,* 7 (1974), 25–27.

Crum, M.A., and N.D. Matkin, "Room Acoustics: The Forgotten Variable," *Language, Speech and Hearing Services in Schools,* 7 (1976), 106–110.

Damashek, M., "Design and Development of Simple, Low Cost Speech Training Devices," *Proceedings of the 47th Meeting of Convention of American Instructors of the Deaf* (CAID), 1975. Document #94–172, U.S. Government Printing Office, Washington, D.C. (1976), 57–63.

Garstecki, D.C., "Survey of Specific Duties and Academic Training Prerequisites of Providers of Audiological Services in Public/Private Schools," Questionnaire of Educational Models and Continuing Education Committee, Academy of Rehabilitative Audiology, November, 1976.

Garwood, V.P., "Audiologic Programs in Public Schools—Another Frontier," Mini Seminar, Annual Meeting, American Speech and Hearing Association, Washington, D.C., 1975.

Garwood, V.P., M. Bergman, J. Dixon, and G. Haspiel, "Task Force 2: Roles Played by Audiologists," *Journal of the Academy of Rehabilitative Audiology*, 5 (1973), 20-21.

Grammatico, L.F., "The Development of Listening Skills," *Volta Review*, 77 (1975), 303-308.

Griffing, B.L., and G.M. Hayes, "Ears: Educational Amplification Response Study," *Ears Monograph #1*. San Diego, Calif., San Diego Speech and Hearing Center, 1968.

Hanners, B.A., and A.B. Sitton, "Ears to Hear: A Daily Hearing Aid Monitor Program," *Volta Review*, 76 (1974), 530-536.

Hoversten, G. (Project Director), *Auditory Skills Instructional Planning System* (an EHA, VI-B project, B.E.I.H., California State Department of Education). Office of the Superintendent, Los Angeles County Schools, personal communication, 1976.

Jeffers, J., *CDQ, Curriculum Development Questionnaire: Audiological Services Needed by Public Schools, and Competencies Needed by Audiologists to Perform Services*. Los Angeles: California State University. Unpublished material, 1973.

Jensema, C.J., "The Distribution of Hearing Loss Among Students in Special Education Programs for the Hearing Impaired," ASHA, 16 (1974), 682-685.

Johnson, M., and E. Forbes, "Bridging the Gap between Education and Audiology," *Audiology and Hearing Education*, 1 (1975), 12.

Joint Committee of American Speech and Hearing Association and Conference of Executives of American Schools for the Deaf, "Guidelines for Audiology Programs in Educational Settings for Hearing Impaired Children," ASHA, 18 (1976), 291-294.

Jones, B.L., "The Audiologist in the Educational Environment," *Bulletin, Division for Children with Communication Disorders* (CED), 10 (1973), 11-17.

Mecham, S.R., "Do-It-Yourself Mini-Loop," *Audiology and Hearing Education*, 2 (1976), 17-20.

Olsen, W.O., "Acoustics and Amplification in Classroom for the Hearing Impaired," in *Childhood Deafness: Causation, Assessment and Management*, edited by F. Bess. New York: Grune and Stratton (in press).

Olsen, W.O., and N.D. Matkin, "Comments on Modern Auditory Training Systems and Their Use," *Bulletin, American Organization for the Education of the Hearing Impaired*, 2 (1971), HI 7-HI 15.

O'Neill, J.J., "The School-Educational Audiologist," *Journal of Academy of Rehabilitative Audiology*, 7 (1974), 31-39.

Randolph, K., "Checking Hearing Aid Operation Using a Cassette Recorder," *Audiology and Hearing Education*, 2 (1976), 28.

Ross, M., "Considerations Underlying the Selection and Utilization of Classroom Amplification Systems," *Journal of the Academy of Rehabilitative Audiology*, 6 (1973), 33-42.

Ross, M., "The Incidence of Hearing Aid Malfunction: A Review and Some Recommendations," mimeographed, 1976.

Ross, M., and T.G. Giolas, "Three Classroom Listening Conditions on Speech Intelligibility," *American Annals of the Deaf*, 116 (1971), 580–584.

Schell, Y.S., "Electro-acoustic Evaluation of Hearing Aids Worn by Public School Children," *Audiology and Hearing Education*, 2 (1976), 7–15.

Sheeley, E.C., and J.E. Hannah, "The Audiologist in the Special School," *Hearing and Speech News*, 42 (1974), 12–14.

Staab, W.J., and E.J. O'Gara, "Auditory Training Systems for the Hearing Impaired," *Telex Audiological Reports*, Sect. 12, Topic 10, 1974. (Reprint from September, 1974 *Hearing Instruments*.)

Zink, G.D., "Rehabilitative and Educational Audiology Programming," *Language, Speech and Hearing Services in Schools*, 4 (1973), 23–36.

SUGGESTED READING

Professional Journals

Audiology and Hearing Education
Journal of the Academy of Rehabilitation Audiology
Language, Speech and Hearing Services in Schools
The Volta Review

State and District Publications

Your state administrative code (particularly sections related to handicapped children)
Your school district policy and procedures manual
Your state laws and regulations relating to licenses, school certificates, or credentials
Job descriptions from school districts

Other Reading

Abeson, A., editor, *A Continuing Summary of Pending and Completed Litigation Regarding the Education of Handicapped Children.* Arlington, Va.: Council for Exceptional Children, 1973.

Amicus, *A Monthly Bulletin of the National Center for Law and the Handicapped, Inc.*, 1235 No. Eddy St., South Bend, Ind. 44617 (Free on request).

Closer Look, *An Occasional Report of National Information Center for the Handicapped*, Box 1492, Washingtin, D.C., #20013 (Free on request).

Northcott, W.N., editor, *The Hearing-Impaired Child in a Regular Classroom.* Washington, D.C.: Alexander Graham Bell Association for the Deaf, 1973.

Author Index

Subject Index